A COMPLETE GUIDE TO
MAGGOT THERAPY

A Complete Guide to Maggot Therapy

Clinical Practice, Therapeutic Principles, Production, Distribution, and Ethics

Edited by Frank Stadler

OpenBook
Publishers

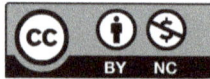

Digital material and resources associated with this volume are available at https://doi.org/10.11647/OBP.0281#resources

ISBN Paperback: 9781800647282
ISBN Hardback: 9781800647299
ISBN Digital (PDF): 9781800647305
ISBN Digital ebook (epub): 9781800647312
ISBN Digital ebook (azw3): 9781800647329
ISBN XML: 9781800647336
ISBN HTML: 9781800647343
DOI: 10.11647/OBP.0300

Cover image: Line drawing of a green bottle blowfly (*Lucilia sericata*) maggot by Frank Stadler (2022), CC BY-NC. Cover design by Katy Saunders.

How to Cite

The book:

Stadler, Frank (ed.), *A Complete Guide to Maggot Therapy: Clinical Practice, Therapeutic Principles, Production, Distribution, and Ethics* (Cambridge: Open Book Publishers, 2022), https://doi.org/10.11647/OBP.0300.

Individual chapters:

Stadler, Frank, 'Introduction', in *A Complete Guide to Maggot Therapy: Clinical Practice, Therapeutic Principles, Production, Distribution, and Ethics*, F. Stadler (ed.). 2022, Cambridge: Open Book Publishers, pp. xx–xx, https://doi.org/10.11647/OBP.0300.01.

Acknowledgements

This book would not have been possible without the in-kind support of the School of Medicine and Dentistry, Griffith University, and a generous financial contribution to the publication costs by the BioTherapeutics, Education & Research (BTER) Foundation. Some contributions made by Dr Stadler were informed by his doctoral research conducted at the Department of International Business and Asian Studies, Griffith University, and supported by a generous scholarship under the Australian Postgraduate Award scheme. Likewise, this book has benefited from images, illustrations, and insights drawn from a research project funded by Creating Hope in Conflict: A Humanitarian Grand Challenge, led by Dr Stadler and his colleagues at Griffith University between 2019 and 2021. The high scientific calibre and integrity on display across the 19 chapters is to a large part due to the fantastic team of expert co-authors as well as the many chapter reviewers we have drawn from both the book co-author team and the independent scientific community. The external independent reviewers included Nazni Wasi Ahmad, Chris Freelance, Martin Hall, Gautham Krishnaraj, Bryan Lessard, Anne Paas, Sebastian Probst, Hitoshi Takase, Tarek Tantawi, Aletha Tippett, Mark Wilson, and Martha Isabel Wolff Echeverri. Thank you, on behalf of the patients who will benefit from your work.

To William S. Baer and fellow pioneers of modern maggot therapy on whose shoulders we stand

Contents

List of Illustrations

List of Boxes and Tables

Contributor Biographies

Frank Stadler is the owner and director of Similitude Pty Ltd and MedMagLabs.[1] He is also the Centre Manager at the ARC Training Centre for the Facilitated Advancement of Australia's Bioactives (FAAB) and Adjunct Fellow at Applied BioSciences, Macquarie University. At Griffith University, Frank holds an Adjunct Research Fellow position with the School of Medicine and Dentistry. For the past eight years he has conducted world-first research on supply chain management for maggot therapy in compromised healthcare settings. Frank has held positions in research, research management, science communication, and project management. He has curated a natural history museum, owned an environmental education business, and managed a multi-million-dollar portfolio of research at the National Climate Change Adaptation Research Facility, Griffith University. Frank has extensive expertise in maggot therapy and its supply chain management, invertebrate biology, and laboratory rearing of invertebrates. He and his colleagues established MedMagLabs, a two-year research and development project funded by Creating Hope in Conflict: A Humanitarian Grand Challenge, to develop medicinal maggot production and maggot therapy solutions for conflict-affected isolated communities. This work has motivated Frank to transition MedMagLabs in 2021 from a university research lab into a for-purpose private enterprise under the governance of Similitude Pty Ltd.

School of Medicine and Dentistry, Griffith University, Brisbane, Queensland, Australia. MedMagLabs, Similitude Pty Ltd, Sydney, New South Wales, Australia.

---

1   https://orcid.org/0000-0002-9158-2792; f.stadler@griffith.edu.au; f.stadler@medmaglabs.com.

Benjamin L. Bullen has contributed to multidisciplinary diabetes foot services throughout Australia and the UK and has a keen clinical and research interest in Charcot foot health literacy and advanced therapies for diabetes foot disease. He is currently a Principal Lecturer in Assessment Skills, Simulation and Interprofessional Education at The University of Wolverhampton's School of Pharmacy, an Honorary Lecturer at Cardiff University's School of Medicine, and a Visiting Lecturer at The Welsh Wound Innovation Centre.

School of Pharmacy, Faculty of Science and Engineering, University of Wolverhampton, Wolverhampton, United Kingdom.

Nathan J. Butterworth is a research fellow at Monash University. He completed his doctoral thesis at the University of Wollongong in 2020, where he studied the evolution of sexual signals in blowflies (Diptera: Calliphoridae). He then worked as a postdoctoral research associate at the University of Technology Sydney, where he investigated how ecological and sexual selection proceeds in natural fly populations. He has published eleven papers in high-ranking journals using blowflies as a model system to answer questions regarding population genetics, animal behaviour, and evolution.

School of Biological Sciences, Monash University, Victoria, Australia.

Paul J. Chadwick has been working as the National Clinical Director for the Royal College of Podiatry for four years. He has led the development and implementation of the Clinical Leadership and Education agenda of the organisation's five-year strategic plan.

Paul qualified in 1990 and gained an MSc (by research) in 2000. He completed a PhD in 2012, looking at the social construction of neuropathic pain. He maintains a clinical role as an honorary consultant podiatrist. He has presented nationally and internationally and published widely in many peer-reviewed journals. He is on the editorial board of a range of journals and is an associate editor of the *Diabetic Foot Journal*. He has a Fellowship from the Royal College of Podiatry and was awarded the meritorious award in 2014 for services to the profession. He also received a Fellowship of the Royal College of Physicians and Surgeons of Glasgow. Paul was appointed a Visiting Professor of Tissue Viability at Birmingham City University in 2018.

Clinical Leadership and Education, Royal College of Podiatry, London, United Kingdom. Faculty of Health, Birmingham City University, Birmingham, United Kingdom.

Kylie J. Elder (RN, BN, Grad Dip Adv Nsg, Grad Dip Nsg Ed, MN) is the Senior Clinical Nurse Advisor in Skin Integrity and Wound Management at Bolton Clarke, an Australian not-for-profit health and aged care provider. She has extensive experience as a clinical leader and educator on wound management, particularly in the area of chronic wounds, their management, and person-centred outcomes. She has served on multiple state and national wound committees, presented nationally and internationally on wound management, contributed to consensus documents, and published in peer-reviewed journals.

Bolton Clarke, Melbourne, Victoria, Australia.

Associate Professor **Michelle L. Harvey** is Associate Dean Teaching and Learning in the Faculty of Science, Engineering and Built Environment at Deakin University, Australia. Her primary field of study is entomology, with her PhD completed in the molecular systematics of the forensically significant blowflies. She has conducted research in Australia, South Africa, the United States and the United Kingdom, supported by prestigious fellowships and academic appointments. Since 2012 she has led the medical entomology laboratory at Deakin University, conducting and directing research largely focussed on the biology of blowflies of medical and veterinary significance. The importance of basic biology and behaviour in understanding blowfly involvement in forensic estimation of postmortem interval, flystrike on sheep, and most recently larval debridement of chronic wounds have been the focus of her publications and presentations. Of key interest is the microbial-insect interaction as a facet of blowfly attraction, oviposition and larval development, and how this may be exploited to improve larval wound debridement and prevent flystrike.

School of Life and Environmental Sciences, Faculty of Science, Engineering and Built Environment, Deakin University, Geelong, Victoria, Australia.

Nikolas P. Johnston is a research fellow at the University of Technology, Sydney. His research is broadly related to the evolutionary biology of flies, with interests in the biodiversity of Australian flies, forensically important flies, carrion ecology, and the role of carrion-breeding flies as mechanical vectors of micro-organisms. Throughout his research he has published revisions of five genera of flesh flies, described fifteen new species of fly, and aided in establishing comprehensive genomic phylogenies for both blowflies and flesh flies.

School of Life Sciences, University of Technology, Ultimo, New South Wales, Australia.

Christopher K. Kibiwott is a Senior Nursing Officer and an Infection Prevention and Control practitioner at Kenyatta National Hospital Infection Prevention Control Unit. He is also a consultant in wound care management in the same institution. His work is focussed on improving patient outcomes through efficacious and affordable medical practices. Christopher was instrumental in the introduction and clinical implementation of a maggot therapy programme in Kenya, in collaboration with KALRO BioRi and Slovak development partners. This included administration of maggot therapy and monitoring and reporting of clinical outcomes. His epidemiological work greatly improved the analysis, reporting and action time of hospital-acquired infections through laboratory surveillance. Christopher was awarded the Order of the Grand Warrior of Kenya (OGW) for his work in maggot therapy. In addition to his day job at Kenyatta National Hospital, he is the owner/operator of the Nairobi Wound Care Centre, where he provides care, including maggot therapy, to private patients with chronic wounds.

Infection Prevention and Control Unit, Wound Care Clinic, Kenyatta National Hospital, Nairobi, Kenya.

Franciéle S. Masiero holds a PhD in Parasitology. She has conducted research related to maggot therapy, including studies concerning the antimicrobial potential of larval excretions and secretions, healing of skin lesions in animal models, and the development of a topical agent with larval excretions and secretions for the healing of skin lesions. She now works as a nurse at the Hospital de Clínicas de Porto Alegre, Brazil.

Hospital de Clínicas de Porto Alegre, Porto Alegre, Brazil.

Grace A. Murilla is Deputy Vice Chancellor at KAG EAST University, Affiliate Staff at Yale University School of Public Health, and Adjunct Professor at Nelson Mandela African Institute of Science and Technology. She is a member of the American Society for the Advancement of Science and the WHO-Africa GLP Network, Director of the ANDI Centre of Excellence in Pre-clinical Development, Associate Editor for *PLOS Neglected Tropical Diseases*, and reviewer for high-impact journals and grant proposals for the Canadian Institutes for Health Research (CIHR) Stars in Global Health Programme, as well as the National Research Fund (Kenya). Grace has published over fifty papers in peer-reviewed journals, and won several scientific awards, including research grants. Previously, she was the Director of the Biotechnology Research Institute at the Kenya Agricultural and Livestock Research Organization and Centre Director of the Trypanosomiasis Research Centre at KARI. She holds a PhD in Pharmacology and Toxicology from the University of Glasgow, and MSc and BSc degrees from the University of Nairobi. Her areas of expertise include Product R&D, product safety/toxicology, drug residues in animal products (public health & trade), drug metabolism, pharmacokinetics/pharmacodynamics, and QA/QC of foods and drugs.

KAG EAST University, Nairobi, Kenya. School of Life Sciences and Bio-engineering, Nelson Mandela African Institute for Science and Technology, Arusha, Tanzania.

Yamni Nigam is a Professor in Biomedical Sciences at Swansea University and a Fellow of the Higher Education Academy. Here, she teaches anatomy, physiology and pathophysiology to a wide range of health professionals including nurses and paramedics. Yamni graduated from Kings College, London and undertook a Master's degree in Applied Parasitology and Medical Entomology at the Liverpool School of Tropical Medicine. After successful completion of her doctorate at Swansea University, she established the Swansea University Maggot

Research Group, focussing on the medicinal maggot, *Lucilia sericata*, and the molecules involved in larval therapy. Her team have published widely on the scientific findings on the antimicrobial activity of larval secretions, and on the wound healing properties of maggots, and have identified a potent new antimicrobial factor, Seraticin®, from maggot secretions. Yamni is leading a project investigating the public understanding and perception of the clinical use of maggots on wounds, has established the "Love a maggot!" campaign, and has featured in numerous media, radio and TV reports and interviews. Yamni has been awarded the National WISE Award for Innovation, presented by HRH The Princess Royal in 2018 and was one of the WISE20 women in 2020. Yamni authored over 75 peer-reviewed articles, book chapters and papers.

Faculty of Medicine, Health and Life Science, Swansea University, Swansea, United Kingdom.

Rajna Ogrin (BSc, BPod (Hons), PhD) is a Senior Research Fellow at Bolton Clarke, an Australian not-for-profit health and aged care provider. Rajna initially trained as a clinical podiatrist, where she identified gaps in the provision of evidence-based clinical practice. This has led to her working and researching in the areas of diabetes, wounds, and community-based, person-centred interprofessional care. She incorporates co-design to better facilitate the translation of evidence into practice, focussing on older people. To further support the dissemination of person-centred and evidence-based care, she has also contributed to national committees and consensus documents, authored publications and presented at national and international conferences, and published in peer-reviewed journals.

Bolton Clarke Research Institute, Bolton Clarke, Melbourne, Victoria, Australia. Department of Business Strategy and Innovation, Griffith University, Brisbane, Queensland, Australia.

Ronald A. Sherman retired from the University of California, Irvine in 2008 in order to devote his time to teaching, research, and patient-care activities using medicinal animals. He has studied maggot therapy for over forty years, and began the first controlled clinical trials of maggot therapy in 1990. In 2004, the Medical Maggots™ which he developed at the University of California became the first living organism to be granted marketing clearance by the U.S. Food and Drug Administration as a medical device. He holds degrees in entomology, medicine, and clinical tropical medicine. Ronald Sherman is Director of the BioTherapeutics, Education and Research (BTER) Foundation, which develops educational and research programmes in biotherapy, and he is Co-Founder and Laboratory Director of Monarch Labs, which produces medicinal animals in North America. He does not accept financial support for either of these positions, nor for any of his maggot therapy teaching or research. Instead, he earns his living working in an unrelated field, as an HIV/AIDS physician for the county health department. His wife, however, is paid a salary for working in the maggot lab, day and night.

BioTherapeutics, Education & Research (BTER) Foundation, Irvine, California, U.S.A. Monarch Labs, Irvine, California, U.S.A. Communicable Diseases, Orange County, Health Care Agency, Santa Ana, California, U.S.A.

Peter Takáč is a senior scientist at the Institute of Zoology, Slovak Academy of Sciences, Slovakia, and at the same time, Managing Director of a private scientific company, Scientica Ltd, Slovakia. His specific fields of interest are entomology, insect physiology and applied entomology. From 1992-95 he participated in the PhD-fellow programme at the Department of Molecular and Cell Biology, University of Connecticut, and the Marine Biology Laboratory, Woods Hole, MA, USA. He worked on the identification and study of methyl farnesoate, the gonad-stimulating hormone in Crustacea. He worked on isolation, identification and synthesis of novel, biologically vasoactive insect peptides in cooperation with the Natural Environment Research Council (NERC) Centre for Ecology and Hydrology, Wallingford, Oxfordshire, UK. Since 2002 he has established in Bratislava, Slovakia with the cooperation of the International Atomic Energy Agency (IAEA) in Vienna (Austria) the largest research and mass-rearing tsetse fly facility in Europe. From 2013-20 Peter was co-founder of the biotherapeutics laboratory of Scientica Ltd, in Bratislava, Slovakia. The laboratory produced medicinal maggots and polymer gels with bioactive compounds for chronic wound therapy, was active in hirudotherapy and ichtyotherapy, and focussed on research and development of biotherapeutic techniques. Currently Peter is interested in the mass-rearing of *Tenebrio molitor* as a new protein source in human and animal nutrition.

Scientica Ltd, Bratislava, Slovakia. Department of Animal Systematics, Institute of Zoology, Slovak Academy of Sciences, Bratislava, Slovakia.

Peter Tatham joined the (UK) Royal Navy in 1970 and served in a variety of logistics appointments during his career of some thirty-five years in which he rose to the rank of Commodore (1*). Following his retirement from the RN, he joined the staff of Cranfield University, UK, and was awarded his PhD in 2009, and subsequently received the 2010 Emerald/EFMD Outstanding Doctoral Research Award. In the same year, Peter joined Griffith University where he taught and researched in the field of supply chain management, specialising in humanitarian logistics. Although recently retired, Peter remains a member of the editorial boards of the *Journal of Humanitarian Logistics and Supply Chain Management*, and the *International Journal of Physical Logistics and Supply Chain Management*.

Department of Business Strategy and Innovation, Griffith University, Brisbane, Queensland, Australia.

Patricia J. Thyssen is an Assistant Professor of Entomology and Parasitology at the University of Campinas (UNICAMP) and a permanent member of the Postgraduate Programs in Animal Biology (in the areas of Anthropic Relations, Environment and Parasitology, and Biodiversity) and Ecology at UNICAMP. She is also a member of the Department of Foot Diseases and Neuropathy and Nursing of the Brazilian Society of Diabetes (2020-21) and author of the chapter 'Interventions to promote the healing of diabetic foot ulcers of the SBD Guidelines' (2021). Her research focusses on the taxonomy, biology and ecology of Neotropical flies (Insecta, Diptera) with an interest in investigations on bioprospecting of blowfly species for therapeutic purposes, the use of blowfly larvae products for microbial control (such as multi-drug resistant bacteria and bacterial biofilms) and *Leishmania* parasites. She develops devices for the transport of larvae and topical agents containing larval products to promote the healing of difficult-to-heal wounds. She is the author or co-author of over seventy papers in the medical and biological literature.

Laboratory of Integrative Entomology, Department of Animal Biology, Institute of Biology, University of Campinas (UNICAMP), São Paulo, Brazil.

James F. Wallman is a professor and the Dean of Science at the University of Technology Sydney (UTS). He is an entomologist with an international reputation in the biology of flies and their forensic application. James has also contributed to science governance in Australia through various leadership roles over many years. Before his appointment as Dean in 2021, James was Head of the School of Life Sciences at UTS, and previously also held academic positions at the University of Wollongong and the University of Adelaide. He is one of Australia's few forensic entomologists, and has long been responsible for the forensic entomology casework for police in New South Wales, Queensland, and South Australia. He has published extensively on fly biology and forensic entomology, and has also brought his expertise to bear on the public understanding of insects through media interviews and television documentaries, in which he has explained the important role of flies in the environment and human affairs.

Faculty of Science, University of Technology, Ultimo, New South Wales, Australia. Centre for Sustainable Ecosystem Solutions, School of Earth, Atmospheric and Life Sciences, University of Wollongong, Wollongong, New South Wales, Australia.

Bernard Wanyonyi Kinyosi is a Research Technologist with BioRI, the Biotechnology Research Institute at the Kenya Agricultural and Livestock Research Organization (KALRO). He attended a four-month training fellowship in 2009 in Bratislava, Slovakia and Seibersdorf, Austria, sponsored by the International Atomic Energy Agency (IAEA), to study mass-rearing of tsetse flies. In 2011, he was sponsored by Slovak Aid to study the rearing of *Lucillia sericata* flies to produce medicinal maggots used to cure both acute and chronic wounds at Kenyatta National Referral Hospital and elsewhere.

KALRO-BioRI, Kenya Agricultural and Livestock Research Organisation, Nairobi, Kenya.

Michael R. Wilson is a researcher with a background in forensic and agricultural entomology. He holds a masters in entomology from Imperial College London and a PhD in Health Science from Swansea University that investigated aspects of maggot therapy. He previously worked in research and quality control at BioMonde, a UK-based company that manufactures maggot therapy products, and as a postdoctoral researcher at Swansea University investigating the antibacterial properties of medical maggots. He currently works as a healthcare market researcher at Life Sciences Hub Wales.

Life Sciences Hub Wales, Cardiff, United Kingdom.

1. Introduction

Frank Stadler

The introductory chapter outlines the global wound burden, explains the basics of maggot therapy, and scopes the content covered by the subsequent 18 chapters. Maggot therapy is the treatment of chronic and infected wounds with living fly larvae commonly known as maggots. When applied to the wound, maggots remove dead tissue, control infection, and promote wound healing. This highly efficacious therapy is not widely available around the world due to actual and perceived social, organisational, economic, logistic, and clinical barriers—all of which can be overcome. This is the first comprehensive book on maggot therapy summarising, beyond clinical practice, the principles of therapeutic action, medicinal maggot production and distribution, and ethical considerations regarding the use of living maggots in wound care. The chapter concludes with reflections on the past, present, and future of maggot therapy.

Maggot Therapy and the Global Wound Burden

There is a large and mostly unmet global need for affordable and efficacious wound care, despite modern-day medicine advancing at break-neck speed. Indeed, the tide of chronic wounds is rising. Modern lifestyle changes, particularly in low- and middle-income countries (LMICs), bring a rapid rise in non-communicable disease including cardiovascular disease, obesity, and diabetes, with the latter leading to

   https://doi.org/10.11647/OBP.0300.01

diabetic ulcers at a lifetime incidence of up to 25% [1]. The cities and urban centres in fast-growing parts of the world are also struggling with ever-increasing motorisation and poor road safety standards while local healthcare systems in many LMICs are ill-prepared for the high traffic accident and injury burden [2, 3]. Likewise, due to population growth and urbanisation in disaster prone regions, the number of people exposed to disaster risk and related injuries is also growing. Where there is conflict there is also injury. Due to changes in the nature of warfare there are now far more casualties among the civilian population than among fighting soldiers [4]. People in such conflict zones and complex humanitarian crises are often isolated and are unable to properly care for the many injured due to limited resources. Acute traumatic war injuries therefore lead to infected chronic wounds and ultimately a high burden of amputation and death. To make matters worse, antibiotic-resistant strains of bacteria are highly prevalent in conflict and LMIC environments due to their mis- and overuse in human and veterinary medicine [5, 6].

Irrespective of the healthcare setting patients find themselves in, chronic wounds make life difficult and people living with chronic wounds struggle on a daily basis with social stigma, isolation, poor self-image, depression, and high treatment costs as explained by Ogrin and Elders in Chapter 1 [7].

With this growing wound burden and its social and socio-economic impact in mind, there is now the need for therapies that provide multiple wound care benefits and accessible, affordable, and effective wound care, regardless of where patients live or how wealthy they are. Contemporary care of acute and chronic wounds as it is practised in resource-rich countries relies heavily on the availability of efficacious antibiotics, sophisticated devices, surgical intervention, and advanced wound dressings. However, in compromised healthcare settings there is often limited or no access to these resources and associated basic consumables, which means that wound care options that are relatively cheap, easy to use, and have multiple therapeutic benefits are required. One such treatment modality is maggot therapy. It is the deliberate therapeutic application of living fly larvae (maggots) to remove dead tissue, control infection, and promote wound healing.

All three therapeutic properties are primarily related to the maggots' ecology and evolutionary history as evident in their nutritional preferences, digestive physiology, and immunology [8]. Medicinal maggots consume dead or devitalised animal tissue and wound fluids. Unlike beetle larvae, for example, maggots do not have mouthparts capable of cutting or biting pieces of solid food. While some food manipulation is achieved with a pair of mouth hooks, maggots need to liquefy their food outside their own body before ingesting this nutrient-rich broth [9]. In order to thrive in a microbe-laden environment of decomposing meat, maggots have also evolved ways to protect themselves from their microbe neighbours [10]. Maggots consume and digest many microbes that are suspended in the liquefied necrotic tissue, and their enzymatic excretions and secretions contain powerful antimicrobial compounds. Finally, maggots have a scrambling feeding habit and constantly probe with their two mouth hooks. This disrupts and prevents microbial communities from forming biofilms that stimy wound healing and evade the immune system and antibiotic treatment. The maggot excretions and secretions also contain growth factors that stimulate the regeneration of blood vessels and the growth of granulation tissue, thus supporting the wound healing process [11]. These principles of maggot-assisted wound healing are under active investigation by numerous research groups and their efficacy has been confirmed both at the bedside and *in vitro*.

Maggot Therapy

The human body is fragile and therefore wounds, acute and chronic, have always been part of the human condition since time immemorial. Likewise, flies have evolved to exploit during larval development the ephemeral cadavers and wounds of living animals (humans included), as Michelle Harvey explains in Chapter 7 [8]. So, it must come as no surprise that people through the ages have also noted the beneficial therapeutic effect maggots can have when they colonise a human wound. It is then only a small step to purposely utilise myiasis for wound care in traditional and tribal medicine as practiced by the Aboriginal Ngemba people in Australia, and the Mayan Indians in South America [12, 13], for example.

Nowhere is human fragility more apparent than on the battlefield where soldiers suffer terrible injury and subsequent infections. There, too, flies have been noted for their wound healing and infection control properties. Recorded accounts date back to the Battle of St Quentin in 1557 and other campaigns thereafter, including the Napoleonic Wars and the American Civil War [14]. However, it was not until after World War I that maggot therapy was formally investigated and introduced to modern medicine. William S. Baer, an orthopaedic surgeon, experienced first-hand the therapeutic benefits of maggots during the Great War. Upon returning to peace-time practice at Johns Hopkins Hospital in Baltimore, U.S.A., he revisited his war experience and commenced the first scientific and clinical studies on maggots and their use in wound therapy, in the first instance for the treatment of osteomyelitis [15]. His work spread like wildfire across North America and Europe, with over a thousand hospitals using maggot therapy to treat chronic wounds in the 1930s and early 1940s [16].

The rapid rise of maggot therapy was followed by an equally rapid decline in the 1940s with the advent of penicillin and other antimicrobials to treat wound infection. However, an increasing chronic wound burden, coupled with the emergence of antibiotic-resistant microorganisms, has resulted in a revival of maggot therapy in research and clinical practice over the past three decades. For a more comprehensive history of maggot therapy, please refer to a couple of early papers by Sherman and Pechter [14, 17] and two articles by Kruglikova and Whitaker, and their colleagues [18, 19].

In modern maggot therapy, as established by Baer [15], medicinal flies are reared in insectaries, and medicinal maggots are prepared aseptically under laboratory conditions with quality control procedures in place [20]. These days, maggot therapy is most commonly carried out with the medicinal fly species *Lucilia sericata* and, to a lesser degree, *L. cuprina* [21], but other species are actively being investigated for their therapeutic and commercial potential [22]. Disinfected maggots are placed on the wound either directly or enclosed in a mesh bag [23]. Most wounds treated with maggot therapy are chronic wounds such as diabetic ulcers, but acute wounds requiring debridement, such as infected traumatic and post-surgical wounds or burns, also respond well to maggot therapy [24, 25].

Why a Book on Maggot Therapy?

Although three or so decades have passed since maggot therapy was rediscovered and re-introduced to mainstream clinical practice, there are many barriers still standing in the way of widespread uptake of maggot therapy in modern and compromised healthcare settings alike. Unfortunately, maggot therapy is still not widely understood as a viable alternative to conventional wound care and therefore much underutilised. Many hospital administrators, physicians, nurses, and allied health practitioners still reject maggot therapy due to unfamiliarity, mistrust, or repulsion. There are also regulatory barriers in ministries of health which are made worse by a lack of international harmonisation of maggot therapy and medicinal maggot production regulations. Each jurisdiction repeats lengthy and costly regulatory processes that are blocking implementation, as is evident in the case of Kenya, presented in Chapter 15 of this book [26]. On a practical level, maggot therapy places specific demands on the supply chain with respect to rapid delivery and cool chain requirements, which is particularly the case in low-resource, compromised healthcare settings. [27].

This book fills the information vacuum, and importantly, it makes the current state of knowledge freely accessible to anyone with an Internet connection. It is the first book to provide sound, evidence-based information beyond the much-discussed therapeutic actions and clinical practice. Particular attention has been paid to the challenges encountered in compromised and low-resource healthcare settings such as disasters, conflict, and poverty. Patients in such settings will benefit greatly from affordable, efficacious, and sustainable maggot therapy. This book is as much a practical guide as a summary of the current state of knowledge in the field. The content has been carefully chosen to build global capacity for maggot debridement therapy services including production, distribution, and treatment.

Content

The next 18 chapters are organised into five parts beginning with Part 1, on the clinical aspects of maggot therapy. The behavioural, physiological, biochemical, and immunological principles of medicinal maggots that bring about debridement, infection control, and wound healing are presented in Part 2. The following three parts are new to the maggot therapy literature as they provide best-practice guidance on medicinal maggot production (Part 3), on medicinal maggot distribution logistics (Part 4), and on the ethics of maggot therapy (Part 5).

Part 1. It is important that we start with the patient. In Chapter 2, Rajna Ogrin and Kylie Elders [7] explain how chronic wounds have a large impact on patients' psycho-social wellbeing. They closely examine what it means to live with a chronic wound. Only if the needs and characteristics of patients and their social environment have been fully appreciated, can medical interventions like maggot therapy be developed and implemented with minimal harm and maximum benefit to the patient. What many clinicians don't realise is that maggot therapy is very versatile and can be used to treat almost any chronic wound. In Chapter 3, Ron Sherman and I [25] present the aetiologies and wound types amenable to maggot therapy. Of course, it is necessary to carefully consider whether patients and their wounds are suitable for maggot therapy. In Chapter 4, Ron [24] develops a typology of factors influencing treatment decisions and explains the recommended indications, contraindications, side-effects, and any interactions between maggot therapy and other treatments or patient behaviour. Practitioners new to maggot therapy will be particularly interested in learning how to apply medicinal maggots to the wound. Ron [23] introduces maggot confinement and containment approaches in Chapter 5 and explains how these dressings are constructed and applied to the wound.

While this clinical knowledge is essential for successful maggot therapy, the biggest hurdle for biotherapists wanting to use maggot therapy is the introduction and integration of the therapy into the healthcare system. To that end, Benjamin L. Bullen, Ronald A. Sherman, Paul J. Chadwick and Frank Stadler [28] explore in Chapter 6 the complexities of such an undertaking and provide guidance on how clinical integration of a maggot therapy programme is best achieved.

Part 2. It is widely acknowledged that medicinal maggots do more than just debride the wound. The second part of this book is concerned with the therapeutic properties of medicinal maggots in the wound. It makes sense to begin this exploration with the natural history of medicinal flies. In Chapter 7, Michelle Harvey [8] scopes the evolutionary history and taxonomic intricacies of calliphorid flies, to which medicinal and many forensically important fly species belong. Michelle reveals how the therapeutic benefits of medicinal maggots can be traced back to the evolutionary history, life history, and ecology of calliphorid flies. The next three chapters by Yamni Nigam and Michael Wilson provide excellent up-to-date reviews of the therapeutic actions of medicinal maggots [9–11]. Chapter 8 is concerned with the outstanding ability of medicinal maggots to remove dead tissue from chronic wounds, Chapter 9 summarises what is known about the antimicrobial properties of medicinal maggots, and Chapter 10 explains our current understanding of how medicinal maggots support and encourage wound healing.

While most maggot therapy around the world is currently conducted with *L. sericata* and *L. cuprina* blowflies, a wide range of other species have also been used for wound care, with varying degrees of clinical evidence supporting their use [21]. With countless potential species to choose from around the world, it is important to have protocols in place for the bioprospecting and testing of new medicinal fly species to ensure their therapeutic efficacy and safety before they can be approved by regulators and used in wound care. In Chapter 11, Patricia Thyssen and colleagues [22] provide a step-by-step guide to the selection and testing of new medicinal fly species, drawing on their own extensive experience in this field.

Part 3. There are only a few publications fully dedicated to the rearing of maggots for medicinal purposes. The earliest papers on the subject are by the fathers of modern maggot therapy, William S. Baer [15] and Duncan C. McKeever [29]. Subsequent publications on medicinal maggot production lean heavily on these seminal works, and mainly offer methodological improvements (e.g. the refinement of rearing techniques) rather than radical changes [27]. The four chapters in Part 3 provide comprehensive guidance on practical aspects of medicinal maggot production. In Chapter 12, I [30] identify the infrastructure and equipment requirements for medicinal fly insectaries and medicinal maggot laboratories. When it comes to sourcing medicinal flies for the establishment of safe maggot therapy programmes, practitioners may need to collect their own stock from the wild especially in situations where they do not have access to research or medical colonies. Nathan Butterworth and colleagues [21] explain in Chapter 13 how to best collect medical fly species, how to select and identify known safe species in each of the major zoogeographic regions of the world, and how to set up a breeding colony for sustainable medicinal maggot production. Although the literature on myiasis involving fly species that specialise exclusively in the consumption of necrotic tissue points clearly to the unintended therapeutic benefits of such infestations [31], it is absolutely necessary to produce maggots for clinical application under controlled and hygienic conditions to avoid adverse treatment outcomes and to inspire the confidence of regulators, health practitioners, and patients. Peter Takáč and I [26] outline in Chapter 14 how to maintain fly colonies in the production insectary and how to produce safe and quality-controlled medicinal maggots for wound treatment. Readers who want to start a maggot therapy programme will find Chapter 15 instructive. Peter and colleagues [26] report on their achievements and challenges encountered when establishing a medicinal maggot production facility and a maggot therapy programme in Kenya.

Part 4. The renaissance in maggot therapy over the past twenty years or so has largely taken place in developed countries with excellent logistics infrastructure such as in western Europe, North America and elsewhere. It appears that the lack of maggot therapy in truly compromised healthcare settings is, apart from social factors, largely brought about by supply-chain management challenges. Indeed, the literature on distribution logistics for medicinal maggots and freight packaging is sparse to non-existent, especially when contemplating distribution under extreme climatic conditions [27]. Therefore, Chapters 16 to 18 are concerned with packaging technology, distribution logistics, and innovative forms of transport. In Chapter 16, I [32] provide guidance on how medicinal maggots ought to be packaged to satisfy regulatory requirements and to ensure safe distribution of highly perishable maggots under unfavourable environmental conditions. Viability of any medicinal maggot production programme is dependent on a sufficiently large market which needs to be reached quickly considering the perishability of medicinal maggots. In Chapter 17, I [33] explain the basics of efficient medicinal maggot distribution systems. With rapid advances in the use of unmanned aerial vehicles (drones) in disaster and development, Peter Tatham and I [34] believe that there is great scope to utilise drones for last-mile delivery of medicinal maggots. Chapter 18 describes the various types of drones, how they may be employed, and what to consider when establishing a distribution partnership with drone operators.

Part 5. While Rajna Ogrin and Kylie Elders [7] begin our complete guide to maggot therapy with a patient's chronic wound journey, the book closes with Chapter 19 where I [35] summarise, for the first time, the ethical dimensions of maggot-assisted wound care from a biomedical and animal ethics point of view. To judge by the animal rights movement and the conscious purchasing choices consumers increasingly make, it is certain that the long-term sustainability and social licence of whole-organism maggot therapy will depend on how producers and health care practitioners treat medicinal flies at all life stages, and their ethical engagement with patients.

Past, Present, and Future

This book was conceived during my research on the supply-chain management for maggot therapy in compromised healthcare settings [36]. It struck me that after almost a hundred years of clinical practice, there was no comprehensive guide on maggot therapy that included guidance on the production of medicinal maggots and maggot therapy supply-chain management. The information that has been published over the years on issues relating to maggot therapy is highly dispersed across a large body of literature and held mostly behind journal paywalls [27]. Consequently, there was a need to both synthesise the literature and make this knowledge accessible to the widest possible readership, including those caring for patients with wounds in low- and middle-income countries, during disasters, and in wartime. It is in these settings where I believe maggot therapy can benefit patients the most because, as Yamni Nigam and Michael Wilson [9–11] explain, medicinal maggots convey several therapeutic properties at once. Besides, maggot therapy itself can be administered in the most austere care settings without diminishing its efficacy.

This book would not have been possible without the contribution of the many expert co-authors and reviewers who followed the highest professional standards. The title of the book claims that it is a complete guide to maggot therapy and related fields. Of course, completeness is wishful thinking and the title has been chosen to tickle the curiosity of readers, but it also signals our aspiration. While scientific or technical knowledge can never be complete, we must nevertheless strive toward completeness. Indeed, there is much that will need to be added to this book—perhaps in future editions. For example, there is recent research published and in press that explores the sociological and psychological dimensions of maggot therapy and builds on earlier work [e.g. 37, 38, 39]. It seeks to clarify what patients and healthcare practitioners really think about maggot therapy, and how psychological barriers can be overcome [40]. Would early education and sensitisation in schools help to shift attitudes toward maggot therapy [41, 42]? With regard to clinical performance, there has been a successful attempt to boost the therapeutic benefit of medicinal maggots with genetic engineering [43] and from the grey zone between whole-organism maggot therapy and drug development, research is emerging that explores the use of maggot-derived living macrophages for chronic wound care [44].

In conclusion, it is safe to say that the heydays for maggot therapy and maggot-inspired biological therapeutics and drugs are still to come. Meanwhile, this first edition of *A Complete Guide to Maggot Therapy: Clinical Practice, Therapeutic Principles, Production, Distribution, and Ethics* provides clinicians, medical entrepreneurs, health administrators, regulators, supply-chain managers, and isolated communities in compromised healthcare settings with the practical knowledge to treat wounds with maggot therapy.

References

1. Singh, N., D.G. Armstrong, and B.A. Lipsky, *Preventing Foot Ulcers in Patients with Diabetes.* JAMA, 2005. 293(2): pp. 217–228, https://doi.org/10.1001/jama.293.2.217.

2. Nsereko, E. and P. Brysiewicz, *Injury Surveillance in a Central Hospital in Kigali, Rwanda.* Journal of Emergency Nursing: JEN: Official Publication Of The Emergency Department Nurses Association, 2010. 36(3): pp. 212–216, https://doi.org/10.1016/j.jen.2009.07.020.

3. Wachira, B. and I.B.K. Martin, *The State of Emergency Care in the Republic of Kenya.* African Journal of Emergency Medicine, 2011. 1(4): pp. 160–165, https://doi.org/10.1016/j.afjem.2011.10.008.

4.   Khorram-Manesh, A., et al., *Estimating the Number of Civilian Casualties in Modern Armed Conflicts–A Systematic Review.* Frontiers in Public Health, 2021. 9: pp. 765261–765261, https://doi.org/10.3389/fpubh.2021.765261.

5.   Nadimpalli, M., et al., *Combating Global Antibiotic Resistance: Emerging One Health Concerns in Lower- and Middle-Income Countries.* Clinical Infectious Diseases, 2018. 66(6): pp. 963–969, https://doi.org/10.1093/cid/cix879.

6.   Älgå, A., et al., *Infection with High Proportion of Multidrug-resistant Bacteria in Conflict-related Injuries Is Associated with Poor Outcomes and Excess Resource Consumption: A Cohort Study of Syrian Patients Treated in Jordan.* BMC Infectious Diseases, 2018. 18(1): pp. 233–233, https://doi.org/10.1186/s12879-018-3149-y.

7.   Ogrin, R. and K. Elders, *Living with a Chronic Wound*, in *A Complete Guide to Maggot Therapy: Clinical Practice, Therapeutic Principles, Production, Distribution, and Ethics*, F. Stadler (ed.). 2022, Cambridge: Open Book Publishers, pp. 17–38, https://doi.org/10.11647/OBP.0300.02.

8.   Harvey, M., *The Natural History of Medicinal Flies*, in *A Complete Guide to Maggot Therapy: Clinical Practice, Therapeutic Principles, Production, Distribution, and Ethics*, F. Stadler (ed.). 2022, Cambridge: Open Book Publishers, pp. 121–142, https://doi.org/10.11647/OBP.0300.07.

9.   Nigam, Y. and M.R. Wilson, *Maggot Debridement*, in *A Complete Guide to Maggot Therapy: Clinical Practice, Therapeutic Principles, Production, Distribution, and Ethics*, F. Stadler (ed.). 2022, Cambridge: Open Book Publishers, pp. 143–152, https://doi.org/10.11647/OBP.0300.08.

10. Nigam, Y. and M.R. Wilson, *The Antimicrobial Activity of Medicinal Maggots*, in *A Complete Guide to Maggot Therapy: Clinical Practice, Therapeutic Principles, Production, Distribution, and Ethics*, F. Stadler (ed.). 2022, Cambridge: Open Book Publishers, pp. 153–174, https://doi.org/10.11647/OBP.0300.09.

11. Nigam, Y. and M.R. Wilson, *Maggot-assisted Wound Healing*, in *A Complete Guide to Maggot Therapy: Clinical Practice, Therapeutic Principles, Production, Distribution, and Ethics*, F. Stadler (ed.). 2022, Cambridge: Open Book Publishers, pp. 175–194, https://doi.org/10.11647/OBP.0300.10.

12. Lee, D.J., *Human Myiasis in Australia.* Medical Journal of Australia, 1968. 1(17): pp. 741–741, https://doi.org/10.5694/j.1326-5377.1968.tb28850.x.

13. Weil, J.C., R.J. Simon, and W.R. Sweadner, *A Biological, Bacteriological and Clinical Study of Larval or Maggot Therapy in the Treatment of Acute and Chronic Pyogenic Infections.* American Journal of Surgery, 1933. 19: p. 36.

14. Pechter, E.A. and R.A. Sherman, *Maggot Therapy: The Surgical Metamorphosis.* Plastic and Reconstructive Surgery, 1983. 72(4): pp. 567–570, https://doi.org/10.1097/00006534-198310000-00032.

15. Baer, W.S., *The Treatment of Chronic Osteomyelitis with the Maggot (Larva of the Blow Fly).* The Journal of Bone & Joint Surgery, 1931. 13(3): pp. 438–475, https://doi.org/10.1007/s11999-010-1416-3.

16. Robinson, W., *Progress of Maggot Therapy in the United States and Canada in the Treatment of Suppurative Diseases*. American Journal of Surgery, 1935. 29: pp. 67–71.

17. Sherman, R.A. and E.A. Pechter, *Maggot Therapy: A Review of the Therapeutic Applications of Fly Larvae in Human Medicine, Especially for Treating Osteomyelitis*. Medical and Veterinary Entomology, 1988. 2(3): pp. 225–230, https://doi.org/10.1111/j.1365-2915.1988.tb00188.x.

18. Kruglikova, A.A. and S.I. Chernysh, *Surgical Maggots and the History of Their Medical Use*. Entomological Review, 2013. 93(6): pp. 667–674, https://doi.org/10.1134/S0013873813060018.

19. Whitaker, I.S., et al., *Larval Therapy from Antiquity to the Present Day: Mechanisms of Action, Clinical Applications and Future Potential*. Postgraduate Medical Journal, 2007. 83(980): pp. 409–413, https://doi.org/10.1136/pgmj.2006.055905.

20. Stadler, F. and P. Takáč, *Medicinal Maggot Production*, in *A Complete Guide to Maggot Therapy: Clinical Practice, Therapeutic Principles, Production, Distribution, and Ethics*, F. Stadler (ed.). 2022, Cambridge: Open Book Publishers, pp. 289–330, https://doi.org/10.11647/OBP.0300.14.

21. Stadler, F., et al., *Fly Colony Establishment*, in *A Complete Guide to Maggot Therapy: Clinical Practice, Therapeutic Principles, Production, Distribution, and Ethics*, F. Stadler (ed.). 2022, Cambridge: Open Book Publishers, pp. 257–288 (p. 269), https://doi.org/10.11647/OBP.0300.13.

22. Thyssen, P.J. and F.S. Masiero, *Bioprospecting and Testing of New Fly Species for Maggot Therapy*, in *A Complete Guide to Maggot Therapy: Clinical Practice, Therapeutic Principles, Production, Distribution, and Ethics*, F. Stadler (ed.). 2022, Cambridge: Open Book Publishers, pp. 195–234, https://doi.org/10.11647/OBP.0300.11.

23. Sherman, R., *Medicinal Maggot Application and Maggot Therapy Dressing Technology*, in *A Complete Guide to Maggot Therapy: Clinical Practice, Therapeutic Principles, Production, Distribution, and Ethics*, F. Stadler (ed.). 2022, Cambridge: Open Book Publishers, pp. 79–96, https://doi.org/10.11647/OBP.0300.05.

24. Sherman, R., *Indications, Contraindications, Interactions, and Side-effects of Maggot Therapy*, in *A Complete Guide to Maggot Therapy: Clinical Practice, Therapeutic Principles, Production, Distribution, and Ethics*, F. Stadler (ed.). 2022, Cambridge: Open Book Publishers, pp. 63–78, https://doi.org/10.11647/OBP.0300.04.

25. Sherman, R. and F. Stadler, *Wound Aetiologies, Patient Characteristics, and Healthcare Settings Amenable to Maggot Therapy*, in *A Complete Guide to Maggot Therapy: Clinical Practice, Therapeutic Principles, Production, Distribution, and Ethics*, F. Stadler (ed.). 2022, Cambridge: Open Book Publishers, pp. 39–62, https://doi.org/10.11647/OBP.0300.03.

26. Takáč, P., et al., and F. Stadler, *Establishment of a Medicinal Maggot Production Facility and Treatment Programme in Kenya* in *A Complete Guide to Maggot Therapy: Clinical Practice, Therapeutic Principles, Production, Distribution, and Ethics*, F. Stadler (ed.). 2022, Cambridge: Open Book Publishers, pp. 331–346, https://doi.org/10.11647/OBP.0300.15.

27. Stadler, F., *The Maggot Therapy Supply Chain: A Review of the Literature and Practice*. Med Vet Entomol, 2020. 34(1): pp. 1–9, https://doi.org/10.1111/mve.12397.

28. Bullen, B. and P. Chadwick, *Clinical Integration of Maggot Therapy*, in *A Complete Guide to Maggot Therapy: Clinical Practice, Therapeutic Principles, Production, Distribution, and Ethics*, F. Stadler (ed.). 2022, Cambridge: Open Book Publishers, pp. 97–118, https://doi.org/10.11647/OBP.0300.06.

29. McKeever, D.C., *Maggots in Treatment of Osteomyelitis: A Simple Inexpensive Method*. The Journal of Bone and Joint Surgery, 1933. 15: pp. 85–93, http://dx.doi.org/10.1007/s11999-008-0240-5.

30. Stadler, F., *Laboratory and Insectary Infrastructure and Equipment*, in *A Complete Guide to Maggot Therapy: Clinical Practice, Therapeutic Principles, Production, Distribution, and Ethics*, F. Stadler (ed.). 2022, Cambridge: Open Book Publishers, pp. 237–256, https://doi.org/10.11647/OBP.0300.12.

31. Terterov, S., et al., *Posttraumatic Human Cerebral Myiasis*. World Neurosurgery, 2010. 73(5): pp. 557–559, https://doi.org/10.1016/j.wneu.2010.01.004.

32. Stadler, F., *Packaging Technology*, in *A Complete Guide to Maggot Therapy: Clinical Practice, Therapeutic Principles, Production, Distribution, and Ethics*, F. Stadler (ed.). 2022, Cambridge: Open Book Publishers, pp. 349–362, https://doi.org/10.11647/OBP.0300.16.

33. Stadler, F., *Distribution Logistics* in *A Complete Guide to Maggot Therapy: Clinical Practice, Therapeutic Principles, Production, Distribution, and Ethics*, F. Stadler (ed.). 2022, Cambridge: Open Book Publishers, pp. 363–382, https://doi.org/10.11647/OBP.0300.17.

34. Stadler, F. and P. Tatham, *Drone-assisted Medicinal Maggot Distribution in Compromised Healthcare Settings*, in *A Complete Guide to Maggot Therapy: Clinical Practice, Therapeutic Principles, Production, Distribution, and Ethics*, F. Stadler (ed.). 2022, Cambridge: Open Book Publishers, pp. 383–402, https://doi.org/10.11647/OBP.0300.18.

35. Stadler, F., *The Ethics of Maggot Therapy*, in *A Complete Guide to Maggot Therapy: Clinical Practice, Therapeutic Principles, Production, Distribution, and Ethics*, F. Stadler (ed.). 2022, Cambridge: Open Book Publishers, pp. 405–430, https://doi.org/10.11647/OBP.0300.19.

36. Stadler, F. *Supply Chain Management for Maggot Debridement Therapy in Compromised Healthcare Settings*. 2018. Unpublished doctoral dissertation, Griffith University, Queensland, https://doi.org/10.25904/1912/3170.

37. Rafter, L., *A Patient's Perceptions of Using Larval Therapy*. Wounds UK, 2010. 6(2): pp. 130–132.

38. Spilsbury, K., et al., *Exploring Patient Perceptions of Larval Therapy as a Potential Treatment for Venous Leg Ulceration*. Health Expectations, 2008. 11(2): pp. 148–159, https://doi.org/10.1111/j.1369-7625.2008.00491.x.

39. Heitkamp, R.A., G.W. Peck, and B.C. Kirkup, *Maggot Debridement Therapy in Modern Army Medicine: Perceptions and Prevalence*. Military Medicine, 2012. 177(11): pp. 1411–1416, https://doi.org/10.7205/milmed-d-12-00200.

40. Pajarillo, C., et al., *Health Professionals' Perceptions of Maggot Debridement Therapy*. Journal of Wound Care, 2021. 30(Sup9a): pp. VIIi–VIIxi, https://doi.org/10.12968/jowc.2021.30.Sup9a.VII.

41. Humphreys, I., P. Lehane, and Y. Nigam, *Could Maggot Therapy Be Taught in Primary Schools?* Journal of Biological Education, 2020: p. 1–11, https://doi.org/10.1080/00219266.2020.1748686.

42. Stadler, F., et al., *Maggot Menageries: High School Student Contributions to Medicinal Maggot Production in Compromised Healthcare Settings*. Citizen Science: Theory and Practice, 2021. 6(1): p. 36, http://doi.org/10.5334/cstp.401.

43. Linger, R.J., et al., *Towards Next Generation Maggot Debridement Therapy: Transgenic Lucilia sericata Larvae that Produce and Secrete a Human Growth Factor*. BMC Biotechnology, 2016. 16: p. 30, https://doi.org/10.1186/s12896-016-0263-z.

44. Yakovlev, A., et al., *The Possibility of Using Xenogeneic Phagocytes in Wound Treatment*. PloS ONE, 2022. 17(1): e0263256-e0263256, https://doi.org/10.1371/journal.pone.0263256.

PART 1

CLINICAL PRACTICE

2. Living with a Chronic Wound

Rajna Ogrin and Kylie J. Elder

Any clinical intervention must be person-centered and maggot therapy is no different. Therefore, it is important to fully understand and appreciate what it means for a person to live with a non-healing wound, often for many years. Using the hypothetical but representative case of Beverly, the authors explore the impact of chronic wounds on the wellbeing of the person. Since wellbeing is a multidimensional concept, the chapter examines psychological, social, as well as spiritual and cultural wellbeing as shaped by the lived experience of a chronic wound. There are feedback loops and interactions between the symptoms and the persons' physical, psychological, social, and spiritual wellbeing.

Introduction

Living with a chronic wound can have a substantial impact on an individual's physical, psychological, social, and spiritual wellbeing. Financial cost can also burden people living with wounds and their families [1]. Maggot therapy can contribute to the better management of chronic wounds and thereby improve the wellbeing of those living with chronic wounds. Medicinal maggots stimulate healthy new granulation tissue in the wound bed [2–4] and reduce the microbiological burden in wounds through their ingestion and digestion of microbes and through the excretion and secretion of antibacterial compounds [5–8]. This supports the management of issues related to chronic wounds,

https://doi.org/10.11647/OBP.0300.02

including healing time [9], need for antibiotics [9], exudate management and odour [10], and cost of treatment [11, 12]. Exudate is defined as "exuded matter; especially the material composed of serum, fibrin, and white blood cells that escapes into a superficial lesion or area of inflammation" [13]. Chapters 8 to 10 of this book give an up-to-date summary of how medicinal maggots achieve debridement, infection control, and wound healing [14–16].

A shared approach to decision making, involving people living with wounds, will encourage optimal treatment outcomes. This should include decisions on the appropriate management of wounds and consideration of the impact of treatment on individuals' wellbeing [17]. This is particularly relevant for consideration and integration of an unusual wound care treatment such as maggot therapy in the care of people with chronic wounds. It is therefore important for stakeholders in the maggot therapy supply chain, whether they be researchers, producers, health insurers, or healthcare providers, to understand what it is like for a person to live with a chronic wound. Using the fictional, albeit entirely representative, case of Beverly who is a person on the chronic wound journey, this chapter will describe the impact of chronic wounds on physical, psychological, social, and spiritual wellbeing as well as the structural aspects of health systems that impact on how people live with chronic wounds.

Wellbeing in People Living with Chronic Wounds

Beverly. Five months ago, while working in her garden, 74-year-old Beverly scratched her lower left leg on a branch, causing her skin to break open. She has diabetes, diagnosed 10 years ago, hypertension, hypercholesteraemia and arthritis in her left knee. Beverly is active in the community, volunteering at the local charity shop twice a week. Her family live an hour's drive away and although she has assistance for house cleaning, she is otherwise self-sufficient. Beverly does not drive but catches the local bus to the charity shop. Social connectedness and staying active are most important to Beverly. When Beverly first developed the wound, she put a clean bandage on it and thought it would go away.

Chronic wounds are simply wounds that do not proceed to heal along the normal wound trajectory [18] which encompasses haemostasis, inflammation, reconstruction, and maturation [19]. Wounds can become chronic for a variety of reasons: physiological, behavioural, societal, and environmental. Chronicity of a wound can also be influenced by the health system structure and ability to access treatment [20]. Because of these factors, once present, chronic wounds are very difficult to heal, and may take considerable time, or not heal at all [18].

The presence of a chronic wound significantly impacts the wellbeing of individuals, with pain, anxiety, and disappointment being common [21]. Those with malignant fungating wounds, in particular, feel a loss of control over their body and their lives [22], with social implications of malodour and other physical symptoms [23]. At first, people with chronic wounds may accept the inconvenience of a wound. However, as the wound duration increases, coping becomes more difficult and withdrawal from their social environment may occur as fears of non-healing increase [21]. Although the goal of care for most people with wounds is healing, for malignant or non-healing wounds, managing the physical symptoms is very important [1, 23, 24], with the aim of living positively with the wound [25]. Palliation goals for non-healing chronic wounds centre around preventing new wounds from developing, preventing existing wounds from deteriorating, and symptom management to address comfort and quality of life [26]. Therefore, the overall wellbeing of the person living with the wound is just as important an outcome as wound healing itself [26].

Wellbeing means that people have the physical, psychological, social, and spiritual resources they need to meet a particular physical, psychological, and/or social challenge [27]. The definition of wellbeing in relation to wound management is outlined in Box 1. The first three interrelated domains of wellbeing have been articulated by the World Health Organization [28] as:

- *Physical wellbeing*: The ability to function independently in activities such as bathing, dressing, eating, and moving around.

- *Psychological wellbeing:* This implies that cognitive faculties are intact and that the person is free from fear, anxiety, stress, depression, or other negative emotions.

- *Social wellbeing:* The ability to participate in and engage with family, society, friends, and workers.

And spiritual wellbeing was added and defined by International Consensus [1]:

- *"Spiritual/cultural wellbeing*: an ability to experience and integrate meaning and purpose in life through connections with one's self and others. This is an integral part of mental, emotional and physical health and may be associated with a specific religion, cultural beliefs or personal values."

Box 1. Wellbeing in relation to wound management.

As defined in *Optimising wellbeing in people living with a wound. An expert working group review* [1]:

Wellbeing is a dynamic matrix of factors, including physical, social psychological and spiritual. The concept of wellbeing is inherently individual, will vary over time, is influenced by culture and context, and is independent of wound type, duration or care setting. Within wound healing, optimising an individual's wellbeing will be the result of collaboration and interactions between clinicians, the person living with a wound, their families and carers, the healthcare system and industry. The ultimate goals are to optimise wellbeing, improve or heal the wound, alleviate/manage symptoms and ensure all parties are fully engaged in this process.

Beverly thought that her wound would heal after a few weeks, but she has had it for over three months and she's so sick of it, and worried it will never heal. The pain has limited her going out and she can only volunteer at the charity shop for a couple of hours a week. She relies on a friend to pick her up and drive her as she can no longer catch public transport. She finds this distressing as she prefers to be self-reliant. Even having to wear the bandages worries her, as it shows that something is wrong. She tries to hide them by wearing long skirts and thick stockings, not able to wear the normal trousers she prefers because she can't fit them over the bandages. Sometimes the wound leaks through the bandage and starts to smell. She has been attending the local doctor's surgery to get some wound advice and dressings but getting there is hard, and she still needs to change the dressing herself.

An attempt has been made to separate the issues associated with living with a chronic wound into physical, psychological, social, and system domains, however, as outlined by Beverly's case, many issues fall under multiple domains. Further, some issues lead to the development of others across the domains. This reinforces how challenging it is to understand the complex impacts of chronic wounds on people's lives. Clinicians must consider the whole person for management to be truly person-centred [29], and thereby more likely to support people to achieve their goals of care. Unfortunately, the majority of existing studies focus on quality of life when living with a wound, which emphasises deficits in peoples' lives, rather than a holistic, asset-based approach associated with wellbeing [17]. We will convey the evidence related to issues affecting the lives of people living with a chronic wound, and show how they impact lives using our case study of Beverly.

Physical Wellbeing

Beverly finds the open wound a bit painful and moving too much hurts. The lack of sleep due to the itchiness and pain in her wound makes her so tired and irritable the next day. She's worried about taking pain medication, as these kinds of tablets can be addictive. She covers her wound with a dressing and bandages, but it leaks quite a lot and the bandages can't contain it all. When the fluid sits for a time it begins to smell and hardens the dressing, which makes the area even more painful to walk with, as well as being very embarrassing. She has had multiple infections, and where previously the wound was clean and red, it now has a persistent smelly grey base and the dressings don't make much of a difference. Beverly stopped volunteering at the charity shop as she doesn't want to be with people for long periods of time in case they notice the leaking or smell. She now relies on a walking frame for mobility as the heavy bandages make her feel as if she will fall. She is beginning to put on weight which is also impacting on her arthritic joints. The ulcer is getting larger and her legs are also swelling. It is hard to shower because she must keep the bandages dry and this is very difficult.

Chronic wounds can impact negatively upon the physical wellbeing of people with wounds, with pain/irritation, wound exudate malodour [25, 30], limitations on mobility and sleep disturbances commonly being raised as issues [31–33]. A poorer quality of life is correlated to dressing change frequency, pain, wound dressing comfort, wound symptom, bleeding, and malodour in individuals with malignant fungating wounds [34]. The effect of each factor can vary, depending on the wound size, depth, location and duration [35]. As shown by Beverly's case, these factors combine to impact on physical functioning. Listed below are issues that have been predominantly identified in the literature. It is important to note this list is not exhaustive, and other issues may also occur:

Pain. Wound pain is reported to vary in type, intensity and duration, and is described in different ways by people with chronic wounds. For example, pain may be experienced as burning, shooting, stabbing, knife-like, throbbing, dull, niggly, gnawing, aching, annoying, hot poker, pins, nerve pain, sticky, or stinging [36]. For some people, pain can be constant, spontaneous, or persistent [37], while others can have pain-free periods interrupted by periods of sudden onset of severe pain with no apparent trigger [36].

Wound pain may be lessened through a number of approaches; however, it can also worsen in the presence of infection, with some treatments, and when undertaking physical activity [36]. It is important to note that if pain is exacerbated or triggered by physical activity, this may also influence the ability of people with chronic wounds to be more active [32, 36]. This, in turn, may lead to further complications that negatively impact physical wellbeing. Pain at dressing changes has been identified as the worst part of having a wound [38].

Finally, pain management may be inadequate in people with chronic wounds [39, 40], with prescription rates and use of analgesia low in people living with wounds [36]. Some individuals are reluctant to use pain medication, concerned they will become addicted [25]. Lack of pain management may impact on attempts at physical activity by virtue of anticipation of the perceived pain [25]. Anxiety can also contribute to this anticipated pain and it is therefore important that this emotion is addressed [41].

Impaired physical mobility. Physical mobility may be impaired either because of ulcer characteristics, the dressing, or self-imposed isolation in response to the impact of symptoms [31]. Limited physical mobility can restrict the ability to undertake activities of daily living including employment, participation in recreational activities, and social interaction [30–32, 36].

- *Ulcer characteristics.* Itchiness, exudate and swelling of the leg are common in people with leg ulcers [32, 36], with itching and pain affecting sleep, leading to increased tiredness during the day, in turn leading to more rest, thereby reducing physical activities [36]. In people with malignant fungating wounds dealing with the physical symptoms of pain, exudate, odour [25], itch, and bleeding is very challenging [23].

- *Dressings.* Undertaking outdoor activities may be off-putting owing to the need for dressing changes in people with chronic wounds as they wait for healthcare professional appointments [32]. Bandages can restrict movement in some people living with chronic wounds [40, 42]. Depending on the dressings used, clothing choice can be restricted, including the ability to wear normal footwear, particularly with bandaging [36, 40, 43]. Bathing can be difficult, as people are advised to keep the dressing dry in between dressing changes, the frequency of which can vary from daily to once a week [40, 43, 44].

- *Self-imposed isolation.* This is particularly evident if people living with a wound are unable to maintain their own hygiene, which is not uncommon, given that they are asked to keep their dressings dry for days at a time, limiting their ability to bathe [40]. The dressings are often cumbersome and unsightly, and if exudate levels are high and sub-optimally managed, people living with chronic wounds are less likely to leave their homes [43–45]. The limitations on what clothing and footwear may be worn may further lead to people living with chronic wounds isolating themselves [36]. If sleep is disturbed by the wound pain and/or itchiness, then resting during the day may contribute to people isolating themselves [32, 36]. Some people living with a wound reduce the amount of activity they undertake, further limiting outside activities because of an expressed fear of falling and traumatic injury which could lead to a worsening of their wound or prevent it from healing [42].

Psychological Wellbeing

Beverly is now unable to get around much at all. During the day she has more time to think about her wound and the pain and this makes her feel down and makes the pain worse. Her anxiety that the wound will never heal consumes her. The added weight gain, loss of mobility, limited hygiene and bulky clothes combined make her feel like she is ugly, and useless as a person.

Psychological and social wellbeing have some overlapping aspects. The psychological includes the emotional impact wounds have on persons living with a wound as well as on their carers and family members. These emotions are pivotal in social wellbeing. This interconnectedness makes it difficult to separate some aspects. For example, when wounds do not heal in the expected timeframe, people may withdraw socially and at the same time, experience increased feelings of fear [21]. In addition, poor psychological health is associated with higher risk of depression, less perceived social support, and greater social isolation [46]. While there are many aspects of chronic wounds that lead to a deterioration in psychosocial wellbeing, it is not all negative. Some people with wounds can find satisfaction in their changed circumstances after accepting their situation and adapting their expectations [36]. Further, while depression is common, some people living with wounds remain hopeful of a positive outcome [31].

The impact of chronic wounds on many peoples' psychological wellbeing is significant [1, 21]. Depression, anxiety [47], low mood, and poor quality of life are common in people living with a chronic wound [31, 33, 34]. Further, changes in mood, acceptance, body image, and issues with self-esteem have been identified in reviews of the literature [36]. Body image and self-esteem are particular issues in malignant fungating wounds [22]. Many of the problems experienced stem from the physical wound characteristics [23, 25, 33], as well as the treatment regimens implemented to manage the wounds [32]. The psychological impact of living with a chronic wound includes, but is not limited to:

Depression

Depression is a common mental condition, "characterized by sadness, loss of interest or pleasure, feelings of guilt or low self-worth, disturbed sleep or appetite, feelings of tiredness and poor concentration" [48]. It is estimated that up to 30% of all people living with chronic wounds develop depression and/or anxiety [49–51]. An international multi-centre study about the psychological burden of skin diseases identified people living with leg ulcers as having the highest odds ratio for depression when compared with other skin conditions. [47]. Feelings of depression, despair and hopelessness were associated with lack of sleep and subsequent fatigue due to the wound [52]. Again, physical symptoms were the main cause of sleep problems, including pain and itching [36].

Negative Emotions

The physical aspects of chronic wounds can trigger stress and other negative emotions. Anxiety was also associated with the fear that others could smell the ulcer or that there would be exudate leakage [39]. Odour and excessive exudate where leakage occurs remind people that they have a wound, and raise feelings of disgust [53], self-loathing and low self-esteem [23, 54]. The ongoing nature of the wound leads to feelings of frustration because the wound appears to be "forever healing" [55] and to concerns that the wound won't ever heal [40] or will deteriorate.

Social Wellbeing

Beverly's family live so far away, so it is difficult for them to help and she is now reliant on neighbours to help her shop and cook. She has also had to accept a carer to shower her because of her poor mobility. She does not feel that she has control over her life. The issues with her wound prevent Beverly from participating in any social activities, and this makes her feel very lonely.

This component involves the ability of people to participate in and engage with family, society, friends, and, if employed, other colleagues at work. The ability to engage with everyday functioning can be restricted either owing to the wound, the dressing or to a self-imposed isolation in response to the impact of symptoms [25, 31].

In the initial stages of developing the wound, people have hope that it will heal in a timely fashion. However, as the wound becomes chronic, relationships with family and friends can become strained as people need to rely on them for help with cooking and cleaning [40, 43]. Further, declining contact with others occurs when people living with wounds lose confidence and hope [56]. They may also hide the true impact of how the wound makes them feel, with some feeling ashamed to talk about their wounds [57].

Self-imposed isolation is common, where people living with wounds may avoid interaction with others because of, either the embarrassing symptoms associated with the wound itself or the physical aspects of the wound and the dressings (or indeed both). The embarrassment can stem from malodour, exudate leakage [25, 58], or blood leakage [25, 37], as well as the unsightly appearance of the dressings [59]. The dressing factors raised previously can negatively impact on body image and life-satisfaction, and contribute to social withdrawal [22, 36, 40, 59–61]. The combination of all of the above factors can also limit mobility, and thereby limit the person's ability to undertake their normal social activities [23, 40, 58].

Spiritual/Cultural Wellbeing

> ***Beverly*** finds solace in her faith. It is hard for her to go to church, with the pain while walking and her worry about the wound leaking, but she makes the effort. She finds she can share her real worries about her leg with the priest, and it gives her some release from her stress.

Spirituality may provide positive and negative contributions to the wellbeing of people living with chronic wounds. In some individuals, they may believe that they are responsible for their wound and consider it a punishment for their actions from a higher being [62]. Conversely, spirituality may provide hope of healing, resilience, and endurance to deal with the symptoms [63]. It is important to understand beliefs, religious and otherwise, of individuals living with their chronic wound, as this impacts on the management of their condition and the support resources available to them [1]. For example, this may involve avoiding appointments on days of religious significance or ensuring permission is sought when using treatments that use animal products [64]. Spirituality and cultural wellbeing are less well studied, and would benefit from more research to identify the way they influence choices and practices related to wound management [1].

How People with Chronic Wounds Seek, Access, and Experience Care

Beverly. The doctor referred Beverly to receive home nursing given that her wound had not progressed and she required closer monitoring of her blood sugar levels. Beverly was embarrassed that she needed help, but she was finding it hard to cope with everything, including paying for all the dressings and the doctors' appointments—everything is so expensive. The nurse attended a full assessment and discovered that Beverly's peripheral vascular system was compromised, meaning she needed to wear compression bandages to support her veins to heal. This was the first time Beverly had been told the reason her wound was not healing. The nurses educated Beverly on wound healing, the importance of nutrition and keeping active. They discussed Beverly's options with her and developed a plan of care that considered Beverly's goals. The nurses continued to visit her to attend to dressings and apply the bandages. The pain and exudate from the wound was reduced and Beverly was able to begin to socialise once more.

In low-income countries, access to healthcare may also be limited due to distance [65], and care is frequently sought from traditional healers, and less from government facilities and private health practitioners [30]. Delays in seeking treatment are very common for a number of reasons. People often turn to the use of traditional medicine first [65, 66] because they strongly believe in their ability to control the disease [67], but also due to social and financial constraints [30, 65] and fear of amputation

[66]. Culture also impacts a person's perception of disease and therefore whether and from whom they seek and accept treatment [68].

Generally, in middle- to high-income countries, the General Practitioner is the most common source of care [69]. Many self-treat, often due to lack of healthcare resources, the cost involved, and dissatisfaction with previously received medical care [70]. Self-treatment may also occur to maintain independence, and for convenience regarding treatment schedules—although most have sought professional healthcare input for assessment and advice at some time [71].

Access to Evidence-based Care

Assessing, diagnosing, and managing wounds are complex activities that need to be enabled by the healthcare system and institutional capacity. In order to be proficient, healthcare workers require significant knowledge, skills, and expertise [72]. There are few healthcare providers in developed countries who have this expertise, let alone in low- and middle-income countries, which means that people with chronic wounds have difficulties accessing quality care [69, 73, 74]

The Cost of Care

Whether in high- or low-income care settings, subsidies for costly dressings, bandages, and footwear are often not available to people living with a wound and their families although they are essential for proper care, wound healing, and prevention of recurrence [20, 75]. Even where these costs are subsidised, full out-of-pocket expenses are not usually recouped [76], making evidence-based care unaffordable and therefore inaccessible [20, 75]. Costs associated with chronic wound treatment also include travel to and from and accommodation for appointments, fees for medical and specialist reviews, loss of wages, equipment purchases or hire, and medication to treat infections [76]. In the end, these factors can lead to significant and even catastrophic healthcare expenditure for people living with chronic wounds.

How People with Chronic Wounds Experience Care

As mentioned earlier, wellbeing is more than just health, and involves the physical, psychological, social, and spiritual domains. Health is only one part of wellbeing, yet our health system focusses almost exclusively on the physical and poorly on psychological, social, and spiritual wellbeing, i.e. the biomedical model [29]. Negative experiences of people seeking care for their chronic wounds from healthcare providers is common. There is a lack of understanding of the priorities of people living with wounds by healthcare providers, limiting effective support [77]. People with chronic wounds can feel that physicians do not understand how they perceive their situation, and that there is the need for improved communication and greater involvement in decisions about their care [78]. Individuals may receive conflicting information [71, 78], need to wait too long for an appointment [71], and perceive poor outcomes from care [65, 70, 71].

The World Health Organization aspires to the biopsychosocial model of care [79] to promote the wellbeing of community members [80]. This approach is person-centred, with the needs of community members driving the care that they require, which includes the physical, psychological and social aspects of wellbeing [1, 28]. Involving people in their care and supporting easy access to the right care with the right person at the right time is essential to achieve optimal outcomes [81].

Summary

Chronic wounds impose all-pervasive physical, psychological, social, and spiritual impacts on individuals, their families, and friends. These are mostly mediated by wound symptoms such as excessive exudate and odour, infection, pain, and lack of healing. As described earlier, there are vicious feedback loops and interactions between the symptoms and peoples' physical, psychological, social, and spiritual wellbeing. Further, there is a widespread knowledge and training deficit regarding appropriate holistic and multidisciplinary wound care, and wounds impose a high financial burden on individuals and society.

Health systems are generally focussed on the medical model, meaning that they consider mostly the disease and not the person living with the disease. Care needs to include a biopsychosocial approach, where effective assessment, diagnosis and management that engages with people living with wounds and considers what is important to them is implemented.

Maggot therapy can play an important role in the provision of such efficacious, affordable and person-centred wound care that improves the physical, psychological, social, and spiritual wellbeing of people living with wounds provided it is properly integrated into the healthcare system. How this may be achieved is discussed in Chapter 6 of this book [82]. Maggot therapy can speed up debridement and promote wound healing, reduce exudate and odour, and control infection, all of which have a significant impact on the wellbeing of people with chronic wounds. Most important, though, in the context of this discussion, maggot therapy requires full consent and acceptance by individuals and their families. This is difficult to achieve if people with wounds are not involved in care decision making. To that end, Chapter 19 [83] examines ethical considerations involved in using medicinal maggots as a wound care therapy, including the importance of consent by the individual for this therapy.

References

1.   International Consensus, *Optimising Wellbeing in People Living with a Wound. An Expert Working Group Review.* 2012, Wounds International: London.   https://www.woundsinternational.com/uploads/resources/ c3a58a73ca934b6989ffdb0e31d2c45d.pdf.

2.   Horobin, A.J., et al., *Maggots and Wound Healing: An Investigation of the Effects of Secretions from Lucilia sericata Larvae upon Interactions between Human Dermal Fibroblasts and Extracellular Matrix Components.* British Journal of Dermatology, 2003. 148(5): pp. 923–933.

3.   Sun, X., et al., *Maggot Debridement Therapy Promotes Diabetic Foot Wound Healing by Up-regulating Endothelial Cell Activity.* Journal of Diabetes and its Complications, 2016. 30(2): pp. 318–322, https://doi.org/10.1016/j. jdiacomp.2015.11.009.

4.   Wollina, U., et al., *Biosurgery Supports Granulation and Debridement in Chronic Wounds — Clinical Data and Remittance Spectroscopy Measurement.* International Journal of Dermatology, 2002. 41(10): pp. 635–639, https:// doi.org/10.1046/j.1365-4362.2002.01354.x.

5.   Bexfield, A., et al., *Detection and Partial Characterisation of Two Antibacterial Factors from the Excretions/Secretions of the Medicinal Maggot Lucilia sericata and Their Activity against Methicillin-Resistant Staphylococcus aureus (MRSA)*. Microbes and Infection, 2004. 6(14): pp. 1297–1304, https://doi.org/10.1016/j.micinf.2004.08.011.

6.   Bohova, J., et al., *Selective Antibiofilm Effects of Lucilia sericata Larvae Secretions/Excretions against Wound Pathogens*. Evidence-Based Complementary and Alternative Medicine, 2014. 2014: pp. 1–9, https://doi.org/10.1155/2014/857360.

7.   Kruglikova, A.A. and S.I. Chernysh, *Antimicrobial Compounds from the Excretions of Surgical Maggots, Lucilia sericata (Meigen) (Diptera, Calliphoridae)*. Entomological Review, 2011. 91(7): pp. 813–819, https://doi.org/10.1134/S0013873811070013.

8.   Lerch, K., et al., *Bacteria Ingestion by Blowfly Larvae: An in vitro Study*. Dermatology, 2003. 207(4): pp. 362–366, https://doi.org/10.1159/000074115.

9.   Sun X, J.K., Chen J, Wu L, Lu H, Wang A, Wang J., *A Systematic Review of Maggot Debridement Therapy for Chronically Infected Wounds and Ulcers*. International Journal of Infectious Diseases, 2014. 25: pp. 32–37, https://doi.org/10.1016/j.ijid.2014.03.1397.

10.   Sig, A.K., O. Koru, and E. Araz, *Maggot Debridement Therapy: Utility in Chronic Wounds and a Perspective Beyond*. Wound Practice & Research, 2018. 26(3): pp. 146–153.

11.   Wilasrusmee, C., et al., *Maggot Therapy for Chronic Ulcer: A Retrospective Cohort and a Meta-analysis*. Asian Journal of Surgery, 2014. 37: pp. 138–147, https://doi.org/10.1016/j.asjsur.2013.09.005.

12.   Gieroń, M., M. Słowik-Rylska, and B. Kręcisz, *Effectiveness of Maggot Debridement Therapy in Treating Chronic Wounds — Review of Current Literature*. Medical Studies/Studia Medyczne, 2018. 34(4): pp. 325–331, https://doi.org/10.5114/ms.2018.80949.

13.   *Merriam-Webster Dictionary*. 2020, www.merriam-webster.com/dictionary/exudate.

14.   Nigam, Y. and M.R. Wilson, *Maggot Debridement*, in *A Complete Guide to Maggot Therapy: Clinical Practice, Therapeutic Principles, Production, Distribution, and Ethics*, F. Stadler (ed.). 2022, Cambridge: Open Book Publishers, pp. 143–152, https://doi.org/10.11647/OBP.0300.

15.   Nigam, Y. and M.R. Wilson, *The Antimicrobial Activity of Medicinal Maggots*, in *A Complete Guide to Maggot Therapy: Clinical Practice, Therapeutic Principles, Production, Distribution, and Ethics*, F. Stadler (ed.). 2022, Cambridge: Open Book Publishers, pp. 153–174, https://doi.org/10.11647/OBP.0300.09.

16.   Nigam, Y. and M.R. Wilson, *Maggot-assisted Wound Healing*, in *A Complete Guide to Maggot Therapy: Clinical Practice, Therapeutic Principles, Production,*

Distribution, and Ethics, F. Stadler (ed.). 2022, Cambridge: Open Book Publishers, pp. 175–194, https://doi.org/10.11647/OBP.0300.10.

17.   Upton, D., A. Andrews, and P. Upton, *Venous Leg Ulcers: What about Well-being?* Journal of Wound Care, 2014. 23(1): pp. 14–17, https://doi.org/10.12968/jowc.2014.23.1.14.

18.   Nunan, R. and P. Martin, *Clinical Challenges of Chronic Wounds: Searching for an Optimal Animal Model to Recapitulate Their Complexity.* Disease Models and Mechanisms, 2014. 7(11): pp. 1205–1213, https://doi.org/10.1242/dmm.016782.

19.   Guo, S. and L.A. Dipietro, *Factors Affecting Wound Healing.* Journal of Dental Research, 2010. 89(3): pp. 219–229, https://doi.org/10.1177/0022034509359125.

20.   Chronic Wounds Solutions Collaborating Group, *Solutions to the Chronic Wounds Problem in Australia: A Call To Action.* 2018, Australian Centre for Health Services Innovation (AusHSI): Kelvin Grove, Queensland.

21.   Marczak, J., et al., *Patient Experiences of Living with Chronic Leg Ulcers and Making the Decision to Seek Professional Health-care.* Journal of Wound Care, 2019. 28(Sup 1): pp. S18-S25, https://doi.org/10.12968/jowc.2019.28.sup1.s18.

22.   Probst, S., A. Arber, and S. Faithfull, *Malignant Fungating Wounds — The Meaning of Living in an Unbounded Body.* European Journal of Oncology Nursing, 2013. 17(1): pp. 38–45, https://doi.org/10.1016/j.ejon.2012.02.001.

23.   Reynolds, H. and G. Gethin, *The Psychological Effects of Malignant Fungating Wounds.* Journal of Wound Management, 2015. 15(2): pp. 29–32.

24.   Probst, S., et al., *Recommendations for the Care of Patients with Malignant Fungating Wounds.* 2015, European Oncology Nursing Society (EONS): London.

25.   Lo, S.-F., et al., *Experiences of Living with a Malignant Fungating Wound: A Qualitative Study.* Journal of Clinical Nursing, 2008. 17(20): pp. 2699–2708, https://doi.org/10.1111/j.1365-2702.2008.02482.x.

26.   Nenna, M., *Pressure Ulcers at End Life: An Overview for Home Care and Hospice Clinicians.* Home Healthcare Nurse, 2011. 29(6): pp. 350–365, https://doi.org/10.1097/nhh.0b013e3182173ac1.

27.   Dodge, R., et al., *The Challenge of Defining Wellbeing.* International Journal of Wellbeing, 2012. 2(3): pp. 222–235, https://doi.org/10.5502/ijw.v2i3.4.

28.   WHO. *Constitution of the World Health Organization.* [Basic works] 2006. https://www.who.int/governance/eb/who_constitution_en.pdf.

29.   Wade, D.T. and P.W. Halligan, *The Biopsychosocial Model of Illness: A Model Whose Time Has Come.* Clinical Rehabilitation, 2017. 31(8): pp. 995–1004, https://doi.org/10.1177/0269215517709890.

30. Ackumey, M.M., et al., *Illness Meanings and Experiences for Pre-ulcer and Ulcer Conditions of Buruli Ulcer in the Ga-West and Ga-South Municipalities of Ghana.* BMC Public Health, 2012. 12(264), https://doi.org/10.1186/1471-2458-12-264.

31. Green, J., et al., *The Impact of Chronic Venous Leg Ulcers: A Systematic Review.* Journal of Wound Care 2014. 23(12): pp. 601–612, https://doi.org/10.12968/jowc.2014.23.12.601.

32. Herber, O.R., W. Schnepp, and M.A. Rieger, *A Systematic Review on the Impact of Leg Ulceration on Patients' Quality of Life.* Health and Quality of Life Outcomes, 2007. 5: 44, https://doi.org/10.1186/1477-7525-5-44.

33. Persoon, A., et al., *Leg Ulcers: A Review of Their Impact on Daily Life.* Journal of Clinical Nursing, 2004. 13(3): pp. 341–354, https://doi.org/10.1046/j.1365-2702.2003.00859.x.

34. Lo, S.-F., et al., *Symptom Burden and Quality of Life in Patients with Malignant Fungating Wounds.* Journal of Advanced Nursing, 2012. 68(6): pp. 1312–1321, https://doi.org/10.1111/j.1365-2648.2011.05839.x.

35. European Wound Management Association, *Hard to Heal Wounds: A Holistic Approach.* 2008, MEP Ltd: London.

36. Phillips, P., et al., *A Systematic Review of Qualitative Research into People's Experiences of Living with Venous Leg Ulcers.* Journal of Advanced Nursing, 2018. 74(3): pp. 550–563, https://doi.org/10.1111/jan.13465.

37. Maida, V., et al., *Symptoms Associated with Malignant Wounds: A Prospective Case Series.* Journal of Pain & Symptom Management, 2009. 37(2): pp. 206–211, https://doi.org/10.1016/j.jpainsymman.2008.01.009.

38. Price, P.E., et al., *Dressing-related Pain in Patients with Chronic Wounds: An International Patient Perspective.* International Wound Journal, 2008. 5(2): pp. 159–171, https://doi.org/10.1111/j.1742-481X.2008.00471.x.

39. Douglas, V., *Living with a Chronic Leg Ulcer: An Insight into Patients' Experiences and Feelings.* Journal of Wound Care, 2001. 10(9): pp. 355–360, https://doi.org/10.12968/jowc.2001.10.9.26318.

40. Hareendran, A., et al., *The Venous Leg Ulcer Quality of Life (VLU-QoL) Questionnaire: Development and Psychometric Validation.* Wound Repair and Regeneration, 2007. 15(4): pp. 465–473, https://doi.org/10.1111/j.1524-475X.2007.00253.x.

41. Woo, K., et al., *Assessment and Management of Persistent (Chronic) and Total Wound Pain.* International Wound Journal, 2008. 5(2): pp. 205–215, https://doi.org/10.1111/j.1742-481X.2008.00483.x.

42. Brown, A., *Chronic Leg Ulcers, Part 2: Do They Affect a Patient's Social Life?* British Journal of Nursing, 2005. 14(18): pp. 986–989, https://doi.org/10.12968/bjon.2005.14.18.19888.

43. Douglas, V., *Living with a Chronic Leg Ulcer: An Insight into Patients' Experiences and Feelings.* Journal of Wound Care, 2001. 10(9): pp. 355–360.

44. Wellborn, J. and J.T. Moceri, *The Lived Experiences of Persons With Chronic Venous Insufficiency and Lower Extremity Ulcers.* Journal of Wound Ostomy & Continence Nursing, 2014. 41(2): pp. 122–126, https://doi.org/10.1097/won.0000000000000010.

45. Charles, H., *Does Leg Ulcer Treatment Improve Patients' Quality of Life? .* Journal of Wound Care, 2004. 13(6): pp. 209–213, https://doi.org/10.12968/jowc.2004.13.6.26670.

46. Moffatt, C.J., et al., *Psychological Factors in Leg Ulceration: A Case–Control Study.* British Journal of Dermatology, 2009. 161(4): pp. 750–756, https://doi.org/10.1111/j.1365-2133.2009.09211.x.

47. Dalgard, F.J., et al., *The Psychological Burden of Skin Diseases: A Cross-Sectional Multicenter Study among Dermatological Out-Patients in 13 European Countries.* Journal of Investigative Dermatology, 2015. 135(4): pp. 984–991, https://doi.org/10.1038/jid.2014.530.

48. WHO. *Depression: Definition.* 2019. http://www.euro.who.int/en/health-topics/noncommunicable-diseases/pages/news/news/2012/10/depression-in-europe/depression-definition.

49. Wachholz, P.A., et al., *Quality of Life Profile and Correlated Factors in Chronic Leg Ulcer Patients in the Mid-west of São Paulo State, Brazil.* Anais Brasileiros de Dermatologia, 2014. 89: pp. 73–81, https://doi.org/10.1590/abd1806-4841.20142156.

50. Magela Salome, G., L. Blanes, and L. Masako Ferreira, *Assessment of Depressive Symptoms in People with Diabetes Mellitus and Foot Ulcers* Revista do Colegio Brasileiro de Cirurgioes, 2011. 38(5): pp. 327–333, https://doi.org/10.1590/s0100-69912011000500008.

51. Renner, R. and C. Erfurt-Berge, *Depression and Quality of Life in Patients with Chronic Wounds: Ways to Measure Their Influence and Their Effect on Daily Life.* Chronic Wound Care Management and Research, 2017. 4: pp. 143–151, https://doi.org/10.2147/CWCMR.S124917.

52. Hopkins, A., *Disrupted Lives: Investigating Coping Strategies for Non-healing Leg Ulcers.* British Journal of Nursing, 2004. 13(9): pp. 556–563, https://doi.org/10.12968/bjon.2004.13.9.12972.

53. Ousey, K. and D. Roberts, *Exploring Nurses' and Patients' Feelings of Disgust Associated with Malodorous Wounds: A Rapid Review.* Journal of Wound Care, 2016. 25(8): pp. 438–442, https://doi.org/10.12968/jowc.2016.25.8.438.

54. Jones, J., et al., *Impact of Exudate and Odour from Chronic Venous Leg Ulceration* Nursing Standard, 2008. 22(45): pp. 53–61 https://journals.rcni.com/nursing-standard/impact-of-exudate-and-odour-from-chronic-venous-leg-ulceration-ns2008.07.22.45.53.c6592.

55. Chase, S., Melloni, M., & Savage, A., *A Forever Healing: The Lived Experience of Venous Ulcer Disease*. Journal of Vascular Nursing, 1997. 15(2): pp. 73–78, https://doi.org/10.1016/s1062-0303(97)90004-2.

56. Lindahl, E., A. Norberg, and A. Söderberg, *The Meaning of Caring for People with Malodorous Exuding Ulcers*. Journal of Advanced Nursing, 2008. 62(2): pp. 163–171, https://doi.org/10.1111/j.1365-2648.2007.04551.x.

57. Ebbeskog, B. and S.-L. Ekman, *Elderly Persons' Experiences of Living with Venous Leg Ulcer: Living in a Dialectal Relationship between Freedom and Imprisonment*. Scandinavian Journal of Caring Sciences, 2001. 15(3): pp. 235–243, https://doi.org/10.1046/j.1471-6712.2001.00018.x.

58. Chase, S., R.Whittemore, N. Crosby, D. Freney, P. Howes, & T. Phillips, *Living with Chronic Venous Leg Ulcers: A Descriptive Study of Patients' Experiences*. Journal of Community Health Nursing, 2000. 17(1): pp. 1–13, https://doi.org/10.1207/s15327655jchn1701_01.

59. Bland, M., *Coping with Leg Ulcers*. Nursing New Zealand, 1996. 2(3): pp. 13–14.

60. Alexander, S., *An Intense and Unforgettable Experience: The Lived Experience of Malignant Wounds from the Perspectives of Patients, Caregivers and Nurses*. International Wound Journal, 2010. 7(6): pp. 456–465, https://doi.org/10.1111/j.1742-481x.2010.00715.x.

61. Hyde, C., B. Ward, J. Horsfall, & G. Winder, *Older Women's Experience of Living with Chronic Leg Ulceration*. International Journal of Nursing Practice, 1999. 5(4): pp. 189–198, https://doi.org/10.1046/j.1440-172x.1999.00170.x.

62. Salome, G.M., V.R. Pereira, and L.M. Ferreira, *Spirituality and Subjective Wellbeing in Patients with Lower Limb Ulceration*. Journal of Wound Care, 2013. 22(5): pp. 230–236.

63. Greenstreet, W., *From Spirituality to Coping Strategy: Making Sense of Chronic Illness*. British Journal of Nursing, 2006. 15(17): pp. 938–942, https://doi.org/10.12968/bjon.2006.15.17.21909.

64. Enoch, S., H. Shaaban, and K.W. Dunn, *Informed Consent Should Be Obtained from Patients to Use Products (Skin Substitutes) and Dressings Containing Biological Material*. Journal of Medical Ethics, 2005. 31: pp. 2–6.

65. Ackumey, M.M., et al., *Help-Seeking for Pre-Ulcer and Ulcer Conditions of Mycobacterium Ulcerans Disease (Buruli Ulcer) in Ghana*. American Journal of Tropical Medicine and Hygiene, 2011. 85(6): pp. 1106–1113, https://doi.org/10.4269/ajtmh.2011.11-0429.

66. Mulder, A.A., et al., *Healthcare Seeking Behaviour for Buruli Ulcer in Benin: A Model to Capture Therapy Choice of Patients and Healthy Community Members*. Transactions of the Royal Society of Tropical Medicine and Hygiene, 2008. 102(9): pp. 912–920, https://doi.org/10.1016/j.trstmh.2008.05.026.

67. Alferink, M., et al., *Perceptions on the Effectiveness of Treatment and the Timeline of Buruli Ulcer Influence Pre-Hospital Delay Reported by Healthy Individuals.* PLoS Neglected Tropical Diseases, 2013. 7(1): p. e2014, https://doi.org/10.1371/journal.pntd.0002014.

68. Zwi, K., et al., *The Impact of Health Perceptions and Beliefs on Access to Care for Migrants and Refugees.* Journal of Cultural Diversity, 2017. 24(3): pp. 63–72.

69. Edwards, H., et al., *Health Service Pathways for Patients with Chronic Leg Ulcers: Identifying Effective Pathways for Facilitation of Evidence Based Wound Care.* BMC Health Services Research, 2013. 13: 86, https://doi.org/10.1186/1472-6963-13-86.

70. Žulec, M.R.-P., D., Z. Puharić, and A. Žulec, *"Wounds Home Alone"—Why and How Venous Leg Ulcer Patients Self-Treat Their Ulcer: A Qualitative Content Study. 2019, 16, 559.* International Journal of Environmental Research and Public Health, 2019. 16(4): 559, https://doi.org/10.3390/ijerph16040559.

71. Kapp, S. and N. Santamaria, *How and Why Patients Self-treat Chronic Wounds.* International Wound Journal, 2017. 14(6): pp. 1269–1275, https://doi.org/10.1111/iwj.12796.

72. World Union of Wound Healing Societies (WUWHS), *Principles of Best Practice: Diagnostics and Wounds. A Consensus Document.* 2008, MEP Ltd.: London.

73. Gray, T.A., et al., *What Factors Influence Community Wound Care in the UK? A Focus Group Study Using the Theoretical Domains Framework.* BMJ Open, 2019. 9(7): e024859, https://doi.org/10.1136/bmjopen-2018-024859.

74. Abbas, Z.G., *Managing the Diabetic Foot in Resource-poor Settings: Challenges and Solutions.* Chronic Wound Care Management and Research, 2017. 4: pp. 135–142, https://doi.org/10.2147/CWCMR.S98762.

75. KPMG, *An Economic Evaluation of Compression Therapy for Venous Leg Ulcers,* 2013, AWMA, Editor, pp. 1–52.

76. Kapp, S. and N. Santamaria, *The Financial and Quality-of-life Cost to Patients Living with a Chronic Wound in the Community.* International Wound Journal, 2017. 14(6): pp. 1108–1119, https://doi.org/10.1111/iwj.12767.

77. Searle, A., et al., *A Qualitative Approach to Understanding the Experience of Ulceration and Healing in the Diabetic Foot: Patient and Podiatrist Perspective.* Wounds, 2005. 17(1): pp. 16–26.

78. Mehica, L., M.A. Gershater, and C.A. Roijer, *Diabetes and Infected Foot Ulcer: A Survey of Patients' Perceptions of Care during the Preoperative and Postoperative Periods.* European Diabetes Nursing, 2013. 10(3): pp. 91–95, https://doi.org/10.1002/edn.235.

79. Engel, G., *The Clinical Application of the Biopsychosocial Model.* American Journal of Psychiatry, 1980. 137(5): pp. 535–544, https://doi.org/10.1176/ajp.137.5.535.

80. WHO. *A Practical Manual for Using the International Classification of Functioning, Disability and Health (ICF)*. 2013. https://www.who.int/classifications/drafticfpracticalmanual2.pdf.

81. Palfreyman, S., *Assessing the Impact of Venous Ulceration on Quality of Life.* Nursing Times, 2008. 104(41): pp. 34–37.

82. Bullen, B. and P. Chadwick, *Clinical Integration of Maggot Therapy*, in *A Complete Guide to Maggot Therapy: Clinical Practice, Therapeutic Principles, Production, Distribution, and Ethics*, F. Stadler (ed.). 2022, Cambridge: Open Book Publishers, pp. 97–118, https://doi.org/10.11647/OBP.0300.06.

83. Stadler, F., *The Ethics of Maggot Therapy*, in *A Complete Guide to Maggot Therapy: Clinical Practice, Therapeutic Principles, Production, Distribution, and Ethics*, F. Stadler (ed.). 2022, Cambridge: Open Book Publishers, pp. 405–430, https://doi.org/10.11647/OBP.0300.19.

3. Wound Aetiologies, Patient Characteristics, and Healthcare Settings Amenable to Maggot Therapy

Ronald A. Sherman and Frank Stadler

It is important for healthcare practitioners to understand when to use maggot therapy. This chapter explains the general factors that determine the choice of wound treatment and how they apply to maggot therapy: i) the wound characteristics, ii) the patient characteristics, iii) the environment, iv) the available resources, and v) the specific characteristics of each available treatment modality. Beyond the regular healthcare setting, maggot therapy can make a significant contribution to the treatment of people with wounds in compromised healthcare settings such as in times of disaster and armed conflict, in underserved populations, or in palliative care.

Introduction

There is a great need for improved wound care in both resourced and compromised healthcare settings. Although not a panacea, maggot therapy can meet many of these pressing wound care needs. It is well-established that medicinal maggots have three major actions on wounds: 1) they dissolve and dislodge dead (necrotic) tissue and debris (debridement), 2) they kill microorganisms ("disinfection"), and 3) they stimulate healthy tissue to grow faster, as explained in Chapters 8

https://doi.org/10.11647/OBP.0300.03

to 10 of this book [1–3]. Therefore, maggot therapy can usually assist in treating wounds that require any of these actions. Notwithstanding this broad spectrum of potential indications, it is important for healthcare policy makers, regulators, and health administrators to understand the contribution maggot therapy can make to wound care in order to support mainstreaming of this therapy [4]. It is also important for healthcare practitioners to understand when to use maggot therapy.

While treatment selection can seem quite complicated at times, the following general factors should always be considered when choosing a wound treatment: i) the wound characteristics, ii) the patient characteristics, iii) the environment, iv) the available resources, and v) the specific characteristics of each available treatment modality. Examples of how these factors might affect treatment decisions can be found in Table 3.1. Using these characteristics as a guiding framework, this chapter explains when maggot therapy is indicated.

It should also be noted that the specific types of wounds and situations that are appropriately treated with a particular method or product are usually based on scientific studies, anecdotal reports, personal experience, and regulatory approvals. Since maggot therapy is not officially regulated in most countries, this discussion of indications for maggot therapy is based primarily on its mechanisms of action and on published experience.

Wounds Amenable to Maggot Therapy

Wound Characteristics

Necrosis. Most wounds on an otherwise healthy person will heal quite well despite our choice of therapy. But when dead tissue covers or fills that wound, then the surrounding healthy tissue cannot fill the void. What's more, microorganisms that live and feed on dead tissue, or under its cover, can multiply and spread beyond these borders, especially if they can also live in the surrounding live tissue. Even if they cannot themselves spread beyond dead tissue, their secretions (called "toxins") may be harmful to the surrounding live tissue, and may cause that tissue, too, to become inflamed and/or die, thereby extending the wound. Although scientific proof is sparse, there is wide agreement that

Table 3.1 Factors to consider when selecting wound treatments.

Factor	Considerations
i) Wound characteristics	• Infection might require specific antimicrobial treatment; aggressive infection might require immediate resection or at least close daily or hourly inspection
	• Dead tissue and debris often require removal (debridement) before healing can fully transpire
	• If the wound cannot be visualised completely, accommodations will need to be made to ensure that even non-visualised surfaces are cleaned and disinfected
	• If vital structures (major vessels, nerves and organs) are involved, accommodations will need to be made to ensure that they are not damaged in the attempt to halt the infection or remove dead tissues
ii) Patient characteristics	• Factors that affect wound healing (i.e., malnutrition, anaemia, diabetes, peripheral vascular disease)
	• Factors that affect a patient's ability to tolerate surgery or other treatments (i.e., underlying heart, kidney, liver disease)
	• Factors that affect a patient's ability to participate in the therapy, to the degree that will be necessary (i.e., ability to consent; physical and mental limitations on the ability to do dressing changes; social support at home; financial limitations; cultural/religious factors)
iii) Environmental characteristics	• Availability of shelter, electricity, refrigeration, clean or sterile water, transportation
	• Weather/temperature extremes can impact the access to or shelf-life of certain products (i.e., medicinal maggots cannot survive extreme cold or hot temperatures unless stored and transported in temperature-resistant containers)
	• Physically/structurally stable environment may be required by certain treatments; this is threatened by ongoing earthquake aftershocks, wildfires, flooding, or civil unrest and conflict

Factor	Considerations
iv) Resource availability	• Financial resources available to the individual
	• Availability of healthcare insurance
	• Level of healthcare resource availability in the country or region
	• Physical ability to access those resources (i.e., transportation and accommodation to access care only available in regional centres; availability of treatment in the home)
	• Availability of adequately trained wound care providers
	• Policies at all levels which affect the availability, provision and financing of various treatment modalities
v) Characteristics of the treatment modality	• Efficacy
	• Safety
	• Cost and likelihood of reimbursement
	• Acceptability to the patient and care provider
	• Indications and contraindications
	• Regulatory status (i.e., whether it is locally considered to be an approved, unapproved, or investigational modality)

a wound with necrotic tissue and debris will not easily heal until the necrotic tissue and debris is removed [5, 6].

Maggots must compete fiercely with other scavengers for limited resources, and many of those competing scavengers would consume the maggots, too, if the maggots were found still on the rotting tissue. The maggots used therapeutically are those that are well-adapted to quickly remove (and ingest) as much of the necrotic tissue and debris as possible, and then leave the area. Maggot therapy debrides the necrotic wound by at least two methods: enzymatic debridement and physical debridement [7]. The maggot's digestive juices, rich with proteolytic enzymes, are excreted into the wound bed and quickly dissolve dead tissue. Meanwhile, as the maggot crawls about the wound bed, its microscopic spines and its modified mandibles ("mouth hooks") physically dislodge some of the debris, helping the digestive juices gain access into the crevices. A more detailed discussion of the maggot's debridement action can be found in Chapter 8 [1].

Infection. Given that medicinal blowflies, if living in the wild, would inhabit corpses, faeces, and other rotting organic matter, it seems logical that the larvae would have a method for killing infectious organisms, or else the microbes might kill the maggots. The mechanisms by which the maggots accomplish microbial killing are covered by Nigam and Wilson in Chapter 9 [2]. For the purpose of this discussion, let it suffice to acknowledge that medicinal maggots kill microbes through a variety of mechanisms including ingestion [8, 9], the secretion of antimicrobial compounds [10–15], dissolving biofilm [12, 16–21] and altering the local environment in ways that make it less hospitable to microbial pathogens [22, 23]. The end result is that microbial populations are reduced or eliminated [24–26] and clinical infections subside [27, 28]. The antimicrobial effect may even endure well beyond the life of the maggots [29].

Wound moisture content. Wounds can vary greatly in wetness. Some wounds are extremely dry; the necrotic tissue covering the wound being like leather ("eschar"). Other wounds may drain serous (watery), sero-sanguinous (bloody), or purulent (pus-filled) liquid profusely. The same wound may switch back and forth over the course of a week. Many dressings are suitable only for moderately dry wounds, or only for very wet wounds. Some dressings will not adhere to a wet wound; others are designed to absorb excess fluid tenaciously, making them superfluous or even dangerous for use with a minimally moist wound. Medicinal maggots have no such limitations, though the dressings used to confine them to the wound may themselves need to be selected or modified to meet the moisture conditions of the wound and surrounding tissue. Dressings will be discussed in detail in Chapter 5 [30].

Absence of healing—the chronic wound. Maggot therapy has been observed to enhance wound healing, even in apparently clean but stagnant wounds, at least as far back as William Baer's time [31]. Subsequent clinicians have described, in controlled studies, the rapid proliferation of granulation tissue and hastened closing of the wound margins in previously stagnant, non-healing wounds [32–35]. The mechanisms known to be involved are described by Nigam and Wilson in Chapter 10 [3]. More and more therapists are using maggot therapy to promote healing and closure of chronic wounds, even though the wounds may not appear grossly necrotic nor infected. Some of the therapists describe this indication as maintenance debridement, others say their intent is growth-stimulation. The desired endpoint is the same: not just a clean (debrided) wound but a clean wound that is healing.

Wounds Treated with Maggot Therapy

Pressure ulcers/injuries. Pressure alone, from lying in the same position for a prolonged time, or in combination with shear force, can starve tissue of oxygenated blood which leads to tissue death. Shear may exacerbate the injury and cause mechanical damage to the compromised tissue [36]. These injuries lead to open necrotic ulcers that often fail to heal (Figure 3.1a). Maggot therapy is frequently used to treat pressure ulcers or injuries, and several controlled studies demonstrate its efficacy [33, 35, 37–39].

Arterial ulcers. Factors other than pressure can also prevent arterial blood from reaching tissue. Primary arterial disease, for example (i.e., vasculitis, arteritis obliterans, or thromboses) can occlude arteries and arterioles, leading to local necrosis of the skin and soft tissue. Many anecdotal reports support the use of maggot therapy for debriding these wounds [40–43]. However, without adequate blood flow, healing cannot occur even in the maggot-debrided wound [40, 41]. Therefore, the arterial flow needs to be assessed prior to maggot therapy. Even if arterial flow cannot be restored, maggot therapy can be administered to palliate ulcer symptoms such as exudate and odour and to prevent infection, thereby maintaining quality of life.

Venous stasis leg ulcers. Venous disease, too, can lead to skin and soft-tissue wounds. Venous insufficiency results in legs, for example, with increased intravascular pressure. The result is that fluid (serum) leaks out of the blood vessels and into the soft tissue, thereby causing swelling, pain, itching (trauma and infection from scratching). Oxygen cannot easily perfuse the fluid-filled (oedematous) leg, and the normal immune mechanisms (i.e., migration of white blood cells) are similarly impaired. In the end, skin breaks down more easily, the body does not fight the infections well, and healing is impaired (Figure 3.1b). Venous ulcers are best prevented by compression and elevation of the affected limb. However, when a person presents with a venous ulcer, then regular debridement is necessary along with compression and elevation of the limb. Multiple controlled and non-controlled maggot therapy studies have described faster debridement (with or without faster healing) of venous ulcers [38, 44–46].

Diabetic foot disease/diabetes related foot ulcers (DFUs). Diabetes results in multi-system disease. Neuropathy can lead to increased trauma, impaired immunity interferes with the body's ability to fight infection, and blood vessel disease greatly inhibits healing (Figures 3.1c, 3.1d). DFUs require timely and expert assessment to identify the aetiology and prompt initiation of tailored management [47]. When aetiology is not ascertained, management will fail to address the underlying cause, which may lead to amputation [48]. Up to 85% of amputations can be prevented [49, 50]. Maggot therapy is often used to debride these wounds and control emerging infections. Several controlled studies [32, 34] and case series [51] have demonstrated significant benefits.

Traumatic and post-surgical wounds. Medicinal maggots are quite useful in debriding traumatic and infected or necrotic post-surgical wounds (Figure 3.1e, 3.1f). In an otherwise healthy individual, these wounds usually heal quite well after initial debridement and infection management.

Burns. Unlike many other necrotic wounds, burns need to be debrided acutely (Figure 3.1g). When the burn area is extensive or when vital structures could be damaged by surgical debridement, maggot debridement has proven to be a good alternative [10, 52–58]. Burn wounds are often painful, and maggot therapy is not likely to be less painful than any other manipulation of the damaged tissue. Therefore, anaesthetics will be just as necessary during maggot debridement as during any other form of debridement, and maybe more so.

Undermining wounds, difficult to reach or visualise. Because medicinal maggots, by nature, crawl into nooks and crannies, they are very appropriate for treating wounds whose boundaries may not be easily visualised. Like miners, the larvae will crawl into the depths of undermined tissue and sinus tracts, debriding within these areas until they need to return to the surface for air, food (assuming that the area no longer contains necrotic tissue or nutritious liquid), or to moult.

Treating undermining wounds with maggot therapy can avoid having to open a deep cavity for accurate visualisation and debridement.

Body cavities. Similar to undermined wounds and sinus tracts, medicinal maggots have been used effectively to debride body cavities with infected necrotic tissue, such as necrotising peritonitis or chronic empyema [56]. If debridement is not needed in the crevices or out-of-sight areas of these cavities, it may be possible and preferable to apply the maggots within sealed mesh bags so that they stay contained and can be more easily removed, as explained in Chapter 5 [30].

Bones and Joints. Bone infections ("osteomyelitis") were a common indication for maggot therapy during the 1930s, when many orthopaedic surgeons used maggot therapy to perform the "fine debridement" after the surgeon removed the grossly infected or dead bone [31, 59, 60]. We now have procedures and antibiotics that make post-operative infections much less common. Maggot therapy is rarely used for osteomyelitis at all anymore; osteomyelitis is generally considered a surgical disease, treated by removing (resecting) the dead bone and by long-term antibiotics to prevent spread or recurrence of the infection. However, when surgical resection and/or antibiotics are inadequate or are not an option, maggot therapy is sometimes used to debride the bone [61–63]. Similarly, infected joints and joint prostheses are generally treated by removing the infected hardware and draining the infection, along with antibiotic coverage. But when the removal of hardware is risky or impossible, maggot therapy has been used alongside the antibiotics to eliminate the infection [64, 65].

Malignancy. Medicinal maggots dissolve necrotic tissue, but not viable tissue. In that regard, they are not useful for killing live cancer cells. However, when a tumour mass outstrips its blood supply and starts to rot, maggot therapy can be a rapid and effective method for removing the necrotic mass (Figure 3.1h). Many cancer patients were able to return to a reasonably normal life in public only after maggot therapy removed their foul-smelling, draining, painfully infected tumours [66–68].

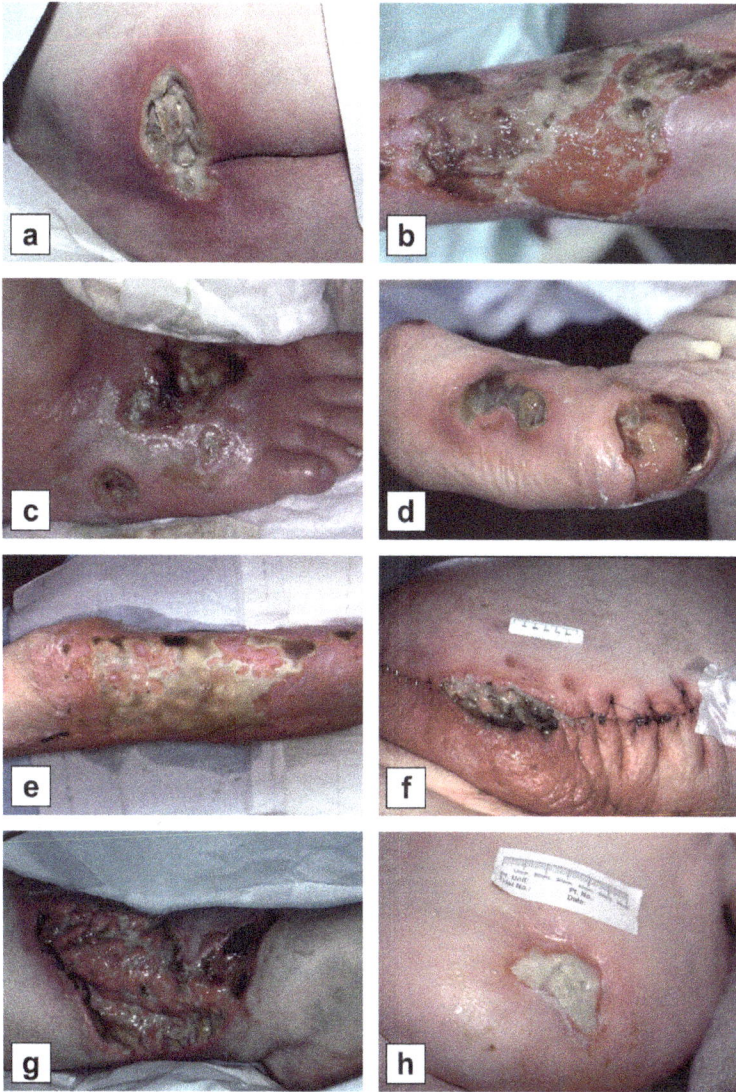

Figure 3.1 Chronic wounds amenable to maggot therapy: a) pressure ulcer, b) venous stasis ulcer, c&d) diabetic foot ulcers, e) burn, f) surgical wound dehiscence, g) orthopaedic wound, h) malignancy. Photos: © Steve Thomas, www.medetec.co.uk.

Specific Infections

Multi-resistant bacteria. Because blowflies kill microbes through mechanisms other than those used by typical antibiotics [2], they are effective in killing pathogens that have developed resistance to those antibiotics, such as methicillin-resistant *Staphylococcus aureus* (MRSA) [66–68]; and multi-resistant *Acinetobacter* [69].

Fungal infections. Maggot secretions kill or inhibit representative fungi in the laboratory [70, 71], though very little clinical experience with fungi has been published [72].

Fasciitis. Several microbes, and especially mixed aerobic and anaerobic infections, can be highly destructive to soft tissue, causing necrosis that rapidly extends down to the deep layers of muscle and bone. Fasciitis is a surgical emergency. Even with immediate resection of the dead tissue, systemic broad-spectrum antibiotics and intensive care, the mortality of these infections can still exceed 40% [73]. Frequently, repeated surgical debridement is required, ultimately leading to destruction or resection of vital structures, and the need for major anatomical reconstruction, if the patient survives at all. Maggot therapy has been used successfully to debride these wounds without unnecessarily harming the remaining viable tissue [74–77]. In a small but prospective study, patients with Fournier's gangrene that were debrided only by maggots if they required more than one initial surgical resection, not only survived their wounds without the need for any additional surgical debridement but also avoided the need for reconstructive surgery [78].

Tropical ulcers (Mycobacteriosis and tropical phagedenic ulcers). The term "tropical ulcers" collectively refers to painful wounds in typically malnourished individuals living in tropical climates. The wounds often follow trauma, and they may be colonised, if not caused, by *Mycobacterium ulcerans* (Buruli ulcer, mycobacteriosis) or *Fusobacterium* and *Borrelia* (Phagedenic ulcers, Naga sores) [79]. These are chronic wounds often with very poor outcomes, though antibiotics and improved nutrition can be curative. Buruli ulcers (*Mycobacterium ulcerans* wounds) often deteriorate following what appears to be appropriate antimicrobial therapy [80]. Medicinal maggots were used extensively in the 1930s as an adjunct to surgical resection, in the treatment of tuberculous osteomyelitis. It is reasonable to assume that maggot therapy should adequately debride tropical ulcer wounds as well, but the efficacy and safety of maggot debridement for these wounds remain undefined.

The wounds commonly seen in patients living with leprosy (caused by *Mycobacterium leprae*) are generally caused by trauma; the leprosy bacterium is not necessarily within the wound [81]. These wounds should also respond to maggot therapy, if needed, just like any other traumatic wound.

Protozoans. Medicinal maggots have demonstrated anti-leishmania activity *in vitro* and in animal models [82–85], though no human studies have been reported. The endemic trepanematoses (i.e., yaws, pinta, and bejel) can also cause problematic soft-tissue wounds, but penicillin and several other readily available antibiotics are generally curative. No experience treating these lesions with maggot therapy has been published to date.

Population and Patient Characteristics

Population Characteristics

Disaster and conflict casualties. During a disaster or military conflict, the number of victims often overwhelms the capacity of first responders. This is the perfect opportunity to recruit fly larvae to assist in wound care [86]. Often there are insufficient facilities or hospital beds, and unreliable electricity and water supplies. Again, maggot therapy is well-suited to these trying circumstances because the larvae require none of those amenities. However, the supply chains for getting medicinal maggots to compromised healthcare settings are hitherto non-existent. Because maggots are highly perishable and cannot be stored for more than a day or two, attention needs to be paid to their production close to the point of care in disasters and conflict, or to reliable logistics solutions that ensure timely and safe delivery of medicinal maggots [87, 88].

Rural, tropical, and medically underserved populations. People living in sparsely populated or medically underserved regions have all the same problems as described above, but often in different proportions. Wounds as a result of infectious and parasitic diseases, burns, and traumatic injury are common, as are increasingly wounds related to cancer, diabetes and cardiovascular disease. Again, maggot therapy is a great resource when there is a severe shortage of medical staff and other healthcare resources, provided that reliable supply chains exist to make maggot therapy accessible to these communities.

End of life and palliative care residents. Death is a part of life whether in a rural part of the world or in a big city. Most people become ill or reach an older age before dying. With aging and chronic illness, organs (including skin) begin to fail. Skin failure is a common pre-terminal occurrence [89]. As already noted, maggot therapy is a simple and effective means of treating necrotic, infected, or chronic wounds in the ill or frail person [90]. Maggot therapy can quickly provide surgical-quality wound care, at home or in long-term/residential care, at a fraction of the cost of a surgeon, and be cost-effective when compared to existing advanced dressings that deliver only limited wound bed improvement.

Characteristics of Persons with Wounds

Age and gender. Many treatment modalities are not available to persons with wounds depending on their particular age, gender, or both. For example, certain antibiotics and other pharmaceuticals should not be used in children or in child-bearing women, or even in women of a particular ("child-bearing") age. Often this is the result of real or theoretical complications that have been observed in humans or in animal models. Other times it is simply because the studies supporting safety and efficacy were performed in populations that excluded these high-risk individuals. Maggot therapy does not need to be withheld from anyone on the basis of gender or age [31, 91].

Frailty. Whether due to age or underlying medical illnesses, some people are unable to endure the physical or mental stress of aggressive medical interventions such as surgery, anaesthesia, or even frequent phlebotomy (needles). Even if their cardiopulmonary status is stable, an underlying problem such as hypertension, obesity, emphysema or sub-optimally managed diabetes may make surgery and/or anaesthesia excessively risky [92]. These conditions are not contraindications to maggot therapy, because maggot therapy does not require general anaesthesia, and does not put any additional physical stress on the body.

Prognosis. Non-healing wounds are often seen in people when they are dying. When managing wounds that cannot heal, including in people who are dying, the focus of holistic management is to optimise quality of life and to maintain optimal dignity. Maggot therapy can be of particular benefit if wounds are infected, foul-smelling, draining, painful, in need of much care and attention. Maggot therapy controls the infection, debrides the necrotic tissue, and thereby diminishes or eliminates the drainage, odour and pain of a necrotic wound or terminal ulcer. Maggot therapy can provide comfort in these ways, without adding additional stress to a patient in their last days of life [77].

Need for other medical interventions. Maggot therapy can be used safely and effectively even in people receiving other drugs and treatments. Medicinal maggots and their debridement efficacy appear to be unaffected by antibiotics [93, 94] and most other drugs in pharmacologic doses, and various medical and life support interventions [56, 95–97]. In fact, maggots have proven to be safe and effective in patients receiving anticoagulants or intensive care that made surgical debridement unsafe [56, 98]. Unpublished anecdotal reports suggest that medicinal maggots may not survive on animals receiving systemic or topical insecticides, such as ivermectin or flea and tick treatments. No work has been published concerning the impact of cancer chemotherapy on medicinal maggots.

Environmental Characteristics

One of the most favourable aspects of maggot therapy is its flexibility regarding the care setting. Patients can be treated as in-patients, as outpatients, in the community, in field hospital situations, and even in the most austere healthcare settings that lack any medical resources [31, 86, 99]. This is because the application of, and treatment with, medicinal maggot dressings does not require energy or sophisticated equipment. Maggots are also well-adapted to unhygienic environments and therefore will perform their therapeutic action equally well in the modern hospital environment, the battlefield, and the disaster zone. The lack of stable shelter is not an impediment to using maggot therapy [86, 99]. Maggot therapy will still be effective, even if exposed to the elements, as long as the maggots receive enough air and the wounds are well-drained to prevent suffocation and drowning. Extreme climatic conditions should not be a deterrent either. In general, if the weather is tolerable to the patient, it will be tolerated by medicinal maggots [100, 101]. Wound temperatures encountered by medicinal maggots will depend on the body region, general condition of the patient and the environmental temperature, but will in most instances not be lower than 30°C or exceed 40°C, which is a temperature range that promotes high activity and rapid growth in medicinal maggots [100, 102] and lies well below the lethal temperature threshold of around 47°C [103]. Environmental temperature is only a concern during transport of young medicinal maggots that are deprived of food until they reach the point of care and patient. To slow down metabolic activity and maintain optimal health, medicinal maggots should be kept at 6 to 25°C and be applied to the wound within 48 hours of dispatch [87]. In other words, most limitations imposed on healthcare provision by the environment, facilities, or equipment will have little to no impact on the work of the maggots.

Resources

Social resources. Social support systems are occasionally called into play to help with medical issues. In some parts of the world, patients are discharged to home while still recovering. Friends and family may need to assist in the care of their loved ones at home or in the hospital. Maggot therapy is simple enough that dressings can be applied, maintained, and/or removed by the patient or the patient's caregivers [104].

Financial resources. Without financial resources, the purchase of specialised medical supplies can seem like an insurmountable problem. Fortunately, medicinal maggots are not very costly to produce (except when regulatory agencies are involved). Many labs provide free or subsidised larvae to patients with limited finances. Some therapists procure larvae themselves when a commercial product is unavailable [99, 105]. Even when financial resources are sparse, maggot therapy remains a viable and cost-effective solution for wound care.

Moreover, the use and application of medicinal maggots requires no electricity, no batteries, no running or sterile water, and no refrigeration [86, 99]. Maggot dressings can be made from materials readily available at any facility that is modestly prepared to manage wounds (e.g. gauze and tape). While specialised or maggot-specific dressing supplies can simplify the application of maggot therapy, such amenities are not required. Please refer to Chapter 5 [30] for a discussion of dressing options.

Summary

While maggot therapy is not a panacea and will not resolve the underlying causes, particularly of chronic wounds, it is appropriate for the treatment of a wide variety of infected, necrotic, non-healing skin and soft-tissue wounds. Maggot therapy may also be used for acute wounds in need of urgent debridement, and non-necrotic wounds that simply will not close. In all of these situations, maggot therapy has proven to be very effective and relatively safe, at a low or reasonable cost. Maggot therapy can make a significant contribution to the treatment of people with wounds in disasters and armed conflict, in underserved populations, and in palliative care. With respect to patient characteristics, maggot therapy is also highly accommodating as it can be used to treat people of all ages, genders and levels of frailty. Indeed, it should be a treatment of choice for debridement and wound maintenance where people are unfit to endure general anaesthesia or are at their end of life. Moreover, medicinal maggots can be deployed in both high- and low-resource care settings irrespective of healthcare infrastructure and hygiene levels as they do not require any special facilities, resources, or highly-skilled personnel. Table 3.2 provides a summary of the ideal wound dressing characteristics, and how maggot therapy compares favourably to that ideal.

Table 3.2 The degree to which maggot therapy compares with the ideal wound dressing.

The ideal wound dressing *****	How maggot therapy compares
Effective for many wound types	*****
Safe for healthy wound tissue	*****
Can be applied by non-healthcare professionals	*****

The ideal wound dressing *****	How maggot therapy compares
Can be applied with minimal training	*****
Low environmental impact	*****
Low cost	*****
Safe for healthy surrounding tissue	****
Low maintenance	****
Simple to discard	****
Patient/cultural acceptability	****
Healthcare provider acceptability	*
Easy availability/convenience	*

References

1. Nigam, Y. and M.R. Wilson, *Maggot Debridement*, in *A Complete Guide to Maggot Therapy: Clinical Practice, Therapeutic Principles, Production, Distribution, and Ethics*, F. Stadler (ed.). 2022, Cambridge: Open Book Publishers, pp. 143–152, https://doi.org/10.11647/OBP.0300.08.

2. Nigam, Y. and M.R. Wilson, *The Antimicrobial Activity of Medicinal Maggots*, in *A Complete Guide to Maggot Therapy: Clinical Practice, Therapeutic Principles, Production, Distribution, and Ethics*, F. Stadler (ed.). 2022, Cambridge: Open Book Publishers, pp. 153–174, https://doi.org/10.11647/OBP.0300.09.

3. Nigam, Y. and M.R. Wilson, *Maggot-assisted Wound Healing*, in *A Complete Guide to Maggot Therapy: Clinical Practice, Therapeutic Principles, Production, Distribution, and Ethics*, F. Stadler (ed.). 2022, Cambridge: Open Book Publishers, pp. 175–194, https://doi.org/10.11647/OBP.0300.10.

4. Bullen, B. and P. Chadwick, *Clinical Integration of Maggot Therapy*, in *A Complete Guide to Maggot Therapy: Clinical Practice, Therapeutic Principles, Production, Distribution, and Ethics*, F. Stadler (ed.). 2022, Cambridge: Open Book Publishers, pp. 97–118, https://doi.org/10.11647/OBP.0300.06.

5. Falabella, A.F., *Debridement and Wound Bed Preparation*. Dermatologic Therapy, 2006. 19(6): pp. 317–325, https://doi.org/10.1111/j.1529-8019.2006.00090.x.

6. Weir, D., P. Scarborough, and J. Niezgoda, *Wound Debridement*, in *Chronic Wound Care: The Essentials*, D.L. Krasner and L. van Rijswijk (eds). 2018, HMP Communications: Malvern, PA, pp. 63–78.

7. Sherman, R.A., *Mechanisms of Maggot-Induced Wound Healing: What Do We Know, and Where Do We Go from Here?* Evidence-based Complementary and Alternative Medicine, 2014. 2014: pp. 1–13, https://doi.org/10.1155/2014/592419.

8. Greenberg, B., *Model for Destruction of Bacteria in the Midgut of Blow Fly Maggots.* Journal of Medical Entomology, 1968. 5(1): pp. 31–38, https://doi.org/10.1093/jmedent/5.1.31.

9. Mumcuoglu, K.Y., et al., *Destruction of Bacteria in the Digestive Tract of the Maggot of Lucilia sericata (Diptera: Calliphoridae).* Journal of Medical Entomology, 2001. 38(2): pp. 161–166, https://doi.org/10.1603/0022-2585-38.2.161.

10. Bian, H., et al., *Beneficial Effects of Extracts from Lucilia sericata Maggots on Burn Wounds in Rats.* Molecular Medicine Reports, 2017. 16(5): pp. 7213–7220, https://doi.org/10.3892/mmr.2017.7566.

11. Erdmann, G.R. and S.K. Khalil, *Isolation and Identification of Two Antibacterial Agents Produced by a Strain of Proteus Mirabilis Isolated from Larvae of the Screwworm (Cochliomyia hominivorax) (Diptera: Calliphoridae).* Journal of Medical Entomology, 1986. 23(2): pp. 208–211, https://doi.org/10.1093/jmedent/23.2.208.

12. Gordya, N., et al., *Natural Antimicrobial Peptide Complexes in the Fighting of Antibiotic Resistant Biofilms: Calliphora Vicina Medicinal Maggots.* PloS ONE, 2017. 12(3): e0173559, https://doi.org/10.1371/journal.pone.0173559.

13. Pöppel, A.-K., et al., *Antimicrobial Peptides Expressed in Medicinal Maggots of the Blow Fly Lucilia sericata Show Combinatorial Activity against Bacteria.* Antimicrobial Agents and Chemotherapy, 2015. 59(5): pp. 2508–2514, https://doi.org/10.1128/AAC.05180-14.

14. Teh, C.H., et al., *Determination of Antibacterial Activity and Minimum Inhibitory Concentration of Larval Extract of Fly via Resazurin-based Turbidometric Assay.* BMC Microbiology, 2017. 17(1): pp. 36–36, https://doi.org/10.1186/s12866-017-0936-3.

15. Wright, E.A. and E.R. Pavillard, *An Antibiotic from Maggots.* Nature, 1957. 180(4592): pp. 916–917, https://doi.org/10.1038/180916b0.

16. Bohova, J., et al., *Selective Antibiofilm Effects of Lucilia sericata Larvae Secretions/ Excretions against Wound Pathogens.* Evidence-Based Complementary and Alternative Medicine, 2014. 2014: pp. 857360–857360, https://doi.org/10.1155/2014/857360.

17. Brown, A., et al., *Blow Fly Lucilia sericata Nuclease Digests DNA Associated with Wound Slough/Eschar and with Pseudomonas aeruginosa Biofilm.* Medical and Veterinary Entomology, 2012. 26(4): pp. 432–439, https://doi.org/10.1111/j.1365-2915.2012.01029.x.

18. Cazander, G., et al., *Maggot Excretions Inhibit Biofilm Formation on Biomaterials*. Clinical Orthopaedics and Related Research, 2010. 468(10): pp. 2789–2796, https://doi.org/10.1007/s11999-010-1309-5.

19. Cazander, G., et al., *The Influence of Maggot Excretions on PAO1 Biofilm Formation on Different Biomaterials*. Clinical Orthopaedics and Related Research, 2009. 467(2): pp. 536–545, https://doi.org/10.1007/s11999-008-0555-2.

20. Harris, L.G., et al., *Disruption of Staphylococcus Epidermidis Biofilms by Medicinal Maggot Lucilia sericata Excretions/Secretions*. International Journal of Artificial Organs, 2009. 32(9): pp. 555–564, https://doi.org/10.1177/039139880903200904.

21. van der Plas, M.J.A., et al., *Maggot Excretions/Secretions Are Differentially Effective against Biofilms of Staphylococcus aureus and Pseudomonas aeruginosa*. Journal of Antimicrobial Chemotherapy, 2008. 61(1): pp. 117–122, https://doi.org/10.1093/jac/dkm407.

22. Davydov, L., *Maggot Therapy in Wound Management in Modern Era and a Review of Published Literature*. 2011, SAGE Publications: Los Angeles, CA, pp. 89–93.

23. Nigam, Y., et al., *Maggot Therapy: The Science and Implication for CAM Part II — Maggots Combat Infection*. Evidence-based Complementary and Alternative Medicine, 2006. 3(3): pp. 303–308, https://doi.org/10.1093/ecam/nel022.

24. Contreras-Ruiz, J., et al., [*Comparative Study of the Efficacy of Larva Therapy for Debridement and Control of Bacterial Burden Compared to Surgical Debridement and Topical Application of an Antimicrobial*]. Gaceta médica de México, 2016. 152(Suppl 2): pp. 78–87, http://www.anmm.org.mx/GMM/2016/s2/GMM_152_2016_S2_78-87.pdf.

25. Malekian, A., et al., *Efficacy of Maggot Therapy on Staphylococcus aureus and Pseudomonas aeruginosa in Diabetic Foot Ulcers: A Randomized Controlled Trial*. Journal of Wound, Ostomy and Continence Nursing, 2019. 46(1): pp. 25–29, https://doi.org/10.1097/WON.0000000000000496.

26. Tantawi, T.I., et al., *Clinical and Microbiological Efficacy of MDT in the Treatment of Diabetic Foot Ulcers*. Journal of Wound Care, 2007. 16(9): pp. 379–383, https://doi.org/10.12968/jowc.2007.16.9.27868.

27. Armstrong, D.G., et al., *Maggot Therapy in "Lower-extremity Hospice" Wound Care: Fewer Amputations and More Antibiotic-free Days*. Journal of the American Podiatric Medical Association, 2005. 95(3): pp. 254–257, https://doi.org/10.7547/0950254.

28. Steenvoorde, P. and J. Oskam, *Use of Larval Therapy to Combat Infection after Breast-conserving Surgery*. Journal of Wound Care, 2005. 14(5): pp. 212–213, https://doi.org/10.12968/jowc.2005.14.5.26778.

29. Sherman, R.A. and K.J. Shimoda, *Presurgical Maggot Debridement of Soft Tissue Wounds Is Associated with Decreased Rates of Postoperative Infection.* Clinical Infectious Diseases, 2004. 39(7): pp. 1067–1070, https://doi.org/10.1086/423806.

30. Sherman, R., *Medicinal Maggot Application and Maggot Therapy Dressing Technology*, in *A Complete Guide to Maggot Therapy: Clinical Practice, Therapeutic Principles, Production, Distribution, and Ethics*, F. Stadler (ed.). 2022, Cambridge: Open Book Publishers, pp. 79–96, https://doi.org/10.11647/OBP.0300.05.

31. Baer, W.S., *The Treatment of Chronic Osteomyelitis with the Maggot (Larva of the Blow Fly).* The Journal of Bone and Joint Surgery. American Volume, 1931. 13: pp. 438–475, https://doi.org/10.1007/s11999-010-1416-3.

32. Markevich, Y.O., et al., *Maggot Therapy for Diabetic Neuropathic Foot Wounds.* Diabetologia, 2000. 43: p. Suppl 1: A15.

33. Sherman, R.A., *Maggot versus Conservative Debridement Therapy for the Treatment of Pressure Ulcers.* Wound Repair and Regeneration, 2002. 10(4): pp. 208–214, https://doi.org/10.1046/j.1524-475X.2002.10403.x.

34. Sherman, R.A., *Maggot Therapy for Treating Diabetic Foot Ulcers Unresponsive to Conventional Therapy.* Diabetes Care, 2003. 26(2): pp. 446–451, https://doi.org/10.2337/diacare.26.2.446.

35. Sherman, R.A., F. Wyle, and M. Vulpe, *Maggot Therapy for Treating Pressure Ulcers in Spinal Cord Injury Patients.* The Journal of Spinal Cord Medicine, 1995. 18(2): pp. 71–74, https://doi.org/10.1080/10790268.1995.11719382.

36. European Pressure Ulcer Advisory Panel. *National Pressure Injury Advisory Panel and Pan Pacific Pressure Injury Alliance. Prevention and Treatment of Pressure Ulcers/Injuries: Clinical Practice Guideline. The International Guideline.* 2019. www.internationalguideline.com/static/pdfs/Quick_Reference_Guide-10Mar2019.pdf.

37. Gilead, L., K.Y. Mumcuoglu, and A. Ingber, *The Use of Maggot Debridement Therapy in the Treatment of Chronic Wounds in Hospitalised and Ambulatory Patients.* Journal of Wound Care, 2012. 21(2): pp. 78–85, https://doi.org/10.12968/jowc.2012.21.2.78.

38. Mumcuoglu, K.Y., et al., *Maggot Therapy for the Treatment of Intractable Wounds: Maggot Therapy for Intractable Wounds Pharmacology and Therapeutics.* International Journal of Dermatology, 1999. 38(8): pp. 623–627, https://doi.org/10.1046/j.1365-4362.1999.00770.x.

39. Polat, E., et al., *Treatment of Pressure Ulcers with Larvae of Lucilia sericata.* Türkiye Fiziksel Tıp ve Rehabilitasyon Dergisi, 2017. 63(4): pp. 307–312, https://doi.org/10.5606/tftrd.2017.851.

40. Fleischmann, W., et al., *Biosurgery — Maggots, Are They Really the Better Surgeons?* Chirurg, 1999. 70(11): pp. 1340–1346, https://doi.org/10.1007/s001040050790.

41. Igari, K., et al., *Maggot Debridement Therapy for Peripheral Arterial Disease.* Annals of Vascular Diseases, 2013. 6(2): pp. 145–149, https://doi.org/10.3400/avd.oa.13-00036.

42. Nishijima, A., et al., *Effective Wound Bed Preparation Using Maggot Debridement Therapy for Patients with Critical Limb Ischaemia.* Journal of Wound Care, 2017. 26(8): pp. 483–489, https://doi.org/10.12968/jowc.2017.26.8.483.

43. Rafter, L., *Larval Therapy Applied to a Large Arterial Ulcer: An Effective Outcome.* British Journal of Nursing, 2013. 22(Sup4): pp. S24-S30, https://doi.org/10.12968/bjon.2013.22.Sup4.S24.

44. Dumville, J.C., et al., *Larval Therapy for Leg Ulcers (VenUS II): Randomised Controlled Trial.* BMJ, 2009. 338(7702): pp. 1047–1050, https://doi.org/10.1136/bmj.b773.

45. Mudge, E., et al., *A Randomized Controlled Trial of Larval Therapy for the Debridement of Leg Ulcers: Results of a Multicenter, Randomized, Controlled, Open, Observer Blind, Parallel Group Study.* Wound Repair and Regeneration, 2014. 22(1): pp. 43–51, https://doi.org/10.1111/wrr.12127.

46. Wayman, J., et al., *The Cost Effectiveness of Larval Therapy in Venous Ulcers.* Journal of Tissue Viability, 2000. 10(3): pp. 91–94, https://doi.org/10.1016/S0965-206X(00)80036-4.

47. Schaper N, et al. *IWGDF Guidelines on the Prevention and Management of Diabetic Foot Disease.* 2019. https://iwgdfguidelines.org/wp-content/uploads/2019/05/IWGDF-Guidelines-2019.pdf.

48. Hingorani, A.M.D., et al., *The Management of Diabetic Foot: A Clinical Practice Guideline by the Society for Vascular Surgery in Collaboration with the American Podiatric Medical Association and the Society for Vascular Medicine.* Journal of Vascular Surgery, 2016. 63(2): pp. 3S-21S, https://doi.org/10.1016/j.jvs.2015.10.003.

49. International Diabetes Federation. *IDF Diabetes Atlas, 7th Edition.* 2015. https://www.idf.org/component/attachments/attachments.html?id=1093&task=download.

50. Krishnan, S., et al., *Reduction in Diabetic Amputations over 11 Years in a Defined U.K. Population: Benefits of Multidisciplinary Team Work and Continuous Prospective Audit.* Diabetes Care, 2008. 31(1): pp. 99–101, https://doi.org/10.2337/dc07-1178.

51. Marineau, M.L., et al., *Maggot Debridement Therapy in the Treatment of Complex Diabetic Wounds.* Hawaii Medical Journal, 2011. 70(6): pp. 121–124, https://www.ncbi.nlm.nih.gov/pmc/articles/PMC3233395/.

52. Jun-cheng, W., et al., *Maggot Therapy for Repairing Serious Infective Wound in a Severely Burned Patient.* Chinese Journal of Traumatology, 2012. 15(2): pp. 124–125, https://doi.org/10.3760/cma.j.issn.1008-1275.2012.02.012.

53. Feng, X., et al., *Evaluation of the Burn Healing Properties of Oil Extraction from Housefly Larva in Mice*. Journal of Ethnopharmacology, 2010. 130(3): pp. 586–592, https://doi.org/10.1016/j.jep.2010.05.044.

54. Li, Q.M.D., et al., *Maggots of Musca Domestica in Treatment of Acute Intractable Wound*. Surgery, 2009. 145(1): pp. 122–123, https://doi.org/10.1016/j.surg.2008.08.016.

55. Namias, N., et al., *Biodebridement: A Case Report of Maggot Therapy for Limb Salvage after Fourth-degree Burns*. Journal of Burn Care & Rehabilitation, 2000. 21(3): pp. 254–257, https://academic.oup.com/jbcr/article-abstract/21/3/254/4758239?redirectedFrom=fulltext.

56. Sherman, R.A., C.E. Shapiro, and R.M. Yang, *Maggot Therapy for Problematic Wounds: Uncommon and Off-label Applications*. Advances in Skin & Wound Care, 2007. 20(11): pp. 602–610, https://doi.org/10.1097/01.ASW.0000284943.70825.a8.

57. Summers, J.B. and J. Kaminski, *Maggot Debridement Therapy (MDT) for Burn Wounds*. Burns: Journal of the International Society for Burn Injuries, 2003. 29(5): pp. 501–502, https://doi.org/10.1016/s0305-4179(03)00059-7.

58. Vistnes, L.M., R. Lee, and G.A. Ksander, *Proteolytic Activity of Blowfly Larvae Secretions in Experimental Burns*. Surgery, 1981. 90(5): pp. 835–841.

59. McKeever, D.C., *Maggots in Treatment of Osteomyelitis: A Simple Inexpensive Method*. The Journal of Bone and Joint Surgery, 1933. 15: pp. 85–93, http://dx.doi.org/10.1007/s11999-008-0240-5.

60. Stewart, M.A., *The Therapeutic Behavior of Lucilia Sericata Meig. Larvae in Osteomyelitis Wounds*. Science (American Association for the Advancement of Science), 1934. 79(2055): pp. 459–460

61. Galeano, M., et al., *Maggot Therapy for Treatment of Osteomyelitis and Deep Wounds: An Old Remedy for an Actual Problem* [8]. Plastic and Reconstructive Surgery (1963), 2001. 108(7): pp. 2178–2179.

62. Horn, K.L., A.H. Cobb, and G.A. Gates, *Maggot Therapy for Subacute Mastoiditis*. Archives of otolaryngology (1960), 1976. 102(6): pp. 377–379, https://doi.org/10.1001/archotol.1976.00780110089013.

63. Mumcuoglu, K.Y., et al., [*Maggot Therapy for Gangrene and Osteomyelitis*]. Harefuah, 1997. 132(5): pp. 323–325, 382.

64. Townley, W.A., A. Jain, and C. Healy, *Maggot Debridement Therapy to Avoid Prosthesis Removal in an Infected Total Knee Arthroplasty*. Journal of Wound Care, 2006. 15(2): pp. 78–79, https://doi.org/10.12968/jowc.2006.15.2.26890.

65. Wollina, U., M. Kinscher, and H. Fengler, *Maggot Therapy in the Treatment of Wounds of Exposed Knee Prostheses*. International Journal of Dermatology, 2005. 44(10): pp. 884–886, https://doi.org/10.1111/j.1365-4632.2005.02366c.x.

66. Beasley, W.D. and G. Hirst, *Making a Meal of MRSA—The Role of Biosurgery in Hospital-acquired Infection*. 2004, Elsevier Ltd: London, pp. 6–9.

67. Bowling, F.L., E.V. Salgami, and A.J.M. Boulton, *Larval Therapy: A Novel Treatment in Eliminating Methicillin-Resistant Staphylococcus aureus from Diabetic Foot Ulcers*. Diabetes Care, 2007. 30(2): pp. 370–371, https://doi.org/10.2337/dc06-2348.

68. Dissemond, J., et al., *Treatment of Methicillin-resistant Staphylococcus aureus (MRSA) as Part of Biosurgical Management of a Chronic Leg Ulcer*. Hautarzt, 2002. 53(9): pp. 608–612, https://doi.org/10.1007/s00105-002-0336-x.

69. Čeřovský, V. and R. Bém, *Lucifensins, the Insect Defensins of Biomedical Importance: The Story behind Maggot Therapy*. Pharmaceuticals, 2014. 7(3): pp. 251–264, https://doi.org/10.3390/ph7030251.

70. Evans, R., E. Dudley, and Y. Nigam, *Detection and Partial Characterization of Antifungal Bioactivity from the Secretions of the Medicinal Maggot, Lucilia sericata*. Wound Repair and Regeneration, 2015. 23(3): pp. 361–368, https://doi.org/10.1111/wrr.12287.

71. Margolin, L. and P. Gialanella, *Assessment of the Antimicrobial Properties of Maggots*. International Wound Journal, 2010. 7(3): pp. 202–204, https://doi.org/10.1111/j.1742-481X.2010.00234.x.

72. Bohac, M., et al., *Maggot Therapy in Treatment of a Complex Hand Injury Complicated by Mycotic Infection*. Bratislava Medical Journal, 2015. 116(11): pp. 671–673, https://doi.org/10.4149/bll_2015_128.

73. Sorensen, M.D. and J.N. Krieger, *Fournier's Gangrene: Epidemiology and Outcomes in the General US Population*. Urologia Internationalis, 2016. 97(3): pp. 249–259, https://doi.org/10.1159/000445695.

74. Angel, K., et al., *Madentherapie bei Fournierscher Gangrän — erste Erfahrungen mit einer neuen Therapie*. Aktuelle Urologie, 2000. 31(07): pp. 440–443.

75. Dunn, C., U. Raghavan, and A.G. Pfleiderer, *The Use of Maggots in Head and Neck Necrotizing Fasciitis*. The Journal of Laryngology & Otology, 2002. 116(1): pp. 70–72, https://doi.org/10.1258/0022215021910212.

76. Preuss, S.F., M.J. Stenzel, and A. Esriti, *The Successful Use of Maggots in Necrotizing Fasciitis of the Neck: A Case Report*. Head & Neck, 2004. 26(8): pp. 747–750, https://doi.org/10.1002/hed.20092.

77. Steenvoorde, P., et al., *Maggot Debridement Therapy in Necrotizing Fasciitis Reduces the Number of Surgical Debridements*. Wounds, 2007. 19(3): pp. 73–78.

78. Fonseca-Muñoz, A., et al., *Clinical Study of Maggot therapy for Fournier's Gangrene*. International Wound Journal, 2020. 17(6): pp. 1642–1649, https://doi.org/10.1111/iwj.13444.

79. Berger, S., *Tropical Skin Ulcers: Global Status*. 2017, Los Angeles: Gideon Informatics, Inc.

80. Frimpong, M., et al., *Paradoxical Reactions in Buruli Ulcer after Initiation of Antibiotic Therapy: Relationship to Bacterial Load*. PLOS Neglected Tropical

Diseases, 2019. 13(8): e0007689-e0007689, https://doi.org/10.1371/journal.pntd.0007689.

81. Eichelmann, K., et al., *Leprosy. An update: Definition, Pathogenesis, Classification, Diagnosis, and Treatment.* Actas Dermo-Sifiliograficas, 2013. 104(7): pp. 554–563, https://doi.org/10.1016/j.ad.2012.03.003.

82. Arrivillaga, J., J. Rodríguez, and M. Oviedo, *Preliminary Evaluation of Maggot (Diptera: Calliphoridae) Therapy as a Potential Treatment for Leishmaniasis Ulcers.* Biomédica, 2008. 28(2): pp. 305–310, https://doi.org/10.7705/biomedica.v28i2.102.

83. Cruz-Saavedra, L., et al., *The Effect of Lucilia sericata- and Sarconesiopsis magellanica-derived Larval Therapy on Leishmania panamensis.* Acta Tropica, 2016. 164: pp. 280–289, https://doi.org/10.1016/j.actatropica.2016.09.020.

84. Polat, E., et al., *Detection of Anti-leishmanial Effect of the Lucilia sericata Larval Secretions in vitro and in vivo on Leishmania tropica: First work.* Experimental Parasitology, 2012. 132(2): pp. 129–134, https://doi.org/10.1016/j.exppara.2012.06.004.

85. Sanei-Dehkordi, A., et al., *Anti Leishmania Activity of Lucilia sericata and Calliphora vicina Maggots in Laboratory Models.* Experimental Parasitology, 2016. 170: pp. 59–65, https://doi.org/10.1016/j.exppara.2016.08.007.

86. Stadler, F., R.Z. Shaban, and P. Tatham, *Maggot Debridement Therapy in Disaster Medicine.* Prehospital and Disaster Medicine, 2016. 31(1): pp. 79–84, https://doi.org/10.1017/S1049023X15005427.

87. Čičková, H., M. Kozánek, and P. Takáč, *Growth and Survival of Blowfly Lucilia sericata Larvae under Simulated Wound Conditions: Implications for Maggot Debridement Therapy.* Medical and Veterinary Entomology, 2015. 29(4): pp. 416–424, https://doi.org/10.1111/mve.12135.

88. Stadler, F. and P. Tatham, *Drone-assisted Medicinal Maggot Distribution in Compromised Healthcare Settings*, in *A Complete Guide to Maggot Therapy: Clinical Practice, Therapeutic Principles, Production, Distribution, and Ethics*, F. Stadler (ed.). 2022, Cambridge: Open Book Publishers, pp. 383–402, https://doi.org/10.11647/OBP.0300.18.

89. Ayello, E.A., et al., *Reexamining the Literature on Terminal Ulcers, SCALE, Skin Failure, and Unavoidable Pressure Injuries.* Advances in Skin & Wound Care, 2019. 32(3): pp. 109–121, https://doi.org/10.1097/01.ASW.0000553112.55505.5f.

90. Steenvoorde, P., et al., *Maggot Debridement Therapy in the Palliative Setting.* American Journal of Hospice & Palliative Medicine, 2007. 24(4): pp. 308–310, https://doi.org/10.1177/1049909107302300.

91. Brüggmann, D., H.R. Tinneberg, and M.T. Zygmunt, [*Maggot Therapy in Gynecology*]. Zentralblatt für Gynäkologie 2006. 128(5): pp. 261–265, https://doi.org/10.1055/s-2006-942121.

92. Wolters, U., et al., *ASA Classification and Perioperative Variables as Predictors of Postoperative Outcome.* British Journal of Anaesthesia, 1996. 77(2): Pp. 217–222, https://doi.org/10.1093/bja/77.2.217.

93. Peck, G.W. and B.C. Kirkup, *Biocompatibility of Antimicrobials to Maggot Debridement Therapy: Medical Maggots Lucilia sericata (Diptera: Calliphoridae) Exhibit Tolerance to Clinical Maximum Doses of Antimicrobials*. Journal of Medical Entomology, 2012. 49(5): pp. 1137–1143, https://doi.org/10.1603/ME12066.

94. Sherman, R.A., F.A. Wyle, and L. Thrupp, *Effects of Seven Antibiotics on the Growth and Development of Phaenicia sericata (Diptera: Calliphoridae) Larvae*. Journal of Medical Entomology, 1995. 32(5): pp. 646–649, https://doi.org/10.1093/jmedent/32.5.646.

95. Felder, J.M., et al., *Increasing the Options for Management of Large and Complex Chronic Wounds with a Scalable, Closed-system Dressing for Maggot Therapy*. Journal of Burn Care & Research, 2012. 33(3): pp. e169-e175, https://doi.org/10.1097/BCR.0b013e318233570d.

96. Sherman, R.A., B. Khavari, and D. Werner, *Effect of Hyperbaric Oxygen on the Growth and Development of Medicinal Maggots*. Undersea and Hyperbaric Medicine, 2013. 40(5): pp. 377–380.

97. Teich, S. and R.A.M. Myers, *Maggot Therapy for Severe Skin Infections*. Southern Medical Journal, 1986. 79(9): pp. 1153–1155.

98. Rojo, S. and S. Geraghty, *Hemophilia and Maggots: From Hospital Admission to Healed Wound*. Ostomy Wound Management, 2004. 50(4): pp. 30, 32, 34.

99. Sherman, R.A. and M.R. Hetzler, *Maggot Therapy for Wound Care in Austere Environments*. Journal of Special Operations Medicine, 2017. 17(2): pp. 154–162.

100. Grassberger, M. and C. Reiter, *Effect of Temperature on Lucilia sericata (Diptera: Calliphoridae) Development with Special Reference to the Isomegalen- and Isomorphen-diagram*. Forensic Science International, 2001. 120(1): pp. 32–36, https://doi.org/10.1016/S0379-0738(01)00413-3.

101. Sherman, R.A., et al., *Effects of Food Storage and Handling on Blow Fly (Lucilia sericata) Eggs and Larvae*. Journal of Food Science, 2006. 71(3): pp. M117-M120, https://doi.org/10.1111/j.1365-2621.2006.tb15634.x.

102. Gallagher, M.B., S. Sandhu, and R. Kimsey, *Variation in Developmental Time for Geographically Distinct Populations of the Common Green Bottle Fly, Lucilia sericata (Meigen)*. Journal of Forensic Sciences, 2010. 55(2): pp. 438–442, https://doi.org/10.1111/j.1556-4029.2009.01285.x.

103. Richards, C.S. and M.H. Villet, *Data Quality in Thermal Summation Development Models for Forensically Important Blowflies*. Medical and Veterinary Entomology, 2009. 23(3): pp. 269–276, https://doi.org/10.1111/j.1365-2915.2009.00819.x.

104. Mirabzadeh, A., et al., *Maggot Therapy for Wound Care in Iran: A Case Series of the First 28 Patients*. Journal of Wound Care, 2017. 26(3): pp. 137–143, https://doi.org/10.12968/jowc.2017.26.3.137.

105. Lin, G., et al., *Hard Times Call for Creative Solutions: Medical Improvisations at the Israel Defense Forces Field Hospital in Haiti*. American Journal of Disaster Medicine, 2010. 5(3): pp. 188–192.

4. Indications, Contraindications, Interactions, and Side-effects of Maggot Therapy

Ronald A. Sherman

Maggot therapy is not regulated in most countries, but in those countries in which it is regulated, indications authorised by regulating bodies are the law of the land. Irrespective of particular jurisdictional limitations, this chapter describes when maggot therapy can be used, when it can't be used, potential adverse events, and when treatment can proceed with caution. The chapter also examines how medicinal maggots interact with concomitant treatments such as systemic antibiotics, anaesthetics and narcotics, or hyperbaric oxygen therapy. Evidence and expert advice suggest that maggot therapy is a safe and widely applicable wound care modality with few side-effects, most of which can be avoided or successfully managed.

Introduction

The terms "indications" and "contraindications" are short-hand for: when should maggot therapy be used and when should it not be used? When deciding whether or not a medical product should be used, it is critical to keep in mind *who* is issuing the recommendations. For the purposes of the following discussion, two groups of authorities will be referenced: regulators and experts. Maggot therapy is not regulated in

https://doi.org/10.11647/OBP.0300.04

most countries, but in those countries in which it is regulated (primarily North America, much of Europe, and several countries in the Middle East and Asia), indications authorised by regulating bodies are the law of the land. Indications issued by regulatory agencies tend to be more restrictive, and the use of maggot therapy for anything other than what is specifically authorised is considered "off-label". Off-label use of a product by a licensed care provider is not illegal, but it does put one at legal or professional risk if it is not in keeping with standard-of-care practice by one's peers and licensing boards. In countries where maggot therapy is not formally regulated, therapists are free to follow the advice of experts. In this chapter, indications recommended by experts but not approved by regulatory agencies will be clearly identified.

Indications for Maggot Therapy

As described in Chapters 8 to 10, medicinal maggots have been found to debride wounds, kill microbes, and stimulate wound healing [1–3]. Therefore, many experts around the world use maggot therapy for any or all of those purposes. In those countries where maggot therapy is regulated by health ministries, maggot therapy is approved only for wound debridement. Specific examples will follow.

Debridement

Wound debridement is the removal of dead (necrotic) tissue and debris from the wound. Sharp debridement with scalpels removes dead tissue mechanically, by cutting it out. Enzymatic debriding ointments remove the dead tissue by enzymatically dissolving it [4]. Necrotic tissue can also be removed by blasting it with a jet of water (hydrosurgery) [5] or with pulses of ultrasound [6]. Autolytic debridement involves dressings which potentiate the body's own mechanisms (mostly enzymatic) to dissolve and discharge the dead tissue [7]. Maggot therapy rids the body of necrotic tissue and debris by both mechanical pathways (the physical action of the maggots' cuticular spines and mouth hooks) and enzymatic pathways (liquefaction of the necrotic tissue by the maggots' secreted and excreted digestive enzymes).

In the U.S., where medicinal maggots are regulated by the Food and Drug Administration (FDA), cleared indications are for "debridement of non-healing necrotic skin and soft-tissue wounds such as pressure ulcers, neuropathic foot ulcers, chronic leg ulcers, or non-healing traumatic or post-operative wounds." These indications broadly cover a variety of necrotic and non-healing wounds, such as those described in Chapter 3 [8]. FDA-cleared indications noticeably exclude the debridement of "hard tissue" (bone) as well as the use of maggots for anything other than debridement. Yet, many experts will sometimes resort to maggot therapy when certain modalities fail to achieve adequate disinfection or wound healing, whether or not debridement is also a major goal.

Disinfection

Microbial infection is a common feature of chronic wounds. If not already infected, most non-healing wounds will eventually become infected by invading bacteria or fungi. After all, necrotic tissue, by definition, has no circulation and no defence against microbial invaders, and it provides a moist, nutrient-rich substrate for microbial growth. As has been discussed in Chapter 9 [2], medicinal maggots kill a wide variety of microbes through ingestion and through the secretion of antimicrobial compounds, which is why maggot therapy is commonly used to debride infected necrotic wounds, and to treat chronic wounds whose primary problem is non-gangrenous infection. Chronically infected wounds are typically characterised by drainage, pain, and bad odour. When treated with maggot therapy, all three of these characteristics substantially decrease or resolve.

Examples of infectious complications that are not easily treated with antibiotics include wounds populated by multi-resistant organisms or biofilm. There are now multiple laboratory studies of maggots' antimicrobial activity, but relatively few controlled clinical studies. Still, a few controlled studies and several case series demonstrate clinically relevant antimicrobial effects of maggot therapy [9–18].

Growth Stimulation

For nearly 100 years, maggot therapy has been observed to enhance wound healing, even in apparently clean but stagnant wounds. Clinicians and researchers have described the rapid proliferation of granulation tissue and hastened closing of the wound margins in previously stagnant, non-healing wounds [19–23]. The mechanisms by which growth stimulation and wound healing are enhanced by maggot therapy are described in Chapter 10 [3]. As a result, some therapists consider non-healing wounds—even those without necrotic tissue or obvious infection—to be appropriate candidates for maggot therapy.

Additional Situations

Maggot therapy is also useful for situations that may not fit neatly into the specific categories of debridement, disinfection and wound healing. Maggot therapy may be used for two or three of these indications simultaneously, and it may be used for non-healing wounds with no obvious infection or gangrene. Often therapists turn to maggot therapy only after conventional therapy has failed or is unavailable. In published studies of patients who failed conventional wound care and were scheduled for amputation but given a trial of maggot therapy instead, at least 50% of those patients healed their wounds and avoided amputation [24]. This has led many therapists to believe that a non-emergency amputation due to a non-healing wound may itself be an appropriate indication for a trial of maggot therapy. Of course, outcomes are even better when wounds are treated with maggot therapy before they progress to the point (and the underlying circulatory status has regressed to the point) that they are earmarked for amputation.

Maggot therapy is useful in treating wounds that are undermined, difficult to visualise, or connected to inner-body cavities [22]. Ordinarily, such wounds might be opened widely ("surgically filleted") to view them completely before cleaning them out. When that is not feasible without significant damage to nearby vital structures, some therapists apply medicinal maggots to the wound entrance so that they will explore the entire inner cavity, looking for and dissolving infected, necrotic tissue. Since medicinal maggots are obligate air breathers and since their natural instinct is to leave the host when satiated or when there is nothing more to eat, they can be considered self-extracting.

Maggot therapy is also indicated for patients who would benefit from surgical debridement but are too frail [22]. Even patients at the end of life or with wounds unlikely to heal can benefit from maggot therapy, if they are suffering from chronic wounds that are painful, draining, malodorous, or require resource-intense treatments [25]. Since maggot therapy can be applied by non-professionals and outside of medical facilities, many patients with non-healing wounds who lack access to such resources are appropriate candidates for maggot therapy [26–28].

Contraindications and Relative Contraindications for Maggot Therapy

There are relatively few absolute contraindications for maggot therapy. One soft-tissue wound to which they must not be applied is a corneal ulcer, because the maggots' cuticle and mouth hooks are likely to scratch and damage the corneal surface. Maggots are obligate air breathers, so they cannot be placed within a closed cavity, such as an abscess. However, if that abscess is opened and allowed to drain, the maggots could be placed on the surface of the drained abscess, if desired. Maggot therapy is generally contraindicated for sterile cavities, but most sterile cavities should have no reason to undergo maggot debridement.

The anatomy and location of the wound can affect dressing selection, but generally is not itself a contraindication, except as described above. For example, a toe or anterior foot wound cannot easily be covered with a sheet of net fabric to confine the maggots because affixing it to the surrounding tissue would result in multiple wrinkles and tunnels through which the maggots might escape. In this case, a stocking-like dressing might be used instead, and affixed proximally to the foot or ankle. Similarly, a wound very near to an orifice might be of concern if the maggots posed a danger to that particular orifice (mouth or tracheostomy, for example). Again, this may be a contraindication to a dressing that requires a sizeable border to adhere to the periphery of the wound, but need not be a contraindication to maggot therapy in general, because a different dressing could be used: maggots contained within a bag [29].

Rapidly advancing, life- or limb-threatening infections are not appropriate for maggot therapy. In these cases, the standard of care is surgical resection and broad-spectrum antibiotics. Maggot therapy is not appropriate, even in combination with first-line surgical and medical therapy, if it will interfere with the critical close and frequent observation of the wound. Once stabilised, maggot therapy may be appropriate to debride the necrotic tissue without harming nearby vital structures [22, 30–34].

Maggot therapy is generally reserved for skin and soft-tissue wounds; maggot secretions do not dissolve tendons, fascia or bone efficiently. That said, when surgical resection is not feasible because of patient frailty, or lack of surgical expertise in compromised healthcare settings, maggot debridement of wounds that include necrotic harder tissues can be quite useful [22, 35–37].

Because maggots are aerobic creatures, they are susceptible to drowning and suffocation. Maggot dressings must be highly permeable to air, and allow the efflux of purulent drainage. Medicinal maggots must not be covered by occlusive dressings (i.e., "semi-permeable" transparent membranes, hydrocolloid and hydrogel pads, etc.) or else they will die. They may also suffocate if applied to wounds along with ointments (petroleum jelly, zinc oxide, silver sulfadiazine, triple antibiotic ointments, etc.), if the oily substance covers the maggots' breathing holes (spiracles).

Interactions between Maggot Therapy and Other Treatment Modalities

The viability and debridement capacity of medicinal maggots have been tested under a wide variety of conditions. Under controlled laboratory conditions, medicinal maggots fed increasing concentrations of antibiotics were found not to be affected by pharmacologic doses of any of the tested antimicrobials [23, 38]. Insecticides, however, can be lethal and should not be used during or within two half-lives prior to application of medicinal maggots. Hyperbaric oxygen therapy (HBOT) has been shown to be lethal to very young larvae, but not to older larvae [39]. Therefore, for patients receiving HBOT, maggot therapy should be administered during the non-diving days or else the larvae should be late-second or early-third instars before the patient re-enters the HBO chamber. As discussed in more detail elsewhere in this chapter, bleeding can sometimes occur with maggot therapy. Blood thinning medication puts those patients at increased risk for more significant blood loss (haemorrhage).

Some drugs—especially drugs of abuse—may be present in the blood or tissue without the awareness of the therapist and maybe even without the complete awareness of the patient. Maggot growth and survival has been assessed in the presence of a variety of narcotics and anaesthetics [40–42]. While most of these will have some effect on the larvae, they are generally not lethal in the doses tested, and medical maggots should still do their job.

Most other contraindications are really "relative contraindications". In other words, the benefits of maggot therapy must be weighed against the risks (which we call "adverse events"). Those risks may be greater in some patients than in others... so great as to be considered a contraindication to maggot therapy. We will discuss such relative contraindications within the context of the underlying adverse effects.

Warnings and Adverse Events Associated with Maggot Therapy

All things considered, there are relatively few serious complications associated with maggot therapy (Table 4.1), and they are certainly not as serious nor as numerous as those that can result from the wounds themselves, in the absence of maggot therapy. The best way to avoid these adverse events is to understand the patient and their medical history, understand the nature of maggot therapy, and to read all package inserts carefully *before* using the products. In this way, adverse events can often be avoided or their risks minimised. For example, by reading the package insert it might be discovered that one of the ingredients is something to which the patient may be allergic. This could be a contraindication to therapy. But if the therapist identifies the problem in advance, a special preparation can probably be made to avoid that ingredient, thereby eliminating the contraindication.

The most common adverse event associated with medicinal maggots is wound pain. Discomfort or pain has been reported in anywhere from 5–30% of patients already experiencing wound pain [21, 43–47]. Maggot-associated pain or discomfort usually does not manifest until about 24 hours into the therapy, but then increases as the larvae grow larger. Patients that are at risk of experiencing pain can easily be identified (and prepared) in advance, because they are the patients with painful wounds

Table 4.1 Adverse events and contributing factors (after Sherman [43]).

Adverse Event or Complication	Contributing Causes	Treatment
Pain	Pre-existing wound pain; large larvae.	Liberal analgaesics; remove the larvae for immediate pain relief.
Infection	Pre-existing wound infection; inadequate maggot dosage; inadequate disinfection of larvae.	Suppress *Pseudomonas aeruginosa* with topical antiseptics prior to maggot therapy; concurrent antibiotics; check adequacy of larval disinfection.
Hepatic encephalopathy or other mental status changes	Underlying hepatic insufficiency; high maggot burden; sepsis.	Check for bacteraemia, serum ammonia; remove maggots.
Excessive bleeding	Coagulopathy; necrosis involving major vessel.	Remove maggots; find and stop source of bleeding.
Hypersensitivity reaction (local or systemic)	Allergy to medicinal maggots (i.e., their media) or the dressings.	Check beforehand; remove immediately and treat reaction.
Tissue invasion	Inappropriate species.	Remove maggots; check species.

who already receive analgaesics during dressing changes or maybe even constantly. Patients should be given liberal access to analgaesics during maggot therapy and offered the opportunity for early removal of dressings upon their request. If systemic analgaesics no longer control the pain, remove the maggot dressing to achieve immediate relief. With these two provisions, patients often cope much better with therapy-related pain and are more satisfied with their experience, even if they do have pain (personal experience).

Patients may be allergic to fly larvae, their media, or the accompanying dressing components. Patients allergic to the maggots or dressing materials may manifest contact dermatitis or more serious immunologic reactions. Patients known to be allergic to media ingredients should not be treated with those constituents; alternatives usually can be substituted. When in doubt, communicate with the manufacturer.

Pseudomonas aeruginosa and some other hardy gram-negative organisms appear to be more resistant to maggot therapy than other microbes [48]. Situations have been reported in which a *P. aeruginosa* infection has actually spread through the wound during maggot therapy. Some experts believe this may occur as a result of maggot-induced killing of the other microbes, leaving the *P. aeruginosa* to grow without competition. When treating wounds with *P. aeruginosa* infection or colonisation, it is recommended that topical anti-pseudomonal antiseptics (i.e., acetic acid, sodium hypochlorite, etc.) be applied for a day or two before maggot debridement, to decrease the *P. aeruginosa* population. Also, a greater density of maggots in the wound is more effective in killing *P. aeruginosa* [48]. Therefore, a high dose of maggots ($10+$ larvae/cm^2) should be applied when treating wounds suspected of harbouring this organism.

Mild bleeding is common during maggot debridement, and it is common that the wound drainage is blood-tinged. However, patients with coagulopathy (inability to form blood clots and halt bleeding) are at risk of more substantial bleeding. Maggot therapy in such individuals should only be performed under close supervision [22, 49]. Maggot debridement of, or around, necrotic blood vessels may also lead to life-threatening blood loss if and when those vessels dissolve under the influence of maggot excretions and secretions [50]. If maggot therapy is attempted for wounds with uncertain vascular integrity, the patient must receive close and continuous observation for bleeding, infection, or thrombosis.

Large maggot burdens in blowfly-infested sheep ($>60,000$ maggots per animal) are associated with serious complications ("blowfly strike"), including elevated serum ammonia levels (presumably due to the large protein breakdown in the wound) and encephalopathy. Similar complications in humans were predicted [43] but not seen until 20,000 larvae were applied (against verbal and written advice) to wounds in a patient with underlying alcoholic hepatic insufficiency [51]. Maggot loads over 6,000 should probably be avoided, even in otherwise healthy individuals. Too many maggots in a tight dressing, especially in a patient with insensate wounds, may exert pressure sufficient to compromise circulation and cause further pressure-related necrosis [43].

Patients with fever or changes in mental status should be evaluated for spread of infection (i.e., cellulitis, bacteraemia, sepsis) or hepatic encephalopathy (check for elevated serum ammonia level). Maggot dressings may need to be removed immediately, even if just to facilitate wound inspection. Patients with infected wounds—especially those with deep or extensive wounds, and those at increased risk of bacteraemia, should receive systemic antibiotic coverage during maggot therapy to prevent sepsis or cellulitis.

The use of maggots that have not been disinfected or were inadequately disinfected has also been found to pose a risk of local and systemic infection [52]. Larvae supplied in a single, primary packaging container are intended for single-use only [53]; they are not to be multi-dosed nor saved for retreatment of the same patient. Firstly, opening and retrieving maggots may contaminate the internal environment and content of the primary packaging container, and secondly, the remaining maggots will have deteriorated beyond therapeutic effectiveness by the time the patient requires a follow-up treatment (usually 48–72 hours later). Medicinal maggots should not be used on more than one patient, nor be allowed to wander away from their host patient. Once they have been applied to a patient, they are contaminated with the patient's wound flora, and must be discarded as infectious ("biohazardous") medical waste.

Summary

Maggot therapy is indicated for the debridement of a wide variety of chronic wounds. Many experts also recommend medicinal maggots for controlling wound infections and the promotion of healthy granulation tissue and reepithelialisation in non-healing wounds. Please refer to Chapter 15, where Takáč and colleagues present examples of successfully treated patients with before-and-after images [54]. Adverse events are very uncommon, with the exception of increased pain in patients with painful wounds. However, a variety of precautions should be taken when treating patients at risk of bleeding, infection, or the complications of liver disease. Patients with inadequate blood flow may never heal their wounds, even if completely debrided by maggot therapy; but we do not yet know how much blood flow is too little because even patients with so little blood flow that they are scheduled for amputation often heal with a trial of maggot therapy.

References

1. Nigam, Y. and M.R. Wilson, *Maggot Debridement*, in *A Complete Guide to Maggot Therapy: Clinical Practice, Therapeutic Principles, Production, Distribution, and Ethics*, F. Stadler (ed.). 2022, Cambridge: Open Book Publishers, pp. 143–152, https://doi.org/10.11647/OBP.0300.08.

2. Nigam, Y. and M.R. Wilson, *The Antimicrobial Activity of Medicinal Maggots*, in *A Complete Guide to Maggot Therapy: Clinical Practice, Therapeutic Principles, Production, Distribution, and Ethics*, F. Stadler (ed.). 2022, Cambridge: Open Book Publishers, pp. 153–174, https://doi.org/10.11647/OBP.0300.09.

3. Nigam, Y. and M.R. Wilson, *Maggot-assisted Wound Healing*, in *A Complete Guide to Maggot Therapy: Clinical Practice, Therapeutic Principles, Production, Distribution, and Ethics*, F. Stadler (ed.). 2022, Cambridge: Open Book Publishers, pp. 175–194, https://doi.org/10.11647/OBP.0300.10.

4. Ramundo, J. and M. Gray, *Enzymatic Wound Debridement.* Journal of Wound, Ostomy, and Continence Nursing, 2008. 35(3): pp. 273–280, https://doi.org/10.1097/01.WON.0000319125.21854.78.

5. Kakagia, D.D. and E.J. Karadimas, *The Efficacy of Versajet™ Hydrosurgery System in Burn Surgery. A Systematic Review.* Journal of burn care & research, 2018. 39(2): pp. 188–200, https://doi.org/10.1097/BCR.0000000000000561.

6. Messa, C.A., et al., *Ultrasonic Debridement Management of Lower Extremity Wounds: Retrospective Analysis of Clinical Outcomes and Cost.* Journal of Wound Care, 2019. 28(Sup5): pp. S30-S40, https://doi.org/10.12968/jowc.2019.28.Sup5.S30.

7. Atkin, L. and M. Rippon, *Autolysis: Mechanisms of Action in the Removal of Devitalised Tissue.* British Journal of Nursing, 2016. 25(20): pp. S40-S47, https://doi.org/10.12968/bjon.2016.25.20.S40.

8. Sherman, R. and F. Stadler, *Wound Aetiologies, Patient Characteristics, and Healthcare Settings Amenable to Maggot Therapy*, in *A Complete Guide to Maggot Therapy: Clinical Practice, Therapeutic Principles, Production, Distribution, and Ethics*, F. Stadler (ed.). 2022, Cambridge: Open Book Publishers, pp. 39–62, https://doi.org/10.11647/OBP.0300.03.

9. Armstrong, D.G., et al., *Maggot Therapy in "Lower-extremity Hospice" Wound Care: Fewer Amputations and More Antibiotic-free Days.* Journal of the American Podiatric Medical Association, 2005. 95(3): pp. 254–257, https://doi.org/10.7547/0950254.

10. Blueman, D. and C. Bousfield, *The Use of Larval Therapy to Reduce the Bacterial Load in Chronic Wounds.* Journal of Wound Care, 2012. 21(5): pp. 244–253, https://doi.org/10.12968/jowc.2012.21.5.244.

11. Bohac, M., et al., *Maggot Therapy in Treatment of a Complex Hand Injury Complicated by Mycotic Infection.* Bratislava Medical Journal, 2015. 116(11): pp. 671–673, https://doi.org/10.4149/bll_2015_128.

12. Bowling, F.L., E.V. Salgami, and A.J.M. Boulton, *Larval Therapy: A Novel Treatment in Eliminating Methicillin-Resistant Staphylococcus aureus from Diabetic Foot Ulcers.* Diabetes Care, 2007. 30(2): pp. 370–371, https://doi.org/10.2337/dc06-2348.

13. Contreras-Ruiz, J., et al., [*Comparative Study of the Efficacy of Larva Therapy for Debridement and Control of Bacterial Burden Compared to Surgical Debridement and Topical Application of an Antimicrobial*]. Gaceta médica de México, 2016. 152(Suppl 2): pp. 78–87 http://www.anmm.org.mx/GMM/2016/s2/GMM_152_2016_S2_78-87.pdf.

14. Dissemond, J., et al., *Treatment of Methicillin-resistant Staphylococcus aureus (MRSA) as Part of Biosurgical Management of a Chronic Leg Ulcer.* [German] Hautarzt, 2002. 53(9): pp. 608–612, https://doi.org/10.1007/s00105-002-0336-x.

15. Kaplun, O., M. Pupiales, and G. Psevdos, *Adjuvant Maggot Debridement Therapy for Deep Wound Infection Due to Methicillin-resistant Staphylococcus aureus.* Journal of Global Infectious Diseases, 2019. 11(4): pp. 165–167, https://doi.org/10.4103/jgid.jgid_30_19.

16. Malekian, A., et al., *Efficacy of Maggot Therapy on Staphylococcus aureus and Pseudomonas aeruginosa in Diabetic Foot Ulcers: A Randomized Controlled Trial.* Journal of Wound, Ostomy and Continence Nursing, 2019. 46(1): pp. 25–29, https://doi.org/10.1097/WON.0000000000000496.

17. Tantawi, T.I., et al., *Clinical and Microbiological Efficacy of MDT in the Treatment of Diabetic Foot Ulcers.* Journal of Wound Care, 2007. 16(9): pp. 379–383, https://doi.org/10.12968/jowc.2007.16.9.27868.

18. Wolff, H. and C. Hansson, *Larval Therapy for a Leg Ulcer with Methicillin-resistant Staphylococcus aureus.* Acta Dermato-Venereologica, 1999. 79(4): pp. 320–321, https://doi.org/10.1080/000155599750010751.

19. Markevich, Y.O., et al., *Maggot Therapy for Diabetic Neuropathic Foot Wounds — a Randomized Study*, in *EASD Annual Conference*. 2000: Jerusalem, Abstract 0059.

20. Sherman, R.A., *Maggot Therapy for Foot and Leg Wounds.* International Journal of Lower Extremity Wounds, 2002. 1(2): pp. 135–142, https://doi.org/10.1177/1534734602001002009.

21. Sherman, R.A., *Maggot Therapy for Treating Diabetic Foot Ulcers Unresponsive to Conventional Therapy.* Diabetes Care, 2003. 26(2): pp. 446–451, https://doi.org/10.2337/diacare.26.2.446.

22. Sherman, R.A., C.E. Shapiro, and R.M. Yang, *Maggot Therapy for Problematic Wounds: Uncommon and Off-label Applications.* Advances in Skin &

Wound Care, 2007. 20(11): pp. 602–610, https://doi.org/10.1097/01.
ASW.0000284943.70825.a8.

23. Sherman, R.A., F.A. Wyle, and L. Thrupp, *Effects of Seven Antibiotics on the Growth and Development of Phaenicia sericata (Diptera: Calliphoridae) Larvae.* Journal of Medical Entomology, 1995. 32(5): pp. 646–649, https://doi.org/10.1093/jmedent/32.5.646.

24. Sherman, R.A., et al., *Maggot Therapy,* in *Biotherapy — History, Principles and Practice,* M. Grassberger, et al. (eds). 2013, Springer: Dordrecht; New York. pp. 5–29.

25. Steenvoorde, P., et al., *Maggot Debridement Therapy in the Palliative Setting.* American Journal of Hospice & Palliative Medicine, 2007. 24(4): pp. 308–310, https://doi.org/10.1177/1049909107302300.

26. Mirabzadeh, A., et al., *Maggot Therapy for Wound Care in Iran: A Case Series of the First 28 Patients.* Journal of Wound Care, 2017. 26(3): pp. 137–143, https://doi.org/10.12968/jowc.2017.26.3.137.

27. Sherman, R.A. and M.R. Hetzler, *Maggot Therapy for Wound Care in Austere Environments.* Journal of Special Operations Medicine, 2017. 17(2): pp. 154–162.

28. Stadler, F., R.Z. Shaban, and P. Tatham, *Maggot Debridement Therapy in Disaster Medicine.* Prehospital and Disaster Medicine, 2016. 31(1): pp. 79–84, https://doi.org/10.1017/S1049023X15005427.

29. Grassberger, M. and W. Fleischmann, *The Biobag — A New Device for the Application of Medicinal Maggots.* Dermatology, 2002. 204(4): p. 306, https://doi.org/10.1159/000063369.

30. Dunn, C., U. Raghavan, and A.G. Pfleiderer, *The Use of Maggots in Head and Neck Necrotizing Fasciitis.* The Journal of Laryngology & Otology, 2002. 116(1): pp. 70–72, https://doi.org/10.1258/0022215021910212.

31. Fonseca-Muñoz, A., et al., *Clinical Study of Maggot Therapy for Fournier's Gangrene.* International Wound Journal, 2020. 17(6): pp. 1642–1649, https://doi.org/10.1111/iwj.13444.

32. Preuss, S.F., M.J. Stenzel, and A. Esriti, *The Successful Use of Maggots in Necrotizing Fasciitis of the Neck: A Case Report.* Head & Neck, 2004. 26(8): pp. 747–750, https://doi.org/10.1002/hed.20092.

33. Steenvoorde, P., et al., *Maggot Debridement Therapy of Infected Ulcers: Patient and Wound Factors Influencing Outcome a Study on 101 Patients with 117 Wounds.* Annals of the Royal College of Surgeons of England, 2007. 89(6): pp. 596–602, https://doi.org/10.1308/003588407X205404.

34. Teich, S. and R.A.M. Myers, *Maggot Therapy for Severe Skin Infections.* Southern Medical Journal, 1986. 79(9): pp. 1153–1155.

35. Baer, W.S., *The Treatment of Chronic Osteomyelitis with the Maggot (Larva of the Blow Fly)*. The Journal of Bone and Joint Surgery. American Volume, 1931. 13: pp. 438–475, https://doi.org/10.1007/s11999-010-1416-3.

36. El-Tawdy, A.H.F., E.A.H. Ibrahim, and T.A. Morsy, *An Overview of Osteomyelitis with Reference to Treatment in Particular Maggot Debridement Therapy (MDT)*. Journal of the Egyptian Society of Parasitology, 2016. 46(3): pp. 613–624.

37. Mumcuoglu, K.Y., et al., [*Maggot Therapy for Gangrene and Osteomyelitis*]. Harefuah 1997. 132: pp. 323–325, 382.

38. Peck, G.W. and B.C. Kirkup, *Biocompatibility of Antimicrobials to Maggot Debridement Therapy: Medical Maggots Lucilia sericata (Diptera: Calliphoridae) Exhibit Tolerance to Clinical Maximum Doses of Antimicrobials*. Journal of Medical Entomology, 2012. 49(5): pp. 1137–1143, https://doi.org/10.1603/ME12066.

39. Sherman, R.A., B. Khavari, and D. Werner, *Effect of Hyperbaric Oxygen on the Growth and Development of Medicinal Maggots*. Undersea and Hyperbaric Medicine, 2013. 40(5): pp. 377–380.

40. Gosselin, M., et al., *Methadone Determination in Puparia and Its Effect on the Development of Lucilia sericata (Diptera, Calliphoridae)*. Forensic Science International, 2011. 209(1): pp. 154–159, https://doi.org/10.1016/j.forsciint.2011.01.020.

41. Kharbouche, H., et al., *Codeine Accumulation and Elimination in Larvae, Pupae, and Imago of the Blowfly Lucilia sericata and Effects on Its Development*. International Journal of Legal Medicine, 2008. 122(3): pp. 205–211, https://doi.org/10.1007/s00414-007-0217-z.

42. Zou, Y., et al., *Effect of Ketamine on the Development of Lucilia sericata (Meigen) (Diptera: Calliphoridae) and Preliminary Pathological Observation of Larvae*. Forensic Science International, 2013. 226(1): pp. 273–281, https://doi.org/10.1016/j.forsciint.2013.01.042.

43. Sherman, R.A., *Maggot versus Conservative Debridement Therapy for the Treatment of Pressure Ulcers*. Wound Repair and Regeneration, 2002. 10(4): pp. 208–214, https://doi.org/10.1046/j.1524-475X.2002.10403.x.

44. Dumville, J.C., et al., *Larval Therapy for Leg Ulcers (VenUS II): Randomised Controlled Trial*. BMJ, 2009. 338(7702): pp. 1047–1050, https://doi.org/10.1136/bmj.b773.

45. Mumcuoglu, K.Y., et al., *Pain Related to Maggot Debridement Therapy*. Journal of Wound Care, 2012. 21(8): pp. 400–405, https://doi.org/10.12968/jowc.2012.21.8.400.

46. Steenvoorde, P., T. Budding, and J. Oskam, *Determining Pain Levels in Patients Treated with Maggot Debridement Therapy*. Journal of Wound Care, 2005. 14(10): pp. 485–488, https://doi.org/10.12968/jowc.2005.14.10.26846.

47. Steenvoorde, P., et al., *Maggot Debridement Therapy in Necrotizing Fasciitis Reduces the Number of Surgical Debridements.* Wounds, 2007. 19(3): pp. 73–78.

48. Andersen, A.S., et al., *Quorum-sensing-regulated Virulence Factors in Pseudomonas aeruginosa Are Toxic to Lucilia sericata Maggots.* Microbiology (Society for General Microbiology), 2010. 156(2): pp. 400–407, https://doi.org/10.1099/mic.0.032730-0.

49. Rojo, S. and S. Geraghty, *Hemophilia and Maggots: From Hospital Admission to Healed Wound.* Ostomy Wound Management, 2004. 50(4): pp. 30, 32, 34.

50. Steenvoorde, P. and L.P. Van Doorn, *Maggot Debridement Therapy: Serious Bleeding Can Occur: Report of a Case.* Journal of Wound, Ostomy, and Continence Nursing, 2008. 35(4): pp. 412–414, https://doi.org/10.1097/01.WON.0000326662.32390.72.

51. Borst, G.M., et al., *Maggot Therapy for Elephantiasis Nostras Verrucosa Reveals New Applications and New Complications: A Case Report.* International Journal of Lower Extremity Wounds, 2014. 13(2): pp. 135–139, https://doi.org/10.1177/1534734614536036.

52. Nuesch, R., et al., *Clustering of Bloodstream Infections during Maggot Debridement Therapy Using Contaminated Larvae of Protophormia terraenovae.* Infection, 2002. 30(5): pp. 306–309, https://doi.org/10.1007/s15010-002-3067-0.

53. Stadler, F., *Packaging Technology,* in *A Complete Guide to Maggot Therapy: Clinical Practice, Therapeutic Principles, Production, Distribution, and Ethics,* F. Stadler (ed.). 2022, Cambridge: Open Book Publishers, pp. 349–362, https://doi.org/10.11647/OBP.0300.16.

54. Takáč, P., et al., and F. Stadler, *Establishment of a medicinal maggot production facility and treatment programme in Kenya* in *A Complete Guide to Maggot Therapy: Clinical Practice, Therapeutic Principles, Production, Distribution, and Ethics,* F. Stadler (ed.). 2022, Cambridge: Open Book Publishers, pp. 331–346, https://doi.org/10.11647/OBP.0300.15.

5. Medicinal Maggot Application and Maggot Therapy Dressing Technology

Ronald A. Sherman

Maggot therapy dressings are intended to keep maggots on the wound during treatment. Some therapists make their own dressings, others use commercially produced dressings, and many use both, depending on their patients' wounds. There are two basic designs for maggot dressings. Maggot confinement dressings confine the maggots to the wound bed and allow them complete access to the wound, while maggot containment dressings totally contain the maggots within a net bag that facilitates easy handling but does not allow full access to the wound. This chapter describes the basic principles and goals of the ideal maggot dressing, and provides examples of how that ideal dressing can be achieved.

Introduction

The first question most people ask about maggot therapy is: "How do you get the maggots off?" In fact, removing the maggots is not difficult because the species employed for maggot therapy are "self-extracting"—their instinctive behaviour is to leave the host as soon as they are satiated or as soon as there is no more nutritious food (necrotic tissue or exudates) left in the wound. Since some of the maggots will become satiated earlier than others, the real problem is how to keep the maggots corralled in one spot until the therapist is ready to remove them all. The solution is the maggot therapy dressing.

There is no one single correct or best maggot dressing. Several techniques exist, each with their advantages and disadvantages. Several

    https://doi.org/10.11647/OBP.0300.05

different commercial dressings are available, but many therapists fashion their own dressings at the bedside. This chapter will describe the basic principles or goals of the ideal maggot dressing, and then provide examples of how that ideal dressing can be achieved.

Maggot Therapy Dressings—Past and Present

The minimal requirements for a maggot dressing are that it be of a porous fabric that allows air to enter and fluid to drain out. This is to prevent the maggots from suffocating or drowning. Also, the dressing should be constructed in such a way that it keeps the maggots from wandering off the wound. Ideally, the dressing should also be comfortable, affordable, and simple to apply, maintain, and remove.

When maggot therapy was commonly used for osteomyelitis and pus-forming wounds in the 1930s, dressings were frequently constructed out of metal screens and/or cloth. Loose-knit gauze does not make an effective barrier because the larvae can easily escape through the large spaces between the woven fibres. The dressing was usually kept in place with an adhesive tape (plaster) and sometimes foam padding was placed between the skin and the maggot dressing [1]. Some dressings were even made to be re-used for repeat applications of maggots to the same wound, with a port to put the young maggots in and take the satiated maggots out.

During the 1990s renaissance of maggot therapy, there was a push to construct maggot dressings from materials readily available on a medical ward [2]. Additionally, many of the patients now receiving therapy are old and frail and have thin sensitive skin prone to tearing. Therefore, efforts were made to identify materials less traumatic to the peri-wound skin, which led to the use of hydrocolloid pads as foundations to which the maggot dressings were then affixed [3]. This and related dressing designs are still commonly used today. Because these dressings confine the maggots to the wound but still provide them with free access to the wound bed and all of its nooks and crannies, they are sometimes called "free-range" or "confined" maggot dressings (Figures 5.1A and 5.1B).

By 2000, Wilhelm Fleischmann developed and patented the concept of containing the maggots within a net bag, which could then be placed over the wound bed without the need for strong tapes or adhesives

[4]. Contained or bagged maggots (also sometimes called "tea-bag maggots") imbibe the liquefied necrotic tissue and wound exudates that enter the net bag, but the maggots cannot leave the bag (Figure 5.1C). Differences between these two dressing designs are described in Tables 5.1 and 5.2.

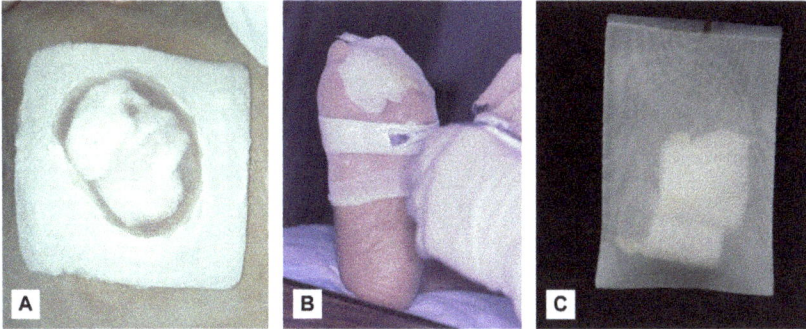

Figure 5.1 Three types of maggot dressings. A) Polyester net fabric was glued to a hydrocolloid pad, the centre of which was cut out to match the wound margins before placing maggot-impregnated gauze over the wound bed. B) Here, a strip of hydrocolloid was placed all around the anterior foot, just proximal to the non-healing toe amputation stump wound. After placing maggot-impregnated gauze over the wound, a nylon stocking (net) was pulled over the anterior foot and glued over the hydrocolloid strip. After covering the adhesive border with water-resistant tape, the excess nylon stocking will be cut off. Many therapists now use only water-resistant tape, not liquid adhesive, to hold the net in place. (Pictures by R.A. Sherman, courtesy of the BioTherapeutics, Education & Research Foundation). C) Maggots are contained within a netted bag. Photos by R. Sherman, Monarch Labs, CC BY.

Table 5.1 Characteristics of confinement and containment dressings.

Characteristic	Confinement Dressing	Containment Dressing
Efficacy	Able to access and more efficiently debride undermined areas, sinus tracks, and other crevices	Valuable for wounds near eyes, mouth, or other sensitive sites where it is imperative to avoid escapes
Debridement Efficiency/Dressing wear-time	Fast, 48–72 hours	Slower, 96 hours (4 days)

Characteristic	Confinement Dressing	Containment Dressing
Wound pain	Most analyses are in patients with confinement dressings; pain occurring in 5%-30%. In the few comparative reports, there has been no significant difference in the frequency or severity of pain between confinement and containment dressings [5–8].	
Escaping maggots	Inexperienced therapists report more escapes from confinement dressings. Experienced therapists report no more escapes from confinement dressings than from containment dressings [7].	
Aesthetics	Less acceptable	More acceptable
Cost	Maggots are less costly to produce, but additional dressing supplies may add cost	Contained maggots are more costly to produce, but few other dressings are required beyond a gauze wrap

Table 5.2 Advantages and disadvantages associated with maggot confinement dressings compared to containment dressings.

	Confined Maggots	Contained Maggots
Advantages	• Maggots have direct contact with the entire wound bed, including undermined areas, sinus tracts, etc. As a result, they are more efficient • Less expensive (less costly to produce)	• Therapist does not touch maggots directly; more aesthetically acceptable to patients and therapists • Faster application • Do not need peri-wound skin to support the dressing

	Confined Maggots	Contained Maggots
Disadvantages	• Therapist may need to see or touch the maggots (gloved, of course); less aesthetically pleasing • Requires a "cage-dressing" to secure the maggots on the wound • Need at least 1cm peri-wound skin to support (adhere) the cage-dressing	• Maggots have limited direct contact with the necrotic tissue; cannot directly access all areas of the wound bed. As a result, they are less efficient • More expensive (more labour-intensive to produce)

Applying Maggot Dressings

The method of dressing application depends on several factors, including the type and location of the wound, the type of dressings to be used (i.e., confinement or containment dressings), and the availability of supplies. Here are descriptions of some common dressing methods, followed by increasingly more complex methods, each intended to address a typical problem or complication.

In its simplest iteration, the maggot dressing might be constructed with a simple breathable or net fabric covering a maggot-laden wound (Figures 5.2, 5.3 and 5.4). The net can be affixed to the peri-wound skin with water-resistant tape. When available, a polyester net fabric is very durable, and provides a known pore size, which is optimally 100 um–160 um: small enough that the larvae cannot escape, but large enough to allow the thick, purulent drainage to drain easily. A fixed-weave fabric prevents these pores from expanding. Other fabrics with similar pore sizes are often described as having a mesh size of approximately 80 to 140. If using a stretchable fabric, the pore size may need to be within the smaller range to prevent the maggots from squeezing through and escaping. If such fabrics are not available, one could use appropriate items of clothing such as a T-shirt, blouse, or shirt (Figure 5.4). But beware: if the pores are too small, the thick purulent drainage that accumulates during therapy may not be able to exit through the fabric.

This could lead to a fluid build-up and drowning of the maggots, or it could block the pores, which in turn would suffocate the maggots.

The optimal dose of maggots is considered to be 5–10 per cm² (the upper range is used for wounds with more necrotic or infected tissue). Medicinal larvae are supplied in primary packaging containers, with or without gauze [9]. Larvae in tubes can be rinsed out with sterile saline or clean water and poured onto a piece of gauze or directly onto the polyester net fabric, which is then inverted and placed over the wound. When using maggot-impregnated gauze, it is not necessary to count individual larvae if the gauze is labelled with the concentration of maggots. Simply apply to the wound bed the amount of gauze that contains the approximate number of maggots needed.

Since the maggots will liquefy the necrotic tissue, one should expect a fair amount of wound drainage. To prevent that drainage from settling on healthy tissue as it flows out of the wound and through the net, the net should be covered with an absorptive material such as cotton gauze. The absorptive gauze should not be too thick or else it could obstruct airflow to the maggots. Wet gauze is not permeable to oxygen, so the absorptive dressings should be changed when soiled. This dressing design is sometimes called a "two-layer" maggot dressing: the "cage layer" on the bottom, and the "absorptive layer" on top.

In order to minimise the risk of peri-wound skin becoming macerated by the drainage, the peri-wound skin can be coated with a skin protectant (liquid, fast-drying). Some therapists coat the peri-wound skin with zinc oxide, being careful to avoid applying it in areas where the adhesive will need to stick to the skin.

Patients with skin integrity problems (i.e., elderly or malnourished patients) may develop skin tears when removing strongly adhered tape (less tacky tapes do not hold the maggot cage layer securely enough to prevent maggots from escaping). Therefore, many therapists do not tape the net directly to the skin. Rather, they first place strips of hydrocolloid, hydrogel, or tissue-friendly tape on the skin, and then tape or glue the net to those strips. Alternatively, a hole is cut in a hydrocolloid pad such that the pad now surrounds the wound and completely covers the skin around the wound, such that the larvae are not able to crawl out of the wound and onto the normally innervated skin (Figure 5.1A). This will prevent the itching, tickling, or pain that sometimes occurs when no such barrier blocks the maggots from accessing healthy skin. Though pre-manufactured maggot therapy confinement dressings can be purchased commercially, they are relatively simple and often less costly to construct at the bedside with locally available materials [2] (see also Figures 5.2, 5.3 and 5.4). While this system works well for flat wounds, the flat fabric does not conform well to circumferential leg wounds or stump and foot wounds. For such three-dimensionally challenging dressings, alternative net fabrics such as net bags (performing a sock or glove function) or nylon stockings (Figure 5.1B) may be used [3], or even clothing items (Figure 5.4). In rare instances, non-permeable dressings may be used [10, 11] as long as a source of fresh oxygen can be passively or actively circulated through the dressing.

Since maggots within a containment bag (bagged maggots) do not require additional confinement, they are faster and simpler to apply. The bags of maggots are simply laid over the wound bed and then held in place with gauze wrap or taped gauze pads. The larvae still require plenty of air, and an absorptive dressing layer will need to be changed daily and whenever soiled. In addition, it is recommended that the larvae be provided with water or saline to prevent dehydration, especially during the first day or two. This hydration can be provided by spraying the bags of larvae during the dressing or re-dressing procedure, or by covering them with moist gauze instead of dry gauze [12].

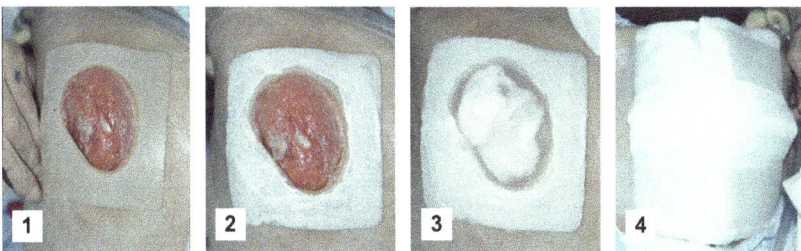

Figure 5.2 How to make a free-range maggot dressing at the bedside using adhesive glue. 1) Place a hydrocolloid pad over the peri-wound skin, with a hole cut out to correspond precisely to the wound perimeter. Alternatively, tape or another simple adhesive could be used to surround the wound. 2) Apply liquid adhesive to the surface of the hydrocolloid pad. 3) As the liquid adhesive sets and becomes tacky, place maggot-impregnated gauze over the wound bed. To prevent escape, apply the net over the wound and hydrocolloid pad immediately thereafter. Apply a second layer of adhesive over the hydrocolloid and net, such that the first and second layers of glue bond through the pores in the net. A layer

of water-resistant tape may then be applied over the still sticky hydrocolloid-glue-net-glue "sandwich", but not on the skin (not shown). 4) Finally, after securing the medicinal maggots within their "cage", place a layer of absorbent gauze on top to collect the wound drainage (liquefied necrotic tissue and wound exudates). Change the outer gauze dressing whenever it becomes soiled with drainage (about every 8 hours) so that fluid does not leak onto the patient's skin, and air can continue to reach the maggots through mostly dry gauze. Photos by R. Sherman, BioTherapeutics, Education & Research Foundation, CC BY.

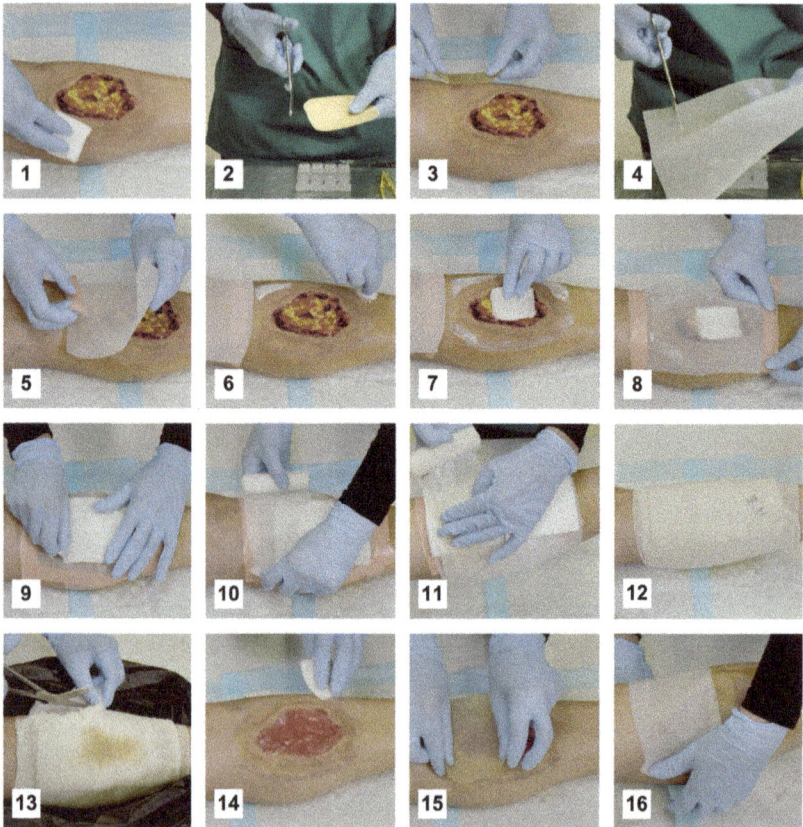

Figure 5.3 Application guidance for a confinement dressing without adhesive glue. 1) Clean the wound and peri-wound area with potable water or saline. 2) Cut hydrocolloid sheets into 2–3 cm-wide strips, perpendicular to the two pieces of plastic film covering the adhesive side of the hydrocolloid. 3) Place hydrocolloid strips around the wound and as close to the wound edge as possible. 4) Cut fine-mesh medical nylon or polyester netting to size. 5) Attach one side of the netting to the hydrocolloid border and flip it out of the way. 6) Apply zinc crème to protect the skin that is not covered by the hydrocolloid. 7) Apply loose medicinal maggots. If the maggots are supplied without a gauze pad, then use some water or saline to wash them out of their primary packaging onto a gauze pad which you apply directly to the wound. 8) Close the netting and secure it on

the hydrocolloid strips using water-proof adhesive strips. Alternatively, you can use fast-curing glue to attach the netting to the hydrocolloid. 9) Place a moistened gauze pad on top of the netting. 10) Secure the gauze pad loosely with a bandage. 11) Place dry absorbing gauze pads on the bandage above the wound to absorb any exudate during treatment. Secure them loosely with another bandage. 12) The wound and dressing must be off-loaded during treatment to protect the medicinal maggots. Replace the outer dressings daily or when heavily soiled with exudate. 13) Removal of dressings and maggots is best done over a large, plastic waste bag to easily capture fast-moving maggots, dressing materials and water/saline you may use to rinse the wound. 14) Wash, wipe, suck or pick maggots off the wound. The most convenient method is determined by the wound morphology, the body region and experience of the clinician. Clean the wound and surrounding skin carefully. 15–16) If the wound is free of necrotic tissue, continue regular wound care, or else repeat maggot therapy. Courtesy MedMagLabs and Creating Hope in Conflict: A Humanitarian Grand Challenge, CC BY.

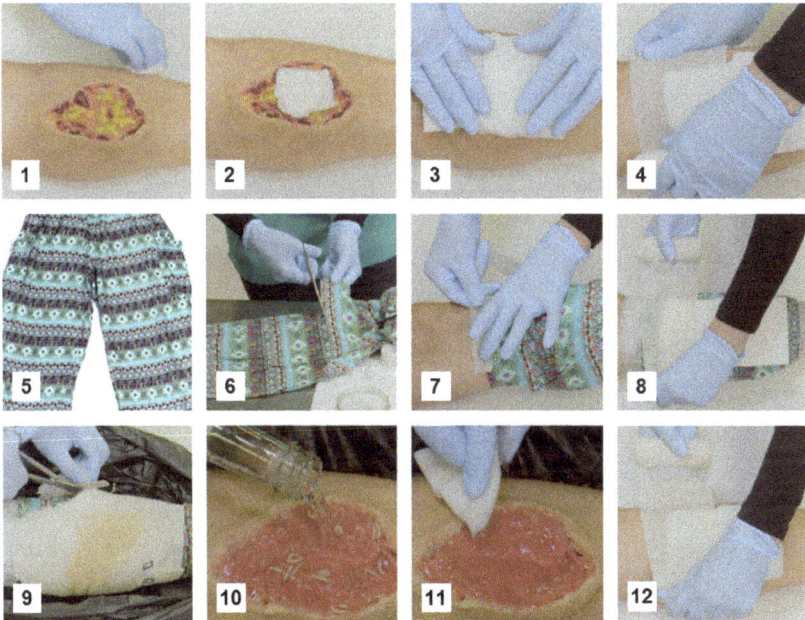

Figure 5.4 Application guidance for a standard confinement dressing in low-resource healthcare settings. 1) Clean the wound and peri-wound area with potable water. You may boil some water for 20 minutes and let it cool before use. 2) Apply loose medicinal maggots. If the maggots are supplied without a gauze pad, you can use some water or saline to wash them out of their primary packaging onto a gauze pad which you apply directly to the wound. Place some larger moistened gauze pads on top of the wound. 4) Secure the gauze pads loosely with a bandage. 5) Use the legs or sleeves of suitable clothing items to confine the maggots on the wound. Make sure the clothing is finely woven to keep maggots in. 6) Cut the leg or sleeve section to size. 7) Tape the fabric tube at the upper and lower end to the leg, making sure there are no gaps for maggots to escape. 8) Place

dry absorbing gauze pads on the confinement fabric above the wound to absorb any exudate during treatment and secure them loosely with another bandage. The wound and dressing must be off-loaded during treatment to protect the medicinal maggots. Replace the outer dressing daily or when heavily soiled with exudate. 9) Removal of dressings and maggots is best done over a large, plastic waste bag to easily capture fast-moving maggots, dressing materials, and water/saline that you may use to rinse the wound. 10) Wash, wipe, or pick maggots off the wound. The most convenient method is determined by the wound morphology, the body region and experience of the clinician. 11) Clean the wound and surrounding skin carefully. 12) If the wound is free of necrotic tissue, continue regular wound care, or else repeat maggot therapy. Courtesy MedMagLabs and Creating Hope in Conflict: A Humanitarian Grand Challenge, CC BY.

Dressing Changes, Maintenance & Repair

Guidance for optimal dressing maintenance should always be sought in the package insert. In general, the goal of maintenance is to ensure that the maggots are healthy, active, and contained or confined to the wound. To that end, many authorities recommend dressing inspection at least once daily, though that inspection need not be done by a health professional as long as the observer knows what s/he is looking for.

If there is a lot of drainage or soiling of the outer absorbent gauze dressing, it should be changed in order to optimise aeration of the maggot dressing and minimise the accumulation or spread of fluids and microorganisms. It is not uncommon for wound exudate to increase during maggot therapy and require 2–6 changes or more per day of the outer gauze dressings. If there is a lot of drainage, the fresh gauze dressings may be reapplied dry. If there was not a lot of drainage—say only one or two dressing changes are required per day—the fresh outer gauze should be moist, in order to keep the maggots hydrated. The outer gauze dressing should be changed at least once daily.

When the outer absorbent dressing is changed, also inspect the netted dressings for signs of loosening. Loosened borders can allow the maggots to escape on their own. Reinforce the dressing with extra tape, or extend the border with transparent membrane dressing (such as negative pressure dressing waste). If a hole in the dressing is discovered and maggots are not seen—especially in a dressing over 48 hours old— assume that the maggots have escaped. Open the net dressings to check. If maggots are found, and if they appear not to be satiated (not full size), then the dressing can be repaired with tape or a new net, and left for another day or two longer.

At the time of the dressing change, check on the status of the maggots. If the dressing is only 24 hours old or less, the larvae may not be visible if they are feeding down on the wound bed. If the dressing is 48 hours old, however, then it should be possible to see movement (undulations) of the maggot dressings, if not the maggots themselves. If no movement or live maggots are visible between 48 and 72 hours, the maggots may have escaped or they may be dead. Look for a break in the netting and repair it, as described in detail, above. If the maggots are found to be dead, take down the dressing and dispose of the maggots, as described in the next section. Leaving non-viable maggots in place serves no benefit and may even increase risks. For example, wound infection may worsen under a dressing of dead maggots. If the dressing is opened and the larvae are found to be alive and healthy, then the dressing can be re-mounted, if desired.

Dressing Duration and Removal

Free-range (confined) maggots mature more quickly than bagged (contained) maggots. Over 50% of free-range maggots will likely be satiated and ready to leave the wound by 48 hours. At that point, they will be near the surface and margins of the maggot dressing, looking for a way out. Many therapists remove the dressings at that point, because leaving them in place for longer increases the risk of pain and escapes. Once satiated, the larvae will spend their time attempting to escape from under the dressings until they are finally removed. In patients without wound pain, some therapists chose to leave the maggot dressings in place for up to 72 hours so that the remaining maggots will provide additional debridement. After 72 hours, all of the free-range maggots should have matured, and will be at the surface trying to escape.

When it is time to remove free-range maggots, remember that the larvae are already lined up at the edges of the dressing, ready and eager to crawl far away. Therefore, have all needed materials at the bedside, including wet gauze to wipe up the larvae, and a receptacle for discarding the larvae. Place a barrier (rubbish bag, incontinence pad, etc.) under the work area (wound) in order to catch maggots that may fall off. Remove the outer absorbent gauze and then gently peel back the netted dressing as though it were a banana peel. Meanwhile, wipe the wound with a water- or saline-moistened gauze pad, closely following the peeled net dressing, sandwiching the maggots between the wet pad and the dressing that is being removed. Then drop the dressing and sandwiched maggots into a biohazardous waste bin. If there are any maggots left behind, they can be removed with the aid of another wet gauze pad, a swab or water irrigation. If the remaining maggots are small and appear to be still working to remove more necrotic tissue, then it would be reasonable to replace a gauze pad over the wound and allow the last few maggots to continue working for another day. The gauze dressing can be removed the following day, by which time the last remaining maggots should be satiated and ready to leave the wound. Thoroughly rinse the wound with sterile water or saline once all of the maggots are removed.

Contained maggots grow more slowly, and typically are not satiated until about 96 hours. Since they are contained, the risk of escape is very low; but the risk of pain still increases with the duration of therapy [5]. There is no benefit to leaving the maggots in place longer than the time that they are feeding, since they will stop secreting their digestive enzymes when they are satiated. Contained maggots are easy to remove because they are not running loose. Simply unwrap the outer absorbent gauze wraps and then remove each sachet of bagged maggots, placing them in a biohazard bag. Thoroughly rinse the wound with sterile water or saline.

When the dressings are opened, if the larvae are found to be dead—or not found at all—pay close attention to the wound bed and the condition of the dressings, for they can reveal what went wrong. If few or no maggots are found and there was a breach in the netted dressing layer, then the maggots likely escaped. If there was no breach in the maggot dressing, look for evidence of dead maggots—either dead bodies or remnants of their mouth hooks (little black dots scattered among the wound bed). If either is found, it is highly likely that most or all of the maggots died all at about the same time, by drowning or suffocation. Crushing is also a possibility, but does not commonly kill all the maggots at the same time.

If very few or no maggot bodies are found—and, again, assuming that no maggots escaped—then the maggots may have died slowly, over the course of 24 hours or more. The causes for this may be more difficult to pinpoint. Again, the first place to start the investigation is with a careful examination of the dressing materials to ensure that the maggots did not suffocate or escape. A clean wound suggests that starvation may have played a role, and this is not an uncommon occurrence when maggots are placed on a relatively clean wound for the purpose of maintenance debridement or growth promotion [13]. The live maggots can survive on the decomposing bodies of the dead ones, but soon some of the survivors may, themselves, starve and die. Starvation is not likely to cause maggots to die unless they are very young. Older maggots, when starved, can survive, but they do not grow as quickly or as large. Hostile environmental factors (chemical or physical) are sometimes invoked to explain mass loss of larvae. A few drugs and wound treatments may be harmful to the maggots [13]. Specific bacterial or viral microbes within the wound might be a cause. This has not been demonstrated clinically, but there is laboratory evidence that certain microbes—at least *Pseudomonas aeruginosa*—can produce maggot-lethal virulence factors [14]. Another possible cause is that the maggots may have been unhealthy to begin with: too old, too starved, exposed to temperature extremes, or contaminated. If poor maggot quality is suspected, look for supporting evidence such as other maggots in the same batch with similar problems.

Often, a definitive cause for widespread maggot death cannot be found. Fortunately, mass maggot death is a rare event when dressings are properly applied, and under these circumstances, a repeat course of therapy will usually proceed without any problem. Some therapists and researchers have speculated that mass maggot death may be due to the host's immunological response. While allergic reactions are known to exist in animals, such reactions should repeat themselves in a maggot-immune wound. As it happens, the rare instance of massive maggot death even more rarely repeats itself in the same patient, except when one of the causes listed above goes uncorrected.

Reapplication or Follow-up Treatment?

Once the maggots have been removed and the wound rinsed, it is time to determine the next course of action. If necrotic tissue still remains, it is usually desirable to reapply another course of maggot therapy. A subsequent course of maggots may be applied straight away (a useful strategy for out-patients, in order to minimise the number and inconvenience of visits to the clinic), or the maggots may be re-applied according to the schedule that best fits the therapist and/or the maggot lab (for example, every "maggot therapy day" on Monday and Thursday, or once weekly). Keep in mind that the sooner the wound is completely debrided, the better the chances for attaining total debridement and, ultimately, wound-healing. Still, sometimes a patient can benefit from a break for a day or two, especially when anxiety or discomfort causes sleepless nights.

It is difficult to define an "average" number of maggot treatments needed to completely debride a wound because the number of treatments is highly dependent on the wound itself. The thicker or deeper the necrotic tissue and the drier that tissue, the greater number of treatments will be required; the greater the number of healthy maggots that are placed on the wound at one time, the fewer will be the number of treatments required. Most wounds can be completely debrided with one or two applications of maggots; some may require four or more applications. One of the most effective ways to hasten the debridement (decrease the number of treatment cycles required) is to remove as much dry necrotic tissue (eschar) as possible before applying the maggots. This can be done with a scalpel, just prior to application of the maggot dressing, or it can be achieved by softening the existing dry tissue with an autolytic dressing technique overnight (occlusive dressing, hydrocolloid, etc.). This process should be fast and simple, done on the day of or the day before applying the maggots. Spending more effort and time than necessary for a very crude thinning or softening of the necrotic tissue is a waste of time and effort, once the decision has already been made that maggot therapy is the best course of action. The maggots will debride the tissue themselves, dry or not, within a few days.

If the wound bed is now well-debrided, it is time to begin the treatment of choice to effect wound closure. Depending on the therapist, patient and resources, treatment choices can vary widely, and are beyond the scope of this chapter. The important thing to note is that there is no need to delay definitive medical or surgical wound closure after maggot therapy. Maggot therapy does not increase the risk of infection or dehiscence, even if wound closure follows immediately [15]. If a decision about the method of closure cannot be made straight away, it is fine to apply a tissue-supportive dressing (i.e., saline-moistened gauze, non-toxic ointments, honey, hydrogels, etc.) until the definitive decision can be made.

Summary

Maggot therapy dressings are intended to keep the maggots on the wound until most are satiated and have stopped feeding. Some therapists make their own dressings; others use commercially produced dressings. Many therapists use both, depending on their patients' wounds. All maggot dressings have at least the following characteristics in common: they prevent the maggots from escaping, they allow adequate amounts of oxygenated air to reach the maggots, and they facilitate the drainage of accumulating liquids (liquefied necrotic tissue and exudates). There are two basic designs for maggot dressings: maggot confinement dressings, which confine the maggots to the wound bed but allow them complete access to the wound; and maggot containment dressings, which totally contain the maggots within a net bag that facilitates easy handling but prevents the maggots from direct contact with all the nooks and crannies of the wound. Each has its advantages and disadvantages. Therapists should use the type of dressing that best meets their needs and their patients' wounds. Once maggot debridement is complete, the appropriate and definitive medical or surgical treatment for closing the wound may begin.

References

1.   Fine, A. and H. Alexander, *Maggot Therapy: Technique and Clinical Application.* The Journal of Bone and Joint Surgery, 1934. 16(3): pp. 572–582.

2.   Sherman, R.A., *A New Dressing Design for Use with Maggot Therapy.* Plastic and Reconstructive Surgery, 1997. 100(2): pp. 451–456, https://doi.org/10.1097/00006534-199708000-00029.

3. Sherman, R.A., J.M. Tran, and R. Sullivan, *Maggot Therapy for Venous Stasis Ulcers*. Archives of Dermatology, 1996. 132(3): pp. 254–256 https://jamanetwork.com/journals/jamadermatology/fullarticle/vol/132/pg/254.

4. Grassberger, M. and W. Fleischmann, *The Biobag — A New Device for the Application of Medicinal Maggots*. Dermatology, 2002. 204(4): p. 306, https://doi.org/10.1159/000063369.

5. Dumville, J.C., et al., *Larval Therapy for Leg Ulcers (VenUS II): Randomised Controlled Trial*. BMJ, 2009. 338(7702): pp. 1047–1050, https://doi.org/10.1136/bmj.b773.

6. Steenvoorde, P., T. Budding, and J. Oskam, *Determining Pain Levels in Patients Treated with Maggot Debridement Therapy*. Journal of Wound Care, 2005. 14(10): pp. 485–488, https://doi.org/10.12968/jowc.2005.14.10.26846.

7. Steenvoorde, P., C.E. Jacobi, and J. Oskam, *Maggot Debridement Therapy: Free-Range or Contained? An in-vivo Study*. Advances in Skin & Wound Care, 2005. 18(8): pp. 430–435, https://doi.org/10.1097/00129334-200510000-00010.

8. Steenvoorde, P., et al., *Maggot Debridement Therapy of Infected Ulcers: Patient and Wound Factors Influencing Outcome — A Study on 101 Patients with 117 Wounds*. Annals of the Royal College of Surgeons of England, 2007. 89(6): pp. 596–602, https://doi.org/10.1308/003588407x205404.

9. Stadler, F., *Packaging Technology*, in *A Complete Guide to Maggot Therapy: Clinical Practice, Therapeutic Principles, Production, Distribution, and Ethics*, F. Stadler (ed.). 2022, Cambridge: Open Book Publishers, pp. 349–362, https://doi.org/10.11647/OBP.0300.16.

10. DeFazio, M.V., et al., *Home Improvement in Maggot Therapy: Designing a Simple, Cost-Effective, Closed-System Habitat to Facilitate Biodébridement of Complex Distal Lower Extremity Wounds*. Plastic and Reconstructive Surgery, 2015. 136(5): pp. 722e–723e, https://doi.org/10.1097/prs.0000000000001685.

11. Felder, J.M., 3rd, et al., *Increasing the Options for Management of Large and Complex Chronic Wounds with a Scalable, Closed-system Dressing for Maggot Therapy*. Journal of Burn Care & Research, 2012. 33(3): pp. e169–175, https://doi.org/10.1097/BCR.0b013e318233570d.

12. All Wales Tissue Viability Nurse Forum. *The All Wales Guidance for the Use of Larval Debridement Therapy (LDT)*. 2013. https://www.wounds-uk.com/download/resource/5850.

13. Sherman, R., *Indications, Contraindications, Interactions, and Side-effects of Maggot Therapy*, in *A Complete Guide to Maggot Therapy: Clinical Practice, Therapeutic Principles, Production, Distribution, and Ethics*, F. Stadler (ed.). 2022, Cambridge: Open Book Publishers, pp. 63–78, https://doi.org/10.11647/OBP.0300.04.

14. Andersen, A.S., et al., *Quorum-sensing-regulated Virulence Factors in Pseudomonas aeruginosa Are Toxic to Lucilia sericata Maggots*. Microbiology

(Society for General Microbiology), 2010. 156(2): pp. 400–407, https://doi.org/10.1099/mic.0.032730-0.

15.   Sherman, R.A. and K.J. Shimoda, *Presurgical Maggot Debridement of Soft Tissue Wounds Is Associated with Decreased Rates of Postoperative Infection.* Clinical Infectious Diseases, 2004. 39(7): pp. 1067–1070, https://doi.org/10.1086/423806.

6. Clinical Integration of Maggot Therapy

Benjamin L. Bullen, Ronald A. Sherman, Paul J. Chadwick and Frank Stadler

The integration of maggot therapy into clinical practice is not a trivial undertaking as it has to overcome social, regulatory, clinical, organisational, financial, and supply-chain-technical barriers. For example, rejection of the therapy by patients due to the 'Yuk' factor is frequently raised as a reason why maggot therapy will not be feasible. Likewise, logistics problems often hamper reliable supply. This chapter identifies these barriers and shows that in some instances they may be more assumed than real, as is the case with the 'Yuk' factor, and that there are tangible solutions for the implementation of maggot therapy programmes, such as supply-chain innovations or socially-minded business models that prioritise patients over profits. In addition, there is a growing body of information and training resources available from medicinal maggot producers, practitioner organisations, and biotherapy advocates that supports the establishment of maggot therapy programmes.

Introduction

This chapter describes a range of factors relevant to the adoption and integration of maggot therapy into clinical practice. Readers of this book are, perhaps, less averse to considering maggot therapy, however there is a well-recognised 'Yuk' factor associated with maggots [1–5]. Distaste for flies or maggots may inhibit healthcare professionals from offering

https://doi.org/10.11647/OBP.0300.06

this therapy as many assume, or claim, that their patients will not accept this therapeutic option.

There are also specific logistical considerations associated with maggot therapy, such as availability, rapid transport of this highly perishable product, temperature and humidity control during transport and storage, clinician training, patient and family-member education, infection control, and waste management, just to mention a few. These and other potential barriers to adoption are considered throughout this chapter, with an emphasis on providing pragmatic solutions and exploring further avenues for implementation.

Fly maggots have been used in wound management 'from antiquity,' as colonisation of the wound by wild maggots (myiasis) was welcome, or maggots were applied to the wound on purpose [6]. Indeed, Mayan tribes in Central America, the Ngemba Aboriginal tribe in Australia and the Hill Peoples of Burma were some of the earliest adopters of maggot therapy [7–9]. Apart from medicinal maggots, there are other examples of invertebrate species that have been used in wound management including ant-heads, bees and honey, leeches, and cobweb [10–12]. While suturing of wounds with ant-heads and cobwebs may have fallen out of common usage, leeches, medical-grade honey, and maggot therapy continue to be employed today.

Despite myiasis of war wounds being considered fortuitous by several military surgeons on far-flung battlefields [8, 13, 14], Western medicine did not see the intentional introduction of larvae until the American orthopaedic surgeon, William Baer (1872–1931), began his landmark studies in the early twentieth century. Baer publicly reported his successful management of chronic osteomyelitis with *L. sericata* at a conference in 1929 [15]. A posthumous publication followed two years later [16], detailing maggot therapy in over a hundred children with complex wounds and osteomyelitis. While clinical results were favourable, secondary infection with *Clostridium tetani* and *Clostridium perfringens* led Baer to further introduce sterilisation procedures [16]. Although the origins of maggot therapy are very much non-sterile, today, medicinal maggots are of high quality and disinfected prior to treatment.

Institutional and Professional Considerations

The establishment of maggot therapy services is commonly frustrated by a lack of support within the wound care team or from administrators [17]. The *Biotherapeutics, Education and Research (BTER) Foundation* [18, 19] produce a wealth of resources to support the adoption of maggot therapy, including template documents to support the development of policies and procedures (https://www.bterfoundation.org/policies-procedures-templates).

Wound care is delivered very differently depending on each country's systems of care, healthcare-provider blend, and clinical settings. For these reasons, the introduction of any new treatment is challenging. Sherman and colleagues [17] identified potential professional boundaries, including insistence that maggot therapy be applied by medical professionals and/or within the in-patient setting. These authors pragmatically recommended compliance and compromise with such requirements in the first instance, with review after successful roll-out.

The *NHS Five Year Forward View* [20] and the *NHS Long-Term Plan* [21] that followed both highlighted the need to use innovations to improve healthcare delivery within the prevailing financial constraints. Whilst the NHS is often seen as a world leader in developing technologies, it has also been criticised for the slow implementation, dissemination and subsequent day-to-day use of innovative technologies. Adoption timescales must also be shortened from an estimated seventeen years for new technologies to be adopted at scale by the NHS [22]. Reasons offered include organisational inertia, local custom and practice. The slow uptake of new therapies poses a significant challenge in the West but in resource-limited settings, adoption of new therapies may take even longer [23]. Patent protection and prohibitive pricing further contribute to a lack of adoption of new therapies in both high- and low-resource settings. Maggot therapy is not a novel therapy and has a long and outstanding safety record and the wealth of supportive evidence should be highlighted when discussing the adoption of maggot therapy and overcoming the *"not in my backyard"* mentality that may prevent lead clinicians and administrators from initiating this therapeutic modality [17, p. 29].

Increased harmonisation and adoption of regulatory approaches between jurisdictions may reduce issues associated with views of maggot therapy as a 'new therapy.' The proof required for new innovations to be adopted into routine clinical use far outweighs the proof required for established practices. New innovations often require conclusive, randomised, controlled studies or meta-analysis evidence before adoption. Whilst at first glance this may appear laudable, the opposite is true of more established clinical routines or innovations. Established clinical practices often have low evidence of efficacy and are instead taken on trust [24].

Regulatory Considerations, Cost and Reimbursement

The cost of maggot therapy treatment and therefore its demand and availability in a particular location is closely linked to the regulatory status of the therapy and whether health insurers subsidise it. It is important for pioneers of maggot therapy in new jurisdictions to consider this interplay of design production and care systems that maximise availability and minimise cost to the patient.

Regulators classify medicinal maggots differently around the world. The Federal Drug Administration (FDA) in the US categorises them as a medical device, "for debriding non-healing necrotic skin and soft tissue wounds, including pressure ulcers, venous stasis ulcers, neuropathic foot ulcers and non-healing traumatic or post-surgical wounds" [25]. Other countries typically regulate medicinal maggots as a drug [26]. Consequently, there is a lack of harmonisation across jurisdictions, which can slow global uptake and implementation of maggot therapy.

How Healthcare Is Paid for

There are four main models that are important to discuss here because they have a significant impact on the integration and delivery of maggot therapy in any particular healthcare setting. These are the Beveridge model, the Bismarck model, the National Health Insurance model, and the Out-of-Pocket model [27]. *The Beveridge model* was first described in *The Beveridge Report: Social Insurance and Allied Services*, paving the way for the development of the 'Welfare State' [28]. This had the core principle of the state being responsible for health and social support. Key amongst these recommendations was the initial outline of the National Health Service (NHS). This model provides universal healthcare for all citizens, free at the point of use, and is financed by the government through tax payments. This model is currently found in Great Britain, Spain and New Zealand. *The Bismarck model* is a non-profit based insurance system where deductions are made from employees' payroll in conjunction with contributions from employers [29]. It must include all citizens and is found in countries such as Germany, Japan and Switzerland. *The National Health Insurance model* is a combination of the Beveridge and Bismarck models. Funding comes from a government-run insurance programme that all citizens fund through a premium or a tax but delivery is through private companies [27]. This model is found in Canada, for example [30]. In the United States of America (USA), Medicare is a government-financed programme, funded through taxation. Medicare is a type of National Health Insurance programme but with age and situation restrictions, unlike the Australian Medicare system. Uptake of private healthcare cover is higher in Australia and the USA than the UK. In the USA, particularly, many individuals also fall into a fourth, *Out-of-Pocket model*, or payment-on-receiving-care model. This model is found in much of the world [27]. In other words, you pay for care as you receive it. It is used in countries that economically and organisationally cannot provide any kind of national healthcare system. In these countries, those that can pay for healthcare can access it and those who cannot afford it remain sick or die. Examples can be found in Africa and South America but self-payment is also applicable for many individuals living in the USA.

Affordability of wound care to the patient is a significant determinant of maggot therapy programme success. For example, in the UK maggot therapy is reimbursed and therefore in demand, which means there is an incentive for a commercial producer to supply medicinal maggots. In Slovakia, by contrast, EU approval for maggot therapy applies but the health insurance system does not reimburse the treatment, thus making the therapy less affordable to patients, in turn making medicinal maggot supply commercially unviable. In other words, the Out-of-Pocket model makes it most difficult to provide maggot therapy services, especially if the producers of medicinal maggots seek to maximise profit. Within the wound care context, the National Institute for Health and Care Excellence [31] states that, in the absence of any robust clinical evidence to guide choice, prescribers should routinely choose the dressing with the *"lowest acquisition cost"* appropriate for the given circumstances. Maggot therapy is certainly more expensive than dry or paraffin gauze bandages, mainstays in low-resource settings. However, compared to other advanced wound therapies, medicinal maggots can be supplied at a very low cost, provided supply chains are efficient and business models do not prioritise profit.

Another consequence of high out-of-pocket costs is that the therapy is seen as a 'last ditch' or 'last resort' [32, 33]. For example, in the United Kingdom larvae are now available on prescription which is due to effective lobbying by the producer and sympathetic clinicians. Courtenay [32, p. 178] conducted telephone interviews with nurses experienced in maggot therapy in the UK. One nurse said, "in the majority of cases, larval therapy was used when all other forms of wound treatment had failed" and another nurse respondent typified this approach by stating "we tend to have tried everything else before the maggots, they are the last-ditch attempt", and yet another said that "originally, maggots were last-ditch. They can be first-line treatment now".

To summarise, in jurisdictions where maggot therapy is approved and subsidised or paid for through national insurance schemes, maggot therapy has become a frequently used wound care modality. Effective lobbying by producers and clinicians who champion the therapy to secure health insurance coverage is therefore a critical part of the introduction of a maggot therapy programme in a new jurisdiction. In places where medicinal maggots are not subsidised, producers must adopt highly efficient business processes or socially-minded business models to make medicinal maggots affordable while still ensuring business viability.

Case Study: Negative Pressure Wound Therapy

There are many differing models of resourcing healthcare and the confounding issues of differing classification of maggot therapy have also led to a multitude of different options and complications for reimbursement. This too has contributed significantly to a lack of standardisation of usage. Compare this to another wound care technology, developed at a similar time, Negative Pressure Wound Therapy (NPWT). Initially, NPWT was dominated by the Vacuum Assisted Closure (VAC) model developed by Kinetics Concepts Incorporated (KCI Medical) for many years. The consistency of one company lobbying and developing the technology led to it becoming embedded as established practice. As a result, they developed standardised guidance and subsequent evidence. This helped establish the practice of NPWT internationally. It is, of course, easier to supply and sell a NPWT device to the global market. While the original VAC units were quite bulky and expensive to hire, recent competitor systems have a simpler pump (PICO) or spring mechanism (SNAP) to apply negative pressure and much smaller dressings and portable containers, respectively, for exudate collection and disposal [34].

In comparison, "there are few commercial producers of medicinal maggots around the world and production is mostly small in scale" [35, p. 2]. The largest commercial producers are *Monarch Labs* in the USA and *BioMonde* in Wales, Belgium, and Germany [6, 36, 37]. *Monarch Labs* and *BioMonde* have established their products and services beyond a niche category, with maggot therapy now a widely-used and accepted therapy in these markets.

Logistics and Distribution

Availability of Local Medicinal Fly Species

Logistics and distribution are, perhaps, the greatest factors for the failure to embed maggot therapy into regular clinical practice, especially in low- and middle-income countries (LMIC) with poor logistics infrastructures. It begins with the availability of suitable species in any particular geographic location. The most commonly used medicinal fly species are *L. sericata* and *Lucilia cuprina* [38], though a wide variety of blowfly species have been used effectively in the past [39]. Safety and efficacy are best documented for *L. sericata*, but in regions of the world where that species is not native, most authorities believe it is best to use a local species for maggot therapy, if possible. This is because despite best efforts, medicinal flies will escape from the lab and from the patient's wound, at some time. From an environmental and regulatory standpoint, it will therefore be much better to use a fly that is native to the area. That is why new blowfly species continue to be investigated. Please refer to Chapter 11 of this book for a detailed discussion of alternative medicinal fly species and the process of bioprospecting and research required for regulatory approval and clinical use [40], and Chapter 13 for guidance on how to collect, identify, and establish laboratory colonies of appropriate species [41].

Distribution Logistics

It is not unusual for physicians and surgeons to order advanced wound therapies in ahead of time. Surgical procedures and certainly sharp debridement can usually be performed at the time of assessment, however. Medicinal maggots need to be ordered 24 (or more) hours ahead of intended treatment, depending on the sophistication of production. As medicinal maggots are perishable and need to be delivered quickly, ideally within the space of 24 to 48 hours from dispatch at 6–25°C [42], the need for temperature control is shared with other advanced wound therapies. Cooling of topical haemoglobin and skin substitutes may require refrigeration, while some graft products, such as xenografts, must be frozen [43–45]. In the case of medicinal maggots, temperature control to within the preferred range during transit and prior to application may be achieved with cool packs [46]. Any transport interruptions jeopardise the health and efficacy of medicinal maggots even if cool-chain packaging is used. This is a problem when servicing rural and remote locations but is particularly limiting in disaster- and war-torn environments where demand for maggot therapy might be high but logistics infrastructure is disrupted or destroyed [47]. Furthermore, a consensus group on the treatment of diabetic ulcers agreed that maggot therapy requires two or three applications to achieve effective debridement, necessitating timely reordering for continuation of the therapy [48]. As a result, a shelf-life of 24–48 hours significantly limits the ability for sufficient quantities to be ordered in advance for such repeat treatment. Seamless reordering and supply over long distances is also more difficult and has limited the ability of any one company to service a large geographic area from a central location.

The perishable nature of larvae raises similar logistical issues to those reported for vaccines and blood products [49, 50]. Cool-chain distribution via couriers remains the most popular method of delivering larvae from production facilities to clinicians. It may or may not include commercial airfreight over long distances. Distribution via military cargo planes and helicopters [51], though physically very demanding on the maggots, has been shown to be feasible, as well as transport via Unmanned Aerial Vehicles (drones) for humanitarian relief missions [52, 53]. For maggot therapy in rural, remote, or compromised healthcare settings, supply chain and logistics innovations are under development that either speed up delivery or locate production at the point of care as described in Chapters 17 and 18 of this book [53, 54].

Treatment Logistics

The application of medicinal maggots and the construction of dressings that keep medicinal maggots in place is highly adaptable to the healthcare setting. Chapter 5 explains the basics of maggot therapy dressings, including the use of ordinary tightly-woven clothing fabrics for maggot dressings, these days a plentiful resource even in compromised healthcare settings [55]. After maggot therapy has been commenced, daily outer dressing changes are necessary to check the viability of the larvae, maintain a moist environment, and facilitate aeration of the wound so that maggots do not suffocate beneath exudate-soaked bandages. Given that a course of maggot therapy takes no longer than 2–4 days, this temporarily increased care burden compares favourably with collagenase, for example, which typically requires ongoing application for months on end.

There may also be additional disposal challenges, particularly in the community setting. After treatment, larvae are usually double-bagged along with soiled dressing materials and disposed of as clinical waste. Stadler [35, p. 5] has explained that clinical safety and infection control are primary considerations rather than "humane treatment of medicinal flies [...] largely because invertebrate animals have not been included in research ethics guidelines, and there has been little research regarding their pain perception, analgesia, anaesthesia and euthanasia." For a detailed discussion of the ethics of maggot therapy, please refer to Chapter 19 [56]. In the community setting, if clinicians are unable to collect and return waste to a hospital with clinical waste disposal, the carefully bagged treatment waste can also be disposed of via the municipal waste stream.

Patient and Practitioner Factors

Perception and Acceptance

Maggot therapy punches above its weight in terms of synonyms that have been devised for the sake of social marketing, motivated by the 'Yuk' factor [3–5], which is a *"perceived squeamishness and disgust of maggots"* [2]. Among a group of UK Open University students, maggots were ranked as the sixth greatest anxiety-inducing animal, behind snakes, wasps, rats, cockroaches and spiders [57]. From a list of 35 animals, maggots were the most disliked, reported among 46% of respondents [57]. Hence the use of terms like 'biosurgery' and 'larval therapy' for this modality instead of the 'M' word. However, fly larvae are maggots and, at the end of the day, that is the most readily understood term. Besides, when it comes to the time patients need to be informed about the therapy, there is no avoiding the fact that biosurgery or larval therapy involves fly maggots. Therefore, in terms of health literacy and informed consent, 'maggot therapy' and 'maggot debridement therapy' are certainly more transparent monikers and have been used in clinical practice and the literature alike [35]. Besides, the 'Yuk' factor is probably far more prominent among healthcare professionals. Qualitative research, conducted by Courtenay [32], found the 'Yuk' factor alive and well among nurses in the UK, with some expressing concerns about escaping larvae. This is why the term 'larval therapy' continues to be used, mainly by the UK and European producer BioMonde, and by researchers from this region. However, phenomenological research by Steenvoorde [4] suggests that the 'Yuk' factor may be tempered among adults when prescribed by a trusted medical professional. Steenvoorde's survey captured the attitudes of 37 individuals receiving maggot therapy, none of whom reported negative pre-conceptions and, having received it, 94% would recommend it to others. This finding is particularly pertinent as it would appear our patients are less averse to this therapeutic option than, perhaps, many healthcare professionals might expect. Recently, Humphreys and colleagues [2] considered the opinions of Welsh schoolteachers concerning the introduction of maggot therapy into primary education to combat the development of fear of larvae. The authors concluded that introducing maggot therapy as a concept earlier in life may reduce the 'Yuk' factor seen among older adults. In the end, the decision as to whether or not maggot therapy should be initiated should consider wound, patient, and healthcare-setting characteristics as discussed in Chapters 3 and 4 [58, 59] and the consent of the patient after factual and unbiased information has been given [56].

For a patient to be able to give informed consent to maggot therapy, all potential risks and the potential expectations and benefits for assessment and treatment must be disclosed, as this will vary for individual patients with differing wounds and medical conditions. Patient and carer guides should also be provided, which patients may wish to share and discuss with members of their family or caregivers. Chapter 19 provides a first-pass discussion of the ethical dimensions of maggot therapy [56].

Clinical Considerations

A full patient assessment must be undertaken prior to initiating maggot therapy, including a full and thorough medical history, comprising i) current medications, ii) known allergies to medications, insects, and products used in the production of medicinal maggots, iii) an assessment of the wound type, underlying diseases, and wound processes, and iv) inspection of the wound bed.

Patients may not be able to accept maggot therapy due to allergies to certain maggot diets or diet-related religious beliefs and customs. Fortunately, there is flexibility in the way medicinal maggots can be produced. Maggots may be fed with meat from a variety of animals other than pork or beef, or even with meat-free diets, thus allowing producers and therapists to tailor maggot therapy to the cultural and religious preferences of the patient [60]. For patients with diabetic ulcers, glycaemic control should be addressed, as must the specific challenges associated with offloading a neuropathic wound on the sole (plantar surface) of the foot or posterior to the heel. Following a complete neurovascular assessment, activity levels and concordance with offloading modalities should be addressed. If pressure cannot be sufficiently relieved from the wound site, larvae may be crushed by unrestrained compressive forces when standing, walking or in bed, in the case of posterior heel ulceration. A range of offloading modalities are available to reduce direct pressure over the wound site and may include, but are not limited to, customisable, apertured, semi-compressed ('Chiropody') felt. The presence and degree of arterial disease must also be considered, and disease-specific national and international guidance should be followed. Examples include National Institute for Health and Care Excellence Guidance in England and Wales [61] and the International Working Group on the Diabetic Foot Guidance [62]. For ischaemic or neuroischaemic foot ulceration, the level and extent of arterial disease should be determined. There is also a need to consider whether critical limb ischaemia is present and to determine if there is a requirement for reconstruction, such as angioplasty or bypass [63, 64]. Venous ulcer assessment also necessitates a thorough investigation for any co-existing arterial disease, before initiation of compression therapy [65]. Pressure ulcers should be staged [66] and further requirements for surgery explored. Pilonidal sinuses, traumatic wounds and necrotising fasciitis may also be suitable for post-surgical maggot therapy, as are post-surgical wounds that are slow to heal or those complicated by MRSA infection [67].

Wound assessment prior to the application of maggot debridement therapy should be carried out by a qualified healthcare practitioner, according to local policy. Application and evaluation, however, may be undertaken by a competent, trained healthcare worker. A freely available position paper by the BioTherapeutics Education and Research Foundation [68] describes the competencies desirable in a clinician treating patients with maggot therapy. It should inform on the training required of new maggot therapy practitioners. In the UK, free training is available via BioMonde's *'Larval Academy'* and accredited by The Royal College of Nursing and approved by The Royal College of Podiatry [69]. The *BioTherapeutics, Education & Research (BTER) Foundation* in the USA and *The Mexican Wound Care Association* also offer informative and helpful education and training resources on their websites and through publications to support maggot therapy in these settings [19, 70]. However, even where trained clinicians are in short supply, it has been shown that lay providers in low-resource environments with only basic instructions can support and perform maggot therapy [71].

Organisational Considerations

When introducing maggot therapy, procedures for prescription, ordering, application and monitoring must be established and key care structures must be in place to support adoption of this modality.

Prescription and ordering. The process for prescribing and ordering larvae in the UK has been described in detail in an *'All Wales Guidance for the Use of Larval Debridement Therapy'* document [72]. Prescription and ordering processes and procedures differ between NHS community and hospital settings. An FP10 prescription order, from a registered prescriber or doctor, must be raised if maggot therapy is initiated in the community setting. Hospital orders, in contrast, are typically included on the patient's prescription sheet. Community or hospital pharmacists then contact the company directly to request the appropriate number and size of maggot containment bags required. Ordering before 2 p.m. will typically permit next-day delivery, from Monday to Saturday. Different countries with different healthcare systems have varying medical goods ordering and procurement practices and medicinal maggot producers need to tailor their production, supply, and sales practices accordingly [73].

Interdisciplinary care and communication. Communication between acute and community services is paramount to ensuring smooth transition of care, both following discharge from hospital or when initiating or continuing collaborative care, guided by acute wound services. Before prescribing and ordering larvae, acute providers must ensure that suitably trained professionals are able to monitor wound progress, maintain optimal moisture conditions and change secondary dressings between pre-scheduled acute service reviews. Daily inspection is typical and should be supported by both written information sheets and verbal handover between healthcare professionals. As part of consent documentation, written information sheets should also be provided to patients and lay carers, to explain maggot therapy and address frequently asked questions. Photographs taken before maggot therapy may further assist in ongoing wound monitoring and community colleagues could be invited to attend the initial larvae application appointment to observe the process and discuss individual requirements. Reapplication of larvae may be performed following assessment by acute expert clinicians. For plantar foot wounds, there is a further imperative to ensure that adequate offloading is maintained through the course of therapy. While larvae may withstand some direct pressure, without appropriate offloading strategies they may simply be crushed and lose viability [48]. Offloading may be achieved with local application of semi-compressed felt, in combination with deflective orthoses and offloading devices or footwear.

Summary

Maggot therapy is highly efficacious in eradicating offending bacterial species, removing tenacious biofilms and slough, and improving outcomes for people with wounds. Administration of the therapy and application of maggot dressings is relatively simple and can even be performed by lay carers provided basic guidance is provided. However, successful implementation of maggot therapy programmes in any jurisdiction depends on whether maggot therapy is affordable to the patient. Affordability may be achieved via health insurance subsidies or low-cost production and supply. It is easier for producers to make a profit from medicinal maggots where treatment is subsidised. Affordable supply elsewhere must resort to socially-minded, for-purpose business models and/or low-cost production.

Because medicinal maggots are perishable goods and have a short shelf-life, it has been difficult to supply them on a reliable basis in places with poor logistics infrastructure. However, it is clear now that these supply-chain barriers can be overcome with innovative technologies and flexible supply-chain architectures as explained at length in this book [41, 53, 54, 74–76].

Rejection of maggot therapy by patients is another often-cited barrier to its wider use. However, there is good reason to believe that patients with chronic debilitating wounds have few reservations and are more than willing to give maggot therapy a try. Rather than assuming a patient's aversion, clinicians should base their decision as to whether to use medicinal maggots on actual patient preferences, medical suitability, local wound factors, and cost considerations.

References

1. Evans, P., *Larvae Therapy and Venous Leg Ulcers: Reducing the 'Yuk Factor'*. Journal of Wound Care, 2002. 11(10): pp. 407–408, https://doi.org/10.12968/jowc.2002.11.10.26445.

2. Humphreys, I., P. Lehane, and Y. Nigam, *Could Maggot Therapy Be Taught in Primary Schools?* Journal of Biological Education, 2020: pp. 1–11, https://doi.org/10.1080/00219266.2020.1748686.

3. Jones, J., J. Green, and A.K. Lillie, *Maggots and Their Role in Wound Care*. British Journal of Community Nursing, 2011. 16: pp. S24-S33.

4. Steenvoorde, P., et al., *Maggot Therapy and the "Yuk" Factor: An Issue for the Patient?* Wound Repair and Regeneration, 2005. 13(3): pp. 350–352, https://doi.org/10.1111/j.1067-1927.2005.130319.x.

5. Sandelowski, M., *What's in a Name? Qualitative Description Revisited*. Research in Nursing and Health, 2010. 33(1): pp. 77–84, https://doi.org/10.1002/nur.20362.

6. Whitaker, I.S., et al., *Larval Therapy from Antiquity to the Present Day: Mechanisms of Action, Clinical Applications and Future Potential*. Postgraduate Medical Journal, 2007. 83(980): pp. 409–413, https://doi.org/10.1136/pgmj.2006.055905.

7. Dunbar, G., *Notes on the Ngemba tribe of the Central Darling River of Western New South Wales*. Mankind, 1944. 81: pp. 199–202.

8. Greenberg, B., *Chapter 1: Flies through History*, in *Flies and Disease: II. Biology and Disease Transmission*, B. Greenberg, Editor. 1973, Princeton University Press: Princeton. pp. 2–18.

9. Weil, J.C., R.J. Simon, and W.R. Sweadner, *A Biological, Bacteriological and Clinical Study of Larval or Maggot Therapy in the Treatment of Acute and Chronic Pyogenic Infections*. American Journal of Surgery, 1933. 19: pp. 36–48.

10. Fonder, M.A., et al., *Treating the Chronic Wound: A Practical Approach to the Cure of Nonhealing Wounds and Wound Care Dressings*. Journal of the American Academy of Dermatology, 2008. 58(2): pp. 185–206, https://doi.org/10.1016/j.jaad.2007.08.048.

11. Saraf, S. and R.S. Parihar, *Sushruta: The First Plastic Surgeon in 600 B.C.* The Internet Journal of Plastic Surgery, 2006. 4(2), https://ispub.com/IJPS/4/2/8232.

12. The University of Nottingham. *We Could Make That!: Chance Meeting Leads to Creation of Antibiotic Spider Silk*. https://www.nottingham.ac.uk/

news/pressreleases/2017/january/chance-meeting-leads-to-creation-of-antibiotic-spider-silk.aspx.

13. Drucker, C.B., *Ambroise Paré and the Birth of the Gentle Art of Surgery*. Yale Journal of Biology and Medicine, 2008. 81(4): pp. 199–202, https://www.ncbi.nlm.nih.gov/pmc/articles/PMC2605308/.

14. Larrey, B.D., *Observations on Wounds, and Their Complications by Erysipelas, Gangrene and Tetanus, etc. [in French]. Translated from French by E.F. Rivinus*. Mielke and Biddle: Philadelphia, 1832.

15. Baer, W.S., *Sacro-iliac Joint-arthritis Deformans-viable Antiseptic in Chronic Osteomyelitis*. Interstate Postgraduate Medical Association of North America, 1929. 371: pp. 365–372.

16. Baer, W.S., *The Treatment of Chronic Osteomyelitis with the Maggot (Larva of the Blow Fly)*. The Journal of Bone and Joint Surgery. American Volume, 1931. 13: pp. 438–475, https://doi.org/10.1007/s11999-010-1416-3.

17. Sherman, R.A., S. Mendez, and C. McMillan. *Using Maggots in Wound Care: Part 2*. 2014, Wound Care Advisor, https://woundcareadvisor.com/using-maggots-in-wound-care-part-2-vol3-no6/.

18. BTER Foundation. *Policies & Procedures Templates*. 2022. https://www.bterfoundation.org/policies-procedures-templates.

19. BTER Foundation. *Welcome to the BTER Foundation*. 2022, https://www.bterfoundation.org.

20. NHS England. *NHS Five Year Forward View*. 2014. https://www.england.nhs.uk/five-year-forward-view.

21. NHS England. *NHS Long Term Plan*. 2019. https://www.england.nhs.uk/long-term-plan.

22. National Health Executive. *The Benefit of Growing at Scale*. 2015. https://www.nationalhealthexecutive.com/Editors-Comment/the-benefit-of-growing-at-scale.

23. Takáč, P., et al., and F. Stadler, *Establishment of a Medicinal Maggot Production Facility and Treatment Programme in Kenya*, in *A Complete Guide to Maggot Therapy: Clinical Practice, Therapeutic Principles, Production, Distribution, and Ethics*, F. Stadler (ed.). 2022, Cambridge: Open Book Publishers, pp. 331–346, https://doi.org/10.11647/OBP.0300.15.

24. Bojke, C., et al. *Economic Evaluation of a Treatment for Non-healing Wounds with Observational Data: An Example of a Topical Haemoglobin Spray for the Treatment of Diabetic Foot Ulcers*. 2019, https://medicinehealth.leeds.ac.uk/download/downloads/id/402/wp19-01_-_b_bojke_et_al_b_-_economic_evaluation_of_a_treatment_for_non-healing_wounds_with_observational_data_%E2%80%93_an_example_of_a_topical_haemoglobin_spray_for_the_treatment.pdf.

25. FDA. *510(k) Summary. Monarch Labs, LLC.* 2007. https://www.accessdata. fda.gov/cdrh_docs/pdf7/K072438.pdf.

26. Sherman, R.A., *Maggot Therapy Takes Us back to the Future of Wound Care: New and Improved Maggot Therapy for the 21st Century.* Journal of Diabetes Science and Technology, 2009. 3(2): pp. 336–344, https://doi.org/10.1177/ 193229680900300215.

27. Alfaro, M., et al., *National Health Systems and COVID-19 Death Toll Doubling Time.* Frontiers in Public Health, 2021. 9, https://doi.org/10.3389/ fpubh.2021.669038.

28. Beveridge, W. *The Beveridge Report: Social Insurance and Allied Services.* 1942. https://dspace.gipe.ac.in/xmlui/bitstream/handle/10973/32621/GIPE-033701-Contents.pdf?sequence=2&isAllowed=y.

29. Wallace, L.S., *A View of Health Care around the World.* Annals of Family Medicine, 2013. 11(1): p. 84, https://doi.org/10.1370/afm.1484.

30. Hanratty, M.J., *Canadian National Health Insurance and Infant Health.* The American Economic Review, 1996. 86(1): pp. 276–284, https://www.jstor. org/stable/2118267.

31. National Institute for Health and Care Excellence. *Chronic Wounds: Advanced Wound Dressings and Antimicrobial Dressings.* 2016. https://www. nice.org.uk/advice/esmpb2/chapter/Key-points-from-the-evidence.

32. Courtenay, M., *The Use of Larval Therapy in Wound Management in the UK.* Journal of Wound Care, 1999. 8(4): pp. 177–179, https://doi.org/10.12968/ jowc.1999.8.4.25866.

33. Evans, H., *A Treatment of Last Resort.* Nursing Times, 1997. 93(23): pp. 62–65.

34. Journal of Wound Care. *Wound Care Handbook: Negative Pressure Wound Therapy.* 2022. https://www.woundcarehandbook.com/configuration/ categories/wound-care/negative-pressure-wound-therapy.

35. Stadler, F., *The Maggot Therapy Supply Chain: A Review of the Literature and Practice.* Med Vet Entomol, 2020. 34(1): pp. 1–9, https://doi.org/10.1111/ mve.12397.

36. BioMonde. *Larval Debridement Therapy: Making Healing Possible.* 2022. https://biomonde.com/en.

37. Monarch Labs. *Monarch Labs: Living Medicine.* 2022. https://www. monarchlabs.com.

38. Paul, A.G., et al., *Maggot Debridement Therapy with Lucilia cuprina: A Comparison with Conventional Debridement in Diabetic Foot Ulcers.* International Wound Journal, 2009. 6(1): pp. 39–46, https://doi. org/10.1111/j.1742-481X.2008.00564.x.

39.   Sherman, R.A., M.J.R. Hall, and S. Thomas, *Medicinal Maggots: An Ancient Remedy for Some Contemporary Afflictions*. Annual Review of Entomology, 2000. 45(1): pp. 55–81, https://doi.org/10.1146/annurev.ento.45.1.55.

40.   Thyssen, P.J. and F.S. Masiero, *Bioprospecting and Testing of New Fly Species for Maggot Therapy*, in *A Complete Guide to Maggot Therapy: Clinical Practice, Therapeutic Principles, Production, Distribution, and Ethics*, F. Stadler (ed.). 2022, Cambridge: Open Book Publishers, pp. 195–234, https://doi.org/10.11647/OBP.0300.11.

41.   Stadler, F., et al., *Fly Colony Establishment*, in *A Complete Guide to Maggot Therapy: Clinical Practice, Therapeutic Principles, Production, Distribution, and Ethics*, F. Stadler (ed.). 2022, Cambridge: Open Book Publishers, pp. 257–288 (p. 269), https://doi.org/10.11647/OBP.0300.13.

42.   Čičková, H., M. Kozánek, and P. Takáč, *Growth and Survival of Blowfly Lucilia sericata Larvae under Simulated Wound Conditions: Implications for Maggot Debridement Therapy*. Medical and Veterinary Entomology, 2015. 29(4): pp. 416–424, https://doi.org/10.1111/mve.12135.

43.   Chadwick, P., et al., *Appropriate Use of Topical Haemoglobin in Chronic Wound Management: Consensus Recommendations*. The Diabetic Foot Journal, 2015. 18(3): pp. 142–146, https://diabetesonthenet.com/diabetic-foot-journal/appropriate-use-of-topical-haemoglobin-in-chronic-wound-management-consensus-recommendations-2/.

44.   Foley, E., A. Robinson, and M. Maloney, *Skin Substitutes and Dermatology: A Review*. Current Dermatology Reports, 2013. 2(2): pp. 101–112.

45.   Snyder, D.L., et al. *Skin Substitutes for Treating Chronic Wounds*. 2020. https://www.ahrq.gov/sites/default/files/wysiwyg/research/findings/ta/comments/skin-substitutes-disposition-of-comments.pdf.

46.   Sherman, R.A. and F.A. Wyle, *Low-cost, Low-maintenance Rearing of Maggots in Hospitals, Clinics, and Schools*. American Journal of Tropical Medicine and Hygiene, 1996. 54(1): pp. 38–41, https://doi.org/10.4269/ajtmh.1996.54.38.

47.   Stadler, F., R.Z. Shaban, and P. Tatham, *Maggot Debridement Therapy in Disaster Medicine*. Prehospital and Disaster Medicine, 2016. 31(1): pp. 79–84, https://doi.org/10.1017/s1049023x15005427.

48.   Chadwick, P., et al., *Appropriate Use of Larval Debridement Therapy in Diabetic Foot Management: Consensus Recommendations*. Diabetic Foot Journal, 2015. 18(1): pp. 37–42, https://diabetesonthenet.com/wp-content/uploads/dfj18-1-37-42-1.pdf.

49.   Beliën, J. and H. Forcé, *Supply Chain Management of Blood Products: A Literature Review*. European Journal of Operational Research, 2012. 217(1): pp. 1–6, https://doi.org/10.2139/ssrn.1974803.

50.   Kumru, O.S., et al., *Vaccine Instability in the Cold Chain: Mechanisms, Analysis and Formulation Strategies*. Biologicals, 2014. 42(5): pp. 237–259, https://doi.org/10.1016/j.biologicals.2014.05.007.

51. Peck, G., et al., *Airworthiness Testing of Medical Maggots*. Military Medicine, 2015. 180(5): pp. 591–596, https://doi.org/10.7205/MILMED-D-14-00548.

52. Tatham, P., et al., *Flying Maggots: A Smart Logistic Solution to an Enduring Medical Challenge*. Journal of Humanitarian Logistics and Supply Chain Management, 2017. 7(2): pp. 172–193, https://dx.doi.org/10.1108/JHLSCM-02-2017-0003.

53. Stadler, F. and P. Tatham, *Drone-assisted Medicinal Maggot Distribution in Compromised Healthcare Settings*, in *A Complete Guide to Maggot Therapy: Clinical Practice, Therapeutic Principles, Production, Distribution, and Ethics*, F. Stadler (ed.). 2022, Cambridge: Open Book Publishers, pp. 383–402, https://doi.org/10.11647/OBP.0300.18.

54. Stadler, F., *Distribution Logistics*, in *A Complete Guide to Maggot Therapy: Clinical Practice, Therapeutic Principles, Production, Distribution, and Ethics*, F. Stadler (ed.). 2022, Cambridge: Open Book Publishers, pp. 363–382, https://doi.org/10.11647/OBP.0300.17.

55. Sherman, R., *Medicinal Maggot Application and Maggot Therapy Dressing Technology*, in *A Complete Guide to Maggot Therapy: Clinical Practice, Therapeutic Principles, Production, Distribution, and Ethics*, F. Stadler (ed.). 2022, Cambridge: Open Book Publishers, pp. 79–96, https://doi.org/10.11647/OBP.0300.05.

56. Stadler, F., *The Ethics of Maggot Therapy*, in *A Complete Guide to Maggot Therapy: Clinical Practice, Therapeutic Principles, Production, Distribution, and Ethics*, F. Stadler (ed.). 2022, Cambridge: Open Book Publishers, pp. 405–430, https://doi.org/10.11647/OBP.0300.19.

57. Davey, G.C., *Self-reported Fears to Common Indigenous Animals in an Adult UK Population: The Role of Disgust Sensitivity*. British Journal of Psychology, 1994. 85 (Pt 4): p. 541–554, https://doi.org/10.1111/j.2044-8295.1994.tb02540.x.

58. Sherman, R. and F. Stadler, *Wound Aetiologies, Patient Characteristics, and Healthcare Settings Amenable to Maggot Therapy*, in *A Complete Guide to Maggot Therapy: Clinical Practice, Therapeutic Principles, Production, Distribution, and Ethics*, F. Stadler (ed.). 2022, Cambridge: Open Book Publishers, pp. 39–62, https://doi.org/10.11647/OBP.0300.03.

59. Sherman, R., *Indications, Contraindications, Interactions, and Side-effects of Maggot Therapy*, in *A Complete Guide to Maggot Therapy: Clinical Practice, Therapeutic Principles, Production, Distribution, and Ethics*, F. Stadler (ed.). 2022, Cambridge: Open Book Publishers, pp. 63–78, https://doi.org/10.11647/OBP.0300.04.

60. Stadler, F., *Supply Chain Management for Maggot Debridement Therapy in Compromised Healthcare Settings*. 2018. Unpublished doctoral dissertation, Griffith University, Queensland, https://doi.org/10.25904/1912/3170.

61. National Institute for Health and Care Excellence. *NG19: The Diabetic Foot (updated 2019)* 2015. https://www.nice.org.uk/guidance/ng19/evidence/full-guideline--august-2015-pdf-15672915543.

62. International Working Group on the Diabetic Foot. *IWGDF Practical Guidelines on the Prevention and Management of Diabetic Foot Disease.* 2019. https://iwgdfguidelines.org/wp-content/uploads/2021/03/IWGDF-2019-final.pdf.

63. Conte, M.S., et al., *Global Vascular Guidelines on the Management of Chronic Limb-Threatening Ischemia.* European Journal of Vascular and Endovascular Surgery, 2019. 58(1s): pp. S1-S109.e33, https://doi.org/10.1016/j.ejvs.2019.05.006.

64. National Institute for Health and Care Excellence. *Lower Limb Pathways.* 2019. https://pathways.nice.org.uk/pathways/lower-limb-peripheral-arterial-disease.

65. National Institute for Health and Care Excellence. *Venous Disease.* 2020. https://cks.nice.org.uk/topics/leg-ulcer-venous/management/venous-leg-ulcers.

66. European Pressure Ulcer Advisory Panel. *New Guidelines.* 2019. https://www.epuap.org/pu-guidelines.

67. Chan, D.C., et al., *Maggot Debridement Therapy in Chronic Wound Care.* Hong Kong Medical Journal, 2007. 13(5): pp. 382–386, https://www.hkmj.org/abstracts/v13n5/382.htm.

68. Sherman, R.A. and R. Chon, *BioTherapeutics, Education and Research Foundation Position Paper: Assessing the Competency of Clinicians Performing Maggot Therapy.* Wound Repair and Regeneration, 2022. 30(1): pp. 100–106, https://doi.org/10.1111/wrr.12986.

69. BioMonde. *Introducing Larval Academy.* 2021. https://biomonde.com/en/hcp/elearning/larval-academy.

70. Mexican Association for Wound Care and Healing. *Clinical Practice Guidelines for the Treatment of Acute and Chronic Wounds with Maggot Debridement Therapy.* 2010. https://s3.amazonaws.com/aawc-new/memberclicks/GPC_larvatherapy.pdf.

71. Mirabzadeh, A., et al., *Maggot Therapy for Wound Care in Iran: A Case Series of the First 28 Patients.* Journal of Wound Care, 2017. 26(3): pp. 137–143, https://doi.org/10.12968/jowc.2017.26.3.137.

72. All Wales Tissue Viability Nurse Forum. *The All Wales Guidance for the Use of Larval Debridement Therapy (LDT).* 2013. https://www.wounds-uk.com/download/resource/5850.

73. Stadler, F. *Supply Chain Management for Maggot Debridement Therapy in Compromised Healthcare Settings.* 2018. Unpublished doctoral dissertation, Griffith University, Queensland, https://doi.org/10.25904/1912/3170.

74. Stadler, F., *Laboratory and Insectary Infrastructure and Equipment*, in *A Complete Guide to Maggot Therapy: Clinical Practice, Therapeutic Principles, Production, Distribution, and Ethics*, F. Stadler (ed.). 2022, Cambridge: Open Book Publishers, pp. 237–256, https://doi.org/10.11647/OBP.0300.12.

75. Stadler, F., *Packaging Technology*, in *A Complete Guide to Maggot Therapy: Clinical Practice, Therapeutic Principles, Production, Distribution, and Ethics*, F. Stadler (ed.). 2022, Cambridge: Open Book Publishers, pp. 349–362, https://doi.org/10.11647/OBP.0300.16.

76. Stadler, F. and P. Takáč, *Medicinal Maggot Production*, in *A Complete Guide to Maggot Therapy: Clinical Practice, Therapeutic Principles, Production, Distribution, and Ethics*, F. Stadler (ed.). 2022, Cambridge: Open Book Publishers, pp. 289–330, https://doi.org/10.11647/OBP.0300.14.

PART 2

THERAPEUTIC PRINCIPLES

7. The Natural History of Medicinal Flies

Michelle L. Harvey

When flies are used for therapeutic purposes to treat wounds (maggot therapy), they may be referred to as medicinal flies. Species that have been used for maggot therapy or which are likely candidates for maggot therapy generally belong to the family Calliphoridae, commonly known as blowflies. These flies have ecological relationships, life-history patterns, physiologies, and nutritional requirements that help them exploit cadavers as well as living bodies. The same adaptations can also be harnessed to treat non-healing necrotic wounds. This chapter first introduces the general features of dipteran diversity, morphology, and biology before a closer examination of the family Calliphoridae.

Introduction

The insect order Diptera is taxonomically and biologically diverse, with in excess of 160,000 described species across 150 families, including a few thousand with medical and veterinary significance [1]. The immense success of the Diptera is evident from their diversity, abundance and virtual omnipresence across habitats, and is a product of highly variable morphology, behaviour, and reproductive biology. Many fly species are closely associated with human activities and settlements. The most thoroughly studied dipteran species comprise those with detrimental effects on society, whether for their biting habits, disease transmission,

https://doi.org/10.11647/OBP.0300.07

or pure nuisance value. A key family recognised for their medical significance is the Calliphoridae or blowflies.

When flies are used for therapeutic purposes to treat wounds (maggot therapy), they may be referred to as medicinal flies. Chapter 11 explains the research process leading to the establishment of a new medicinal fly species [2]. Species that have been used for maggot therapy or which are likely candidates for maggot therapy generally belong to the Calliphoridae, with the exception of *Wohlfahrtia nuba* (Sarcophagidae) [3] and *Musca domestica* (Muscidae). The latter species was successfully used by Chinese physicians to treat a catastrophic hot-crush injury [4]. Blowflies have ecological relationships, life-history patterns, physiologies, and nutritional requirements that help them exploit cadavers as well as living bodies. The same adaptations can also be harnessed to treat non-healing necrotic wounds.

This chapter will first introduce the general features of dipteran diversity, morphology, and biology before a closer examination of the family Calliphoridae.

Life Histories

Broadly divided into two suborders, the lower Diptera and the Brachycera, the order Diptera is highly diverse in morphology, biology, and behaviour. Diverse feeding strategies and optimal microenvironments enable dipterans to invade a large range of habitats. Their holometabolous life history further contributes to their taxonomic and numerical abundance. Holometabolous insects exhibit a complete metamorphosis, a strategy that sees larvae and adults occupy often disparate habitats with differing feeding preferences, allowing immatures and adults to avoid competition for a single food substrate [5]. Metamorphosis from larva to adult generally takes place within an immobile pupa, with often complete remodelling of external and internal morphological structures, including digestive and reproductive systems.

Morphology

Morphology of the Diptera

Morphology in the Diptera is highly variable and reflective of the diversity of taxa present in the order [6–8]. The Diptera includes such divergent taxa as fruit flies, mosquitoes, blowflies, sand flies, bee flies, crane flies and midges, and their individual life histories, habitats, feeding and reproductive specialisations necessitate adaptation of morphology to adequately support their respective biology.

Dipteran adults are nearly all characterised by a single pair of functional, mesothoracic forewings and modified, club-like, metathoracic hindwings known as halteres, used largely for balancing and stabilisation [6], but some may be apterous (wingless). Their mobile head bears large compound eyes equipped for strong sight in active flight, and mouthparts often modified into a proboscis or sucking structure and directed ventrally beneath the insect [1]. Mouthpart organisation may be highly modified in taxa equipped for biting and/or blood feeding, with adaptation for rasping, sawing, tearing and injection of mouthparts into the skin all observed in blood feeders. Antennae may be variable and exhibit sexual dimorphism (variation between the sexes) [6]. Legs always bear five tarsomeres and adult genitalia may differ greatly between taxa, which allows differentiation between species.

Larvae are apodous (lacking true legs), but prolegs may be present [6]. The larval form may be variously modified for aquatic habitats in some families (e.g. Culicidae, Simuliidae). Head morphology varies from a sclerotised head capsule in some taxa through to acephaly (no head capsule) and an internal skeleton in others. Larvae lack true articulated mandibles (adecticous), and may metamorphose in a cocoon with appendages glued to the body wall (obtect pupa) or without forming a cocoon and with free appendages (exarate pupa) [1]. A sub-group of the exarate pupae are coarctate, meaning the pupa is contained within the hardened cuticle of the last larval instar and thus retains physical characteristics of the last larval form. This includes the Calliphoridae or blowflies, the subject of this chapter.

Suborder Morphology

The lower Diptera tend to be more delicate, including the mosquitoes, crane flies and midges, with long, slender antennae, and some taxa with aquatic larvae. Larvae of the lower Diptera are usually eucephalic (with a complete head capsule) [6]. The Brachycera are recognised as having more robust adult flies, with shorter, aristate antennae. A characteristic of the cyclorrhaphan flies (a grouping within the Brachycera and focus of this chapter) is the presence of a ptilinum. This is an eversible, bladder-like structure situated between the eyes of the adult [6], used to rupture the pupal casing and allow the emergence of the adult. Following eclosion of the adult, the ptilinum is retracted but evidence of its former presence and purpose is retained in the form of the ptilinal fissure. The bulk of the medically significant Diptera are found within the Brachycera (Table 7.1). The focus of the remainder of this chapter will be the family Calliphoridae.

Morphology of the Calliphoridae

Calliphorid adults vary greatly in size and colouration, and this diversity is reflected numerically with close to 1,500 described species [9]. Adults are often shiny with metallic colouring or dusted with a luminescent sheen referred to as pollinosity or pruinosity [10], which is best observed in bright sunlight. Three-segmented horned antennae, with a plumose arista and well developed calypters (lobes at the rear of the forewings) are additional classifying features. Within the family, key distinguishing taxonomic features include wing venation and chaetotaxy (bristle arrangement) [10, 11]. Features such as colouration and size of an individual should be treated cautiously when identifying a species. Individuals of the same species may be larger or smaller or look different in other ways because of geographical separation and adaptation to local conditions, or perhaps because their larvae had greater or lesser access to food.

Eggs are cylindrical in shape with rounded ends, and are pale white or yellow-coloured. The chorion ("shell") bears a median groove referred to as the plastron, which serves as the respiratory surface of the organism, and is also the point of weakness from which first-instar larvae emerge at hatching [5].

Table 7.1 Key dipteran taxa recognised for medical and/or veterinary significance.

Suborder	Taxon	Family	Synanthropic Nature
Lower Diptera	Mosquitoes	Culicidae	Nuisance value from biting; disease transmission (malaria, dengue, yellow fever, Ross River Fever, various forms of Encephalitis, filariasis)
	Black flies	Simuliidae	Nuisance value from biting; vector for transmission of onchocerciasis (river blindness)
	Biting Midges	Ceratopogonidae	Nuisance value from biting
Brachycera	Tsetse flies	Glossinidae	Myiasis; transmission of trypanosomiasis (sleeping sickness)
	Bot flies	Oestridae	Myiasis (including humans)
	Soldier flies	Stratiomyidae	Nuisance value; mechanical vectors of disease; forensic use
	Louse flies	Hippoboscidae	Obligate parasites of vertebrates
	Horse flies	Tabanidae	Biting nuisance, plus potential vectors of blood-borne disease
	House/bush flies	Muscidae	Nuisance value, plus biting in some taxa; forensic use
	Flesh flies	Sarcophagidae	Nuisance value; some parasitoids; some involvement in myiasis; forensic use
	Blowflies	Calliphoridae	Nuisance value; involvement in myiasis; forensic use

Larvae have a pointed anterior end and a blunt posterior end (Figures 7.1 and 7.2). They are apodous and lack a head capsule, instead housing an internal cephalopharyngeal skeleton that may be visible through their relatively translucent integument. Larvae lack mandibulate mouthparts but the mouth hooks are visibly extended from the head, and are used to loosen and separate food particles and for crawling. The structure of the cephalopharyngeal skeleton and associated sclerites may be of taxonomic value [5, 10]. In terrestrial insects, oxygen exchange occurs using breathing structures called spiracles, and these are borne in two places on calliphorid larvae. A pair of anterior spiracles can be found on the second segment, and a pair of posterior spiracles on the twelfth segment. The anterior spiracles are absent, or at least non-functional, in first-instar larvae [10]. The posterior spiracles are taxonomically important, and their structure may be used to distinguish between the three instars. The first-instars bear simple spiracles with a single simple hole, while the second- and third-instars bear two or three pairs of spiracular slits respectively (Figure 7.1) [7, 10]. The spiracular structure is considerably more reliable for distinguishing the relative development of a larva than the use of larval length, width or weight. The integument is ornamented with spines or scales that circle the insect in bands, and may be used taxonomically. Between each larval instar, a moult occurs, enabling larvae to shed their constrictive integument and continue to feed and increase in size in the next stage.

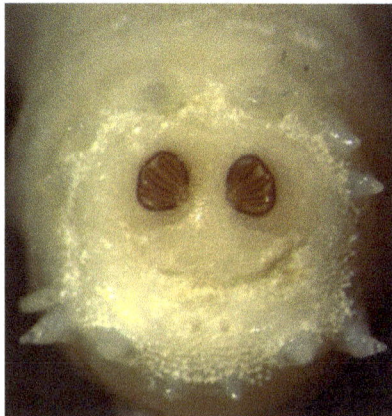

Figure 7.1 Posterior spiracles of third-instar calliphorid larva, showing three pairs of spiracular slits. Photo by M. Harvey, CC BY-NC.

Pupae of calliphorid flies are coarctate, which means that they are retained within the last larval cuticle. At the end of the third-instar phase, this cuticle sclerotises (hardens) and becomes a dark brown colour (Figure 7.2), providing a tough, hydrophobic casing called the puparium. Within the puparium, the larva undergoes extensive remodelling of tissues and organ systems in order to transform into an adult fly (metamorphosis). During this stage, taxonomically important features of the larva are retained on the outside of the puparium [10], and the mouth hooks do not fuse with the puparium.

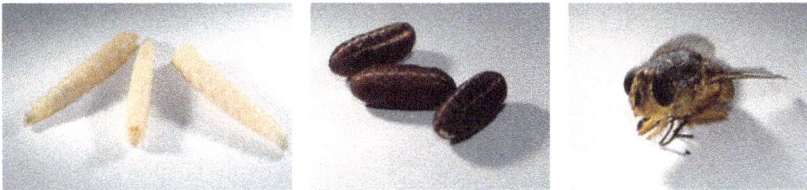

Figure 7.2 Larvae, pupae and adult calliphorid flies. Photos by M. Harvey, CC BY-NC.

Life-cycle and Developmental Traits of Calliphorid Flies

Adults: Attraction and Oviposition Behaviour

Calliphorid females lay eggs in batches of varying size on a nutritionally attractive substrate; frequently a microbially dense, moist surface suitable as a food source for offspring. Individual species have geographical ranges that reflect their species' biology, generally governed by availability of potential food sources, ambient temperature range, and humidity. When seeking a suitable surface upon which to lay, females are attracted to matter in a particular state of decay, and other factors such as indoor/outdoor/direct sunlight and the presence of fleece/hair on the body surface of the host may also be relevant [5]. How attractive a food source is may also be dependent on microbial contamination of that food. Volatile (easily evaporating) compounds taken from substrate colonised by non-sterile larvae are highly attractive to *Lucilia cuprina*, compared to volatiles from substrate infested with microbe-free larvae [12].

The females locate a suitable larval food source using highly developed chemoreceptors located on their antennae [5]. These receptors enable the flies to detect a food source from a considerable distance—some studies have indicated attraction of gravid (ready to deposit offspring) females from up to 63km away [13], demonstrating their ability to locate an ephemeral resource with high efficiency. Individual species may exhibit preference for substrate in a particular state of decay, as reflected by its odour, thus the condition of the substrate will determine which species is likely to colonise it. Dry substrate generally lacks appeal [5].

Females may also be attracted to a suitable substrate by pheromones from females of the same species, resulting in an accumulation of eggs in a single spot. Thus, the attraction of a single female to a suitable site may result in large aggregations of eggs [14]. As eggs are laid on top of each other, they protect each other from drying out [5]. The number of eggs laid by a female is thought to vary for different resources depending on the level of competition anticipated and other environmental factors, with the obvious goal being to maximize offspring fitness [15]. It has further been shown that female flies may be attracted by interkingdom bacterial swarming which signals the presence of a suitable food source. For example, swarming *Proteus mirabilis* attract female greenbottle blowflies (*Lucilia sericata*) [16].

Not all calliphorid fly species lay eggs. Indeed, there is a bewildering variety of reproductive strategies. While some (oviparous) species lay eggs directly on the food source in batches up to several hundred per fly [17], other species, particularly those found in more extreme climates, may be larviparous and deposit live larvae or ovoviviparous and deposit live larvae ensheathed in a chorion that hatch almost immediately on deposition. Such species exhibit lower batch sizes due to increased maternal investment, but egg desiccation is avoided and larvae can immediately commence feeding. This allows species to capitalise quickly on the presence of an ephemeral and high-value resource, thus providing a competitive edge to their offspring as they commence development ahead of egg-laying species [18, 19]. Oviparous females have been shown to lay approximately 150–180 eggs per oviposition event, with larviparous species producing approximately 50 offspring per event [5, 20, 21]. Some species exhibit both larviparous and oviparous reproduction. [17, 20]. In a study of *Calliphora dubia*, 70% of females laid only live larvae, 14% laid eggs and larvae concurrently, and 16% laid only eggs, with all eggs nonviable due to the females being too immature [17]. Mackerras [20] also reported that *Calliphora augur* eggs were produced before females were ready to larviposit and the eggs were consequently not viable. Furthermore, ovoviviparous females have the ability to resorb larvae when no suitable laying site is present [17]. To make matters even more complicated, oviparous females can lay live "precocious" larvae that develop within the oviduct and are consequently many hours older than all other offspring [5, 22].

Female flies must consume protein-rich food soon after their emergence as an adult. This is referred to as anautogeny [5]. Without such provision, their ovaries do not mature to produce fertile eggs but males are fertile regardless of diet [20]. It costs a lot of energy to fly and therefore adults must consume copious amounts of sugary food in the form of nectar, which makes them important pollinators of crops [23, 24].

Larval Development

Larvae digest food externally by secreting enzymes and bacteria that breakdown and liquefy the food source which is then ingested [5]. This is critical given the simplicity of their mouthparts and modification of their digestive system into a straight-forward, tube-like structure. Ammonia is their primary excretory product. Larvae push deep into flesh, necrotic tissue or other substrate while their back ends remain exposed. This allows them to breathe through the posterior spiracles while feeding in liquid anoxic substrates. For larvae to be able to grow, they need to periodically shed their cuticle, which does not expand along with the growing larva. Food sources harbouring bacteria and yeasts will support larval growth more effectively than sterile substrate [25], but it is also well-established that larvae produce antimicrobial substances that inhibit growth of microbes. It is thus likely that suppression of bacterial growth may be selective against particular species, regulating the overall density of microbes.

Pupal Metamorphosis

Larvae empty their gut at the cessation of feeding in the third instar [5], and this most likely occurs by digestion of consumed substrate which

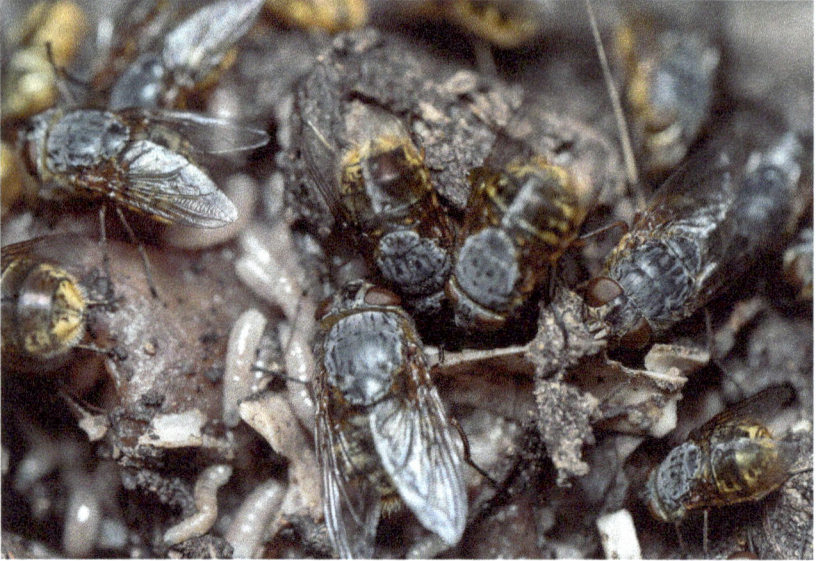

Figure 7.3 *Calliphora stygia* adult flies and their larvae (maggots) feeding on carrion. Photo by Ash Powell CC BY-NC-ND.

further adds to energy stores that have been accumulated for the long-lasting quiescent pupal phase that follows. Larvae burrow into soil or under objects where they develop the hardened cuticle (puparium) that protects the metamorphosing insect within (pupa). Pupae breathe through respiratory horns on the fifth segment of the puparium. During metamorphosis, complete remodelling of internal systems occurs, as well as development of external appendages and the segmented body plan (tagmosis). The adult fly emerges using the expansion and contraction of the ptilinum between the eyes, a haemolymph-filled sac that pulsates to break the operculum, a lid-like structure, from the anterior end of the puparium [5]. Over an approximately 24-hour period the newly eclosed fly unfurls its wings, develops pigmentation, and prepares for flight.

Environmental Factors Affecting Calliphorid Fly Behaviour

Because flies are poikilothermic organisms (having varying body temperatures), the activity level, oviposition behaviour, and the developmental rate of immatures are fundamentally dependent on ambient temperatures. Thus, development of immatures proceeds when the ambient temperature is within species-specific temperature thresholds. For *L. sericata* larvae the optimal temperature for development is 33°C. [20], which corresponds closely to the surface temperature of a human or livestock wound which they frequently colonise. It is common for calliphorid fly larvae to form large aggregations counting many thousands of individuals. This massing generates heat and increases the ambient temperatures that larvae experience, which are sometimes upwards of 50°C. Larvae survive exposure to such potentially lethal temperatures by cycling from the centre to the periphery of aggregations [5, 26]. The exothermic nature of larval masses is a critical issue when estimating the age of larvae in forensic investigations, and when predicting the growth of individuals in research or clinical studies, or laboratory-rearing contexts. Pupal development is also temperature dependent, but the effect of aggregations is not relevant in this stage.

The lower temperature threshold for development is of considerable relevance, because below this temperature, development largely ceases. Adult flies of some species are known to overwinter with the ability to become active on warm winter days—the cold-adapted *Calliphora vicina* and *Calliphora stygia* are two examples [20]. Immature flies may suspend their development under unfavourable climatic conditions (diapause) either as larvae, pre-pupae, or pupae [20, 21], only to resume development when triggered by changes in daylength and/ or temperature that promise more favourable conditions. Larvae have been observed to successfully feed at both high and low temperature extremes, but may not pupate successfully [27].

Furthermore, ambient temperature affects oviposition behaviour, thus affecting the "colonisation interval" for a suitable substrate. Suitable food sources for colonisation are highly ephemeral, necessitating rapid colonisation by blowflies. This may be highly variable and dependent on humidity, rainfall, wind, light, sun exposure and, fundamentally, temperature [5, 28]. Adults are generally active during daylight hours, although warm evenings have been reported to promote adult activity [29, 30]. When days are mild then flies tend to show a unimodal activity pattern, getting more active as the morning progresses and temperature rises and slowing down again in the afternoon hours when it gets cooler.

When days are very hot, a bimodal activity pattern is not uncommon with flies being most active in the morning and afternoon [5]. Having said that, optimal temperatures for adult flight are highly species-dependent and generally dictate species distributions and population density in a given location [31], but the optimal air temperature range for species colonising decomposing remains is considered to lie between 10 and 30°C [5, 29, 31]. For the cold-tolerant *Calliphora vicina*, egg-laying was shown to occur between 10 and 35°C, while the more temperate *L. sericata* was shown to lay eggs between 16 and 40°C [32]. Furthermore, adult flight and oviposition behaviours appear to be innately regulated in many species by circadian rhythms. Environmental and climatic conditions aside, reproduction in flies is fundamentally determined by the location and availability of suitable food for the development of offspring. Through the ages, human activity has supplied flies with plentiful organic waste to breed in. For calliphorid flies this has developed into a close (synanthropic) relationship with humans and their settlements.

Calliphorid Interactions with Humans and Domesticated Animals

The requirement for high protein substrate for larval development makes the association of calliphorids with humans and associated animals a natural interaction. Attracted to rubbish and decomposing matter, blowflies have naturally become nuisances when they occur in high abundance. Well-adapted to life associated with humans and our domesticated animals, blowflies are easily spread through human transport within vehicles [5] which helps in the expansion of their natural ranges.

Since calliphorid species will readily feed on a range of proteinaceous, microbially-rich food sources, they are easily maintained taxa for laboratory-rearing, which facilitates research into their biology. A large amount of this research has been in the field of forensic entomology. It has been established that the arrival of species is predictable and can be correlated to particular decomposition stages. This information can be combined with previously established developmental characteristics of the fly species to calculate the postmortem interval, which is the time that has passed since death occurred. Forensic investigators use ambient temperatures to calculate how long it would have taken for the blowfly species that were found on or near the cadaver to develop to the stage at which they were collected. This, combined with the particular colonisation speed for each species, permits fairly accurate determination of the time a person died. In this way, humans have exploited the attraction of flies to protein-rich and microbially-dense environments to provide information in legal investigations.

While often recognised for their role as important nutrient recyclers of dead matter, blowfly larvae may also colonise living organisms (myiasis). Living tissues may be infested by larvae which may be painful and result in the death of the host [5]. Among the cyclorrhaphan flies there are both facultative and obligate parasites of animals. Facultative parasites are species that develop in carrion but will occasionally become parasites in living tissue, while obligate parasites must inhabit a living animal to successfully develop. Obligate parasites include species such as *Chrysomya bezziana*, the Old World screwworm fly, which requires living flesh for larval development. Most blowfly species are facultative parasites, recognised for their role in forensic science as colonisers of human carrion. The ability to exploit living tissue when it is accessible is a highly successful adaptation [19]. Levot et al. (1979) cite rapid growth through short feeding periods, effective digestive enzymes, few larval instars, and the early colonisation of lucrative decomposing remains as reasons for the immense success of cyclorrhaphan larvae, and the calliphorids are no exception.

Key species recognised as inhabiting carrion include members of the genera *Phormia*, *Protophormia*, *Cordylobia*, *Calliphora*, *Lucilia*, *Chrysomya* and *Cochliomyia*, and many of these species are also recognised for their role as facultative parasites of living animals. This easy shift likely reflects the microbially rich nature of the food source in both situations. Mackerras & Mackerras [33] indicate that carrion is more attractive to facultative parasites than the flesh of living animals.

Primary colonising larvae secrete proteolytic enzymes including collagenases that externally digest the cutaneous tissue through liquefaction, and larvae gradually invade the subcutaneous tissues, causing shock and septicaemia in hosts [34]. Although *L. sericata* and *L. cuprina* are most often responsible for flystrike (myiasis in sheep and other domestic animals), *Chrysomya rufifacies*, *C. stygia*, and *C. augur* were all recorded to also cause myiasis in sheep [20]. In one study, *Calliphora augur* and sister species *C. dubia* were recorded to be present in 15% of single species strikes on sheep and in 35% of 1088 strikes in total [35].

Lucilia—Friend or Foe?

Lucilia sericata and *L. cuprina* are sister species with interesting behavioural inconsistencies, as well as geographically-based differences that make them of significant interest to entomologists. *Lucilia cuprina* was thought to have originated in the Oriental or Afrotropical regions, while *L. sericata* was endemic to the Palearctic [36], but they have spread considerably with movement of humans and livestock. They are now both cosmopolitan blowfly species and both are recognised for their role in the colonisation of carrion, although *L. sericata* more so than *L. cuprina*. However, this affinity to carrion does not prevent these species from switching to living animals when the opportunity arises.

In Australia, *L. sericata* is mainly an urban species attracted to refuse. It has limited relevance with regard to flystrike, and was considered by Waterhouse and Paramonov [37] to be "economically unimportant". Their experiments showed that *L. sericata* displayed limited oviposition on sheep as compared to *L. cuprina* [37]. However, in Britain, *L. sericata* readily laid eggs on live sheep in field experiments [38], and is recognised as the main myiasis-causing blowfly species in sheep in the United Kingdom. *Lucilia cuprina* is known as the Australian Sheep Blowfly, and is attracted to livestock and generally found in rural areas [37], where it is the primary agent of flystrike. Females lay eggs in the soiled fleece of the animals [5] and larvae feed on the animals' flesh. Affected livestock may suffer from a large burden of larvae and initial infestation by *L. cuprina* is often followed by secondary blowfly species. Severe infestations may result in the animal dying and the economic loss to Australian farmers from fly strike is estimated to be in the vicinity of $280 million per annum [39].

Interestingly, *L. cuprina* females are readily attracted to sheep with clean fleece, but will not lay unless the fleece is soiled with faeces or urine [5]. Fleece-rot results from bacterial infections of *Pseudomonas aeruginosa* proliferation in moist fleece, causing a green colouration and subsequently becoming highly attractive to female *L. cuprina* [40, 41]. Thus, it is the bacterial presence that attracts female flies to the area, as seen with the attraction of *L. sericata* to swarming *P. mirabilis* on carrion [16]

While myiasis is well-documented to be of detriment in the case of flystrike, there is also a beneficial application of myiasis. Maggot therapy involves the deliberate application of larvae to non-healing human wounds in an effort to debride necrotic tissue, flush the wound with antimicrobial compounds, and stimulate the growth of new tissue [42–44]. *Lucilia sericata* is commonly the species utilised for this purpose, but *L. cuprina* has been applied both accidentally [45] and deliberately [46], yielding similar results to its sister species. Thus, the interchangeability of the two species is again established.

Genetic studies have supported the separate species status of both *L. cuprina* and *L. sericata*, in spite of strong similarities in morphology and ecology [47]. Hawaiian flies morphologically identified as *L. cuprina*, however, have been shown to possess *L. sericata*-type mitochondrial DNA sequences across the COI and COII regions of mitochondrial DNA, which are maternally inherited [48]. According to Stevens and Wall [48] this may suggest a hybridisation event that has become fixed in *L. cuprina* within Hawaii by lineage sorting. Although hybrids of the two species have been produced in the laboratory but were not highly fertile [37], there have been no reports of true hybrids in the field.

There are two subspecies of *L. cuprina*. *Lucilia cuprina dorsalis* is the subspecies dominant throughout sub-Saharan Africa and the Australasian regions [37, 49]. The second subspecies, *L. cuprina cuprina* has been shown to readily interbreed with *L. c. dorsalis* in the wild, indicating that despite their varying morphology and behaviour, they taxonomically comprise a single species [49]. This said, varying behaviour and biology between the subspecies may be highly important in the consideration of use of *L. cuprina* in maggot therapy, but this has not been considered yet given the focus on *L. sericata*. Future studies investigating the use of *L. cuprina* in maggot therapy will need to consider possible differences in efficacy and risk.

Summary

The Diptera is a highly diverse insect order but it is the family Calliphoridae (blowflies) that has been the focus of this chapter because many calliphorid species are of great medical and veterinary importance. Calliphorid flies utilise a variety of food sources both as adults and during larval development. Adult blowflies seek the nectar and pollen of flowering plants and are consequently important pollinators. They also visit dung, carrion, and living animals to feed. This means they can potentially spread germs. Generally, calliphorid flies prefer to breed in dead and decomposing organic matter, including carrion, but living animals are also utilised as a food source for larvae. Myiasis, the colonisation of living animals and humans by fly larvae, may be the only way a species of blowfly reproduces, but other species are more flexible and able to utilise both carrion and living animals depending on availability and resource competition.

While blowflies are a nuisance to people and responsible for disease in humans and livestock, many species are also of significant benefit to people beyond their widely-recognised ecosystem services (decomposition, pollination, and food for other animals). Some species that colonise wounds such as *L. sericata* have a benign and even beneficial impact on wound healing. It is this therapeutic benefit that has led people for thousands of years to use fly larvae (maggots) for the treatment of infected and chronic wounds. Chapters 3 to 6 provide guidance on clinical aspects of maggot therapy and its integration into the healthcare setting [50–53]. In forensic science, it is the knowledge of female colonisation and oviposition habits and species developmental rates that allows law-enforcement to estimate the time of death in coronial or murder inquests.

References

1.   Gullan, P. and P. Cranston, *The Insects: An Outline of Entomology*. 2014: Jihn Wiley & Sons, Incorporated.

2.   Thyssen, P.J. and F.S. Masiero, *Bioprospecting and Testing of New Fly Species for Maggot Therapy*, in *A Complete Guide to Maggot Therapy: Clinical Practice, Therapeutic Principles, Production, Distribution, and Ethics*, F. Stadler (ed.).

2022, Cambridge: Open Book Publishers, pp. 195–234, https://doi. org/10.11647/OBP.0300.11.

3.   Grantham-Hill, C., *Preliminary Note on the Treatment of Infected Wounds with the Larva of Wohlfahrtia Nuba*. Transactions of the Royal Society of Tropical Medicine and Hygiene, 1933. 27: pp. 93–98.

4.   Wu, J.C., et al., *Maggot Therapy for Repairing Serious Infective Wound in a Severely Burned Patient*. Chinese Journal of Traumatology, 2012. 15(2): pp. 124–125, https://linkinghub.elsevier.com/retrieve/pii/S1008-1275(15)30283-2.

5.   Erzinclioglu, Z., *Blow Flies*. 1996, Slough: The Richmond Publishing Co Ltd.

6.   Colless, D. and D. McAlpine, *39: Diptera (Flies)*, in *The Insects of Australia: A Textbook for Students and Research Workers*, C.S.a.I.R.O. Division of Entomology (ed.). 1991, Melbourne University Press: Australia, pp. 717–786.

7.   Cumming, J.M., et al., *Manual of Central American Diptera*. 2009, Ottawa: National Research Council Press.

8.   Bertone, M.A., *Manual of Afrotropical Diptera, Volume 1: Introductory Chapters and Keys to Diptera Families*. American Entomologist, 2019. 65(1): pp. 69–70, https://doi.org/10.1093/ae/tmz011.

9.   Species2000. *Calliphoridae*. 2020. https://www.catalogueoflife.org/data/ taxon/7KK.

10.   Zumpt, F., *Myiasis in Man and Animals in the Old World: A Textbook for Physicians, Veterinarians and Zoologists*. 1965, London: Butterworths.

11.   Wallman, J.F., *A Key to the Adults of Species of Blowflies in Southern Australia Known or Suspected to Breed in Carrion*. Medical and Veterinary Entomology, 2001. 15(4): pp. 433–437, https://doi.org/10.1046/j.0269-283x.2001.00331.x.

12.   Eisemann, C.H. and M.J. Rice, *The Origin of Sheep Blowfly, Lucilia cuprina (Wiedemann) (Diptera: Calliphoridae), Attractants in Media Infested with Larvae*. Bulletin of Entomological Research, 1987. 77: pp. 287–294, https:// dx.doi.org/10.1017/S0007485300011767.

13.   Braack, L.E. and P.F. Retief, *Dispersal, Density and Habitat Preference of the Blow-flies Chrysomyia Albiceps (Wd.) and Chrysomyia Marginalis (Wd.) (Diptera: Calliphoridae)*. Onderstepoort Journal of Veterinary Research, 1986. 53(1): pp. 13–18.

14.   Barton Browne, L., R.J. Bartell, and H.H. Shorey, *Pheromone-mediated Behaviour Leading to Group Oviposition in the Blowfly, Lucilia cuprina*. Journal of Insect Physiology, 1969. 15: pp. 1003–1014.

15.   Brockelman, W.Y., *Competition, the Fitness of Offspring, and Optimal Clutch Size*. American Naturalist, 1975. 109: pp. 677–699.

16. Ma, Q., et al., *Proteus Mirabilis Interkingdom Swarming Signals Attract Blow Flies*. The ISME Journal, 2012. 6(7): pp. 1356–1366, https://dx.doi.org/10.1038/ismej.2011.210.

17. Cook, D.F. and I.R. Dadour, *Larviposition in the Ovoviviparous Blowfly Calliphora Dubia*. Medical and Veterinary Entomology, 2011. 25: pp. 53–57, https://doi.org/10.1111/j.1365-2915.2010.00894.x.

18. Norris, K.R., *The Ecology of Sheep Blowflies in Australia*, in *Monographiae Biologicae: Biogeography and Ecology in Australia*, A. Keast, R.L. Crocker, and C.S. Christian (eds). 1959, Junk: The Hague, pp. 514–544.

19. Levot, G.W., K.R. Brown, and E. Shipp, *Larval Growth of Some Calliphorid and Sarcophagid Diptera*. Bulletin of Entomological Research, 1979. 69: pp. 469–475, https://dx.doi.org/10.1017/S0007485300018976.

20. Mackerras, M.J., *Observations on the Life-histories, Nutritional Requirements and Fecundity of Blowflies*. Bulletin of Entomological Research, 1933. 24: pp. 353–362, https://dx.doi.org/10.1017/S0007485300031680.

21. Callinan, A.P.L., *Aspects of the Ecology of Calliphora Augur (Fabricius) (Diptera: Callaiphoridae), a Native Australian Blowfly*. Australian Journal of Zoology, 1980. 28: pp. 679–684, https://dx.doi.org/10.1071/ZO9800679.

22. Davies, K. and M. Harvey, *Precocious Egg Development in the Blowfly Calliphora Vicina: Implications for Developmental Studies and Post-mortem Interval Estimation*. Medical and Veterinary Entomology, 2012. 26(3): pp. 300–306, https://doi.org/10.1111/j.1365-2915.2011.01004.x.

23. Cook, D.F., et al., *Yield of Southern Highbush Blueberry (Vaccinium Corymbosum) Using the Fly Calliphora Albifrontalis (Diptera: Calliphoridae) as a Pollinator*. Austral Entomology, 2020. 59(2): pp. 345–352, https://doi.org/10.1111/aen.12455.

24. Cook, D.F., et al., *The Role of Flies as Pollinators of Horticultural Crops: An Australian Case Study with Worldwide Relevance*. Insects, 2020. 11(6): p. 341, https://doi.org/10.3390/insects11060341.

25. Hobson, R.P., *Studies on the Nutrition of the Blow-fly Larvae. III. The Liquefaction of Muscle*. Journal of Experimental Biology, 1932. 9: pp. 359–365.

26. Johnson, A.P. and J.F. Wallman, *Infrared Imaging as a Non-invasive Tool for Documenting Maggot Mass Temperatures*. Australian Journal of Forensic Sciences, 2014. 46(1): pp. 73–79, https://doi.org/10.1080/00450618.2013.793740.

27. O'Flynn, M.A., *The Succession and Rate of Development of Blowflies in Carrion in Southern Queensland and the Application of these Data to Forensic Entomology*. Journal of the Australian Entomological Society, 1983. 22: pp. 137–148, https://dx.doi.org/10.1111/j.1440-6055.1983.tb01860.x.

28. Dickson, G.C., et al., *Marine Bacterial Succession as a Potential Indicator of Postmortem Submersion Interval*. Forensic Science International, 2011. 209(1–3): pp. 1–10, https://doi.org/10.1016/j.forsciint.2010.10.016.

29. Amendt, J., R. Zehner, and F. Reckel, *The Nocturnal Oviposition Behaviour of Blow Flies (Diptera: Calliphoridae) in Central Europe and Its Forensic Implications*. Forensic Science INternational, 2008. 175: pp. 61–84, https://doi.org/10.1016/j.forsciint.2007.05.010.

30. George, K.A., M.S. Archer, and T. Toop, *Nocturnal Colonisation Behaviour of Blowflies (Diptera: Calliphoridae) in Southeastern Australia*. Journal of Forensic Science, 2013. 58: pp. S112-S116, https://doi.org/10.1111/j.1556-4029.2012.02277.x.

31. Brundage, A., S. Bros, and J. Honda, *Seasonal and Habitat Abundance and Distribution of some Forensically Important Blowflies (Diptera: Calliphoridae) in Central California*. Forensic Science International, 2011. 212(1–3): pp. 115–120, https://dx.doi.org/10.1016/j.forsciint.2011.05.023.

32. Ody, H., M.T. Bulling, and K.M. Barnes, *Effects of Environmental Temperature on Oviposition Behaviour in Three Blow Fly Species of Forensic Importance*. Forensic Science International, 2017. 275: pp. 138–143, https://dx.doi.org/10.1016/j.forsciint.2017.03.001.

33. Mackerras, I.M. and M.J. Mackerras, *Sheep Blowfly Investigations. The Attractiveness of Sheep for Lucilia cuprina*. Bulletin of the Council for Scientific and Industrial Research, 1944. 181: pp. 1–44.

34. Mauldin, E.A. and J.P. Peters-Kennedy, *Chapter 6 — Integumentary System*, in *Jubb, Kennedy and Palmer's Pathology of Domestic Animals: Volume 1*, M.G. Maxie (ed.). 2016, Saunders Ltd, pp. 509–736.

35. Mackerras, I.M. and M.E. Fuller, *A Survey of the Australian Sheep Blowflies*. Journal of the Council of Scientific and Industrial Research in Australia, 1937. 10: pp. 261–270.

36. Aubertin, D., *Revision of the Genus Lucilia R.-D. (Diptera, Calliphoridae)*. Linnean Society Journal of Zoology, 1933. 38: pp. 389–463.

37. Waterhouse, D.F. and S.J. Paramonov, *The Status of the Two Species of Lucilia (Diptera: Calliphoridae) Attacking Sheep in Australia*. Australian Journal of Scientific Research, 1950. 3: pp. 310–336, http://dx.doi.org/10.1071/BI9500310.

38. Cragg, J.B., *The Reactions of Lucilia sericata (Mg.) to Various Substances Placed on Sheep*. Parasitology, 1950. 40: pp. 179–186, https://doi.org/10.1017/s0031182000018011.

39. Department of Primary Industries and Regional Development, G.o.W.A. *Managing Flystrike in Sheep*. 2017. https://www.agric.wa.gov.au/livestock-parasites/managing-flystrike-sheep.

40.   Emmens, R.L. and M.D. Murray, *The Role of Bacterial Odours in Oviposition by Lucilia cuprina (Wiedemann) (Diptera: Calliphoridae), the Australian Sheep Blowfly*. Bulletin of Entomological Research, 1982. 72: pp. 367–375, https://dx.doi.org/10.1017/S0007485300013547.

41.   Emmens, R.L. and M.D. Murray, *Bacterial Odours as Oviosition Stimulants for Lucilia cuprina (Wiedemann) (Diptera: Calliphoridae), the Australian Sheep Blowfly*. Bulletin of Entomological Research, 1983. 73: pp. 411–415, https://dx.doi.org/10.1017/S0007485300009019.

42.   Nigam, Y. and M.R. Wilson, *Maggot Debridement*, in *A Complete Guide to Maggot Therapy: Clinical Practice, Therapeutic Principles, Production, Distribution, and Ethics*, F. Stadler (ed.). 2022, Cambridge: Open Book Publishers, pp. 143–152, https://doi.org/10.11647/OBP.0300.08.

43.   Nigam, Y. and M.R. Wilson, *The Antimicrobial Activity of Medicinal Maggots*, in *A Complete Guide to Maggot Therapy: Clinical Practice, Therapeutic Principles, Production, Distribution, and Ethics*, F. Stadler (ed.). 2022, Cambridge: Open Book Publishers, pp. 153–174, https://doi.org/10.11647/OBP.0300.09.

44.   Nigam, Y. and M.R. Wilson, *Maggot-assisted Wound Healing*, in *A Complete Guide to Maggot Therapy: Clinical Practice, Therapeutic Principles, Production, Distribution, and Ethics*, F. Stadler (ed.). 2022, Cambridge: Open Book Publishers, pp. 175–194, https://doi.org/10.11647/OBP.0300.10.

45.   Tantawi, T.I., K.A. Williams, and M.H. Villet, *An Accidental but Safe and Effective Use of Lucilia Cuprina (Diptera: Calliphoridae) in Maggot Debridement Therapy in Alexandria, Egypt*. Journal of Medical Entomology, 2010. 47(3): pp. 491–494, https://doi.org/10.1093/jmedent/47.3.491.

46.   Paul, A.G., et al., *Maggot Debridement Therapy With Lucilia Cuprina: A Comparison With Conventional Debridement in Diabetic Foot Ulcers*. International Wound Journal, 2009. 6(1): pp. 39–46, https://doi.org/10.1111/j.1742-481x.2008.00564.x.

47.   Stevens, J. and R. Wall, *Genetic Variation in Populations of the Blowflies Lucilia cuprina and Lucilia sericata: Random Amplified Polymorphic DNA Analysis and Mitochondrial DNA Sequences*. Biochemical Systematics and Ecology, 1997. 25: pp. 81–97, https://doi.org/10.1017/S0007485300033058.

48.   Stevens, J.R., R. Wall, and J.D. Wells, *Paraphyly in Hawaiian Hybrid Blowfly Populations and the Evolutionary History of Anthropophilic Species*. Insect Molecular Biology, 2002. 11(2): pp. 141–148, https://dx.doi.org/10.1046/j.1365-2583.2002.00318.x.

49.   Norris, K.R., *Evidence for the Multiple Exotic Origin of Australian Populations of the Sheep Blowfly, Lucilia-Cuprina (Wiedemann) (Diptera, Calliphoridae)*. Australian Journal of Zoology, 1990. 38(6): pp. 635–648, https://dx.doi.org/10.1071/ZO9900635.

50.   Bullen, B. and P. Chadwick, *Clinical integration of Maggot Therapy*, in *A Complete Guide to Maggot Therapy: Clinical Practice, Therapeutic Principles,*

Production, Distribution, and Ethics, F. Stadler (ed.). 2022, Cambridge: Open Book Publishers, pp. 97–118, https://doi.org/10.11647/OBP.0300.06.

51.   Sherman, R., *Indications, Contraindications, Interactions, and Side-effects of Maggot Therapy*, in *A Complete Guide to Maggot Therapy: Clinical Practice, Therapeutic Principles, Production, Distribution, and Ethics*, F. Stadler (ed.). 2022, Cambridge: Open Book Publishers, pp. 63–78, https://doi.org/10.11647/OBP.0300.04.

52.   Sherman, R., *Medicinal Maggot Application and Maggot Therapy Dressing Technology*, in *A Complete Guide to Maggot Therapy: Clinical Practice, Therapeutic Principles, Production, Distribution, and Ethics*, F. Stadler (ed.). 2022, Cambridge: Open Book Publishers, pp. 79–96, https://doi.org/10.11647/OBP.0300.05.

53.   Sherman, R. and F. Stadler, *Wound Aetiologies, Patient Characteristics, and Healthcare Settings Amenable to Maggot Therapy*, in *A Complete Guide to Maggot Therapy: Clinical Practice, Therapeutic Principles, Production, Distribution, and Ethics*, F. Stadler (ed.). 2022, Cambridge: Open Book Publishers, pp. 39–62, https://doi.org/10.11647/OBP.0300.03.

8. Maggot Debridement

Yamni Nigam and Michael R. Wilson

For non-healing wounds to progress past the inflammatory stage, it is vital that necrotic tissue is quickly and effectively removed, a treatment that is known as debridement. Maggot therapy is the treatment of wounds with living fly larvae (maggots) to remove necrotic tissue. In recent years, much progress has been made in understanding the therapeutic principles of maggot-assisted debridement. This chapter describes the physiological and biochemical principles underpinning the extraordinary ability of medicinal maggots to precisely debride highly necrotic wounds in a matter of days without the need for surgical intervention.

Introduction

Non-healing wounds containing necrotic tissue can be attributed to a variety of factors including chronic disease, vascular insufficiencies, advanced age, neurological defects, nutritional deficiencies, or local factors such as infection, pressure, and oedema [1]. In these wounds, the normal healing process stalls, typically in a chronic state of inflammation, causing a cascade of abnormal tissue responses which can generate and amplify a hostile microenvironment inside the wound. This results in accumulation of cellular debris on the wound surface and damage to surrounding tissue, leading to infection and necrosis [2, 3]. To aid the process of wound healing and allow it to progress past the inflammatory stage, it is vital that this necrotic tissue is quickly and effectively removed, a treatment that is known as debridement [4, 5].

https://doi.org/10.11647/OBP.0300.08

Maggot therapy is the treatment of wounds with living fly larvae (maggots) in need of debridement. The ability of *Lucilia sericata* and other fly species to debride is attributed to their necrophagous nature. This is to say that their primary source of nutrition in the wild is dead and rotting tissue [6]. The larvae of *L. sericata* consume the necrotic tissue, and it is their voracious appetite for this material that makes them so effective in this process (Figure 8.1).

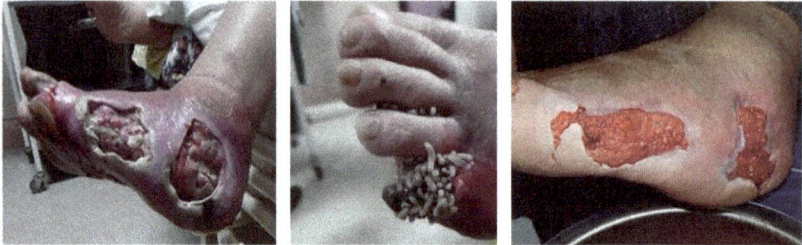

Figure 8.1 Maggot therapy with free-range larvae (Photos by Parizad *et al*. 2021, https://doi.org/10.1016/j.ijscr.2021.105931 [7], CC BY-NC.

Efficacy of Maggot Therapy for Wound Debridement

Since its resurgence in the USA and UK in the 1990s, a number of clinical studies have been conducted to compare the efficacy of larval therapy to conventional treatment methods in debriding chronic wounds. A systematic review of the clinical studies of larval therapy incorporated twelve comparative studies, including six randomised controlled trials, from the years 2000–2014 [8]. Based on the analysis of these twelve studies, the authors concluded that larval therapy was both more effective and more efficient in the debridement of chronic ulcers when compared with conventional treatments. They also associated larval therapy with other benefits, including quicker healing rate of chronic wounds, a shortened time to healing in ulcers, a longer antibiotic-free time period, decreased amputation risk, and similar antibiotic usage compared with conventional therapies [8]. A subsequent review of clinical studies of maggot therapy from 2000–2015 corroborated the positive debridement results, showing a significantly higher rate of successful debridement compared with conventional treatments and a significantly faster time for wounds to heal [9].

The Feeding Process and Maggot Enzymatic Action

In the wild, carrion is a nutritive but ephemeral resource, and there is intense competition among arthropods to acquire these resources before they are depleted. Therefore, like many other species of Calliphoridae, L. sericata larvae have adapted some particularly effective mechanisms to satisfy their nutritional requirements and ensure rapid development [10–12]. Chapter 7 of this book explains the natural history of calliphorid flies, including their feeding strategies [6]. The primary feeding mechanism of larvae is extracorporeal digestion, a process that was first demonstrated in the 1930s [13]. The food is digested externally by larval excretions/secretions which contain a potent mixture of proteolytic enzymes, deoxyribonuclease, ammonia, and antimicrobial substances. The movement of the larvae over the food then facilitates the penetration of these secretions into the necrotic tissue, causing it to break down and liquefy into a nutrient-rich fluid that the larvae subsequently ingest [14, 15]. This method of feeding is particularly well-suited to individuals feeding together in large populations such as those seen in blowfly larvae as it enables them to share and combine the enzymatic secretions they release, allowing them to feed more efficiently [16, 17]. Additionally, the secretions produced by maggots work to increase pH in the wound environment, making it more conducive to the action of the proteolytic enzymes [15, 18, 19]. It is also believed that the secretions help to irrigate bacteria from the wound environment [20] as discussed in more detail in Chapter 9 [21]. These initial debridement and disinfection processes are vital for wound healing to proceed [22].

As well as the enzymatic action, it is also thought that debridement in larval therapy is aided by the physical action of the larvae themselves. Each larva possesses a set of mouth hooks which they use to scrape and tear at the surface tissue, and it is thought that the most significant function of this action is to facilitate the penetration of their secretions into the tissue, thereby making it easier to break down [23, 24]. The mouth hooks are also used for locomotion as they help to pull the body forward when maggots crawl [25]. Additionally, larvae seek out areas containing necrotic tissue and thus ensure that debridement activity is focussed on the areas of greatest need [26].

Identification of Maggot Enzymes in Debridement

The enzymes that are contained in larval secretions are key to wound debridement. Therefore, identifying those enzymes responsible would be very helpful in further understanding the action of larvae in the chronic wound. Initial work looked at characterising the types of enzymes at work. Using class specific substrates and inhibitors, Chambers and Woodrow [15] identified three classes of proteolytic enzymes at work in the process of larval debridement: serine proteases, aspartyl proteases, and metalloproteases. Of these enzymes, the most significant activity was attributed to serine proteases of two different sub-classes, trypsin-like and chymotrypsin-like. Larvae also provide the optimal conditions for the serine and metalloproteases to act within the wound, secreting ammonia to increase the pH in the wound bed and thus allowing activation of trypsin-like proteases (which have a role in cell proliferation, cytokine secretion and ultimately wound healing) and chymotrypsin-like proteases that degrade the extracellular matrix components laminin, fibronectin and collagen types I and III [15].

Serine proteases were also subsequently identified in larval secretions in a separate study, indicating the role of these enzymes in wound debridement [27]. A recent, novel investigation using a physical model corroborated this idea. The work involved the incorporation of trypsin inhibitors in the feed of larvae so that enzymes that were produced by the larvae were inhibited. The result of this was a significant decrease in consumption rates and a severe stunting of larval growth [28]. This work confirmed that larvae did indeed utilise trypsin proteases for extracorporeal digestions and subsequent consumption of dead tissue. Trypsin inhibitors have also been successfully incorporated into the diets of other insect species, which has resulted in similarly detrimental effects on both feeding and development [29–32]. This means that the use of serine proteases in digestion is not unique to *L. sericata*.

There has also been work to identify the individual enzymes at work. It had been demonstrated that a chymotrypsin-like serine protease was able to degrade extracellular matrix components in wounds and aid fibroblast migration through this action. The three major components in extracellular matrix that were degraded by this chymotrypsin were fibronectin, laminin and collagen [15]. This chymotrypsin was subsequently identified and characterised from *L. sericata* larvae and a recombinant form (named "chymotrypsin I") was shown to be effective in degrading venous leg wound eschar *ex vivo* [33–35]. Utilising various techniques including 2D gel electrophoresis and the monitoring of the release of 7-amino-4-methyl coumarin from the chymotrypsin substrate, it was concluded that the active recombinant chymotrypsin I degraded the wound eschar more efficiently than commercially available chymotrypsin from bovine and human sources [35].

Additionally, chymotrypsin I was found not to be restrained by endogenous inhibitors that were found in high concentrations within wound slough (α-1-antichymotrypsin and α-1-antitrypsin), indicating a means by which the activity of the enzyme is able to survive within the wound and contribute to debridement [36]. The protease is, however, inhibited by α-2-macroglobulin which is significant because it is a macromolecule found in blood plasma which in turn is abundant in healthy and blood-perfused tissue. It is hypothesised that the specificity of *L. sericata* larvae for digesting only necrotic tissue may be explained by this inhibitory effect of α-2-macroglobulin [37].

Larval secretions have also been found to contain deoxyribonuclease, capable of degrading genomic and extracellular bacterial DNA, as well as DNA from wound slough, indicating a potential to aid in wound debridement and inhibition of the growth of bacteria and biofilm [14]. In another study, a complementary DNA library was constructed from the salivary glands of medicinal larvae and five full-length and several incomplete complimentary DNAs encoding for serine proteases were identified [38]. Further work to characterise the active enzymes in larval secretions resulted in the identification of a chymotrypsin-like serine protease known as "Jonah$_\text{m}$" which was found to digest certain extracellular matrix components normally present in the chronic wound environment [39]. However, this enzyme was found not to digest certain other components, suggesting that it is a complex mix of enzymes in larval secretions that facilitate debridement. This was confirmed in another study where a comprehensive analysis of the proteolytic enzymes released from larval tissues—including the salivary glands, crop, and gut—identified hundreds of clusters representing five classes of enzyme: aspartic, cysteine, threonine, serine, and metallopeptidases [40]. Serine peptidases represented the largest group of peptidases identified from

L. sericata, and in addition to the previously characterised proteases, dozens more were identified with roles in digestion, immunity, blood coagulation, and others whose roles are still unclear [40].

The significance of uncovering the therapeutically active substances in larval secretions lies not only in gaining a greater understanding of how larval therapy works, but also in aiding the possible development of new treatments. Whilst the efficacy of larval therapy is well proven, its widespread adoption is limited by practical problems associated with using live organisms. These include a short shelf-life, the need for an advanced logistics network to allow for express delivery, and the need for extra training to ensure that dressings are applied and maintained correctly [33]. By uncovering the active components of larvae secretions, it is envisioned that these molecules could be synthesised and then delivered by a suitable device or mechanism without having to use live larvae.

Summary

Maggot therapy is made possible by the extraordinary life-history characteristics of medicinal flies, and by the feeding behaviour and physiology of their larvae. Adapted to the exploitation of ephemeral cadavers, they have evolved the capacity to rapidly consume decaying flesh and complete their larval growth in just a few days. A cocktail of digestive enzymes is secreted to dissolve only necrotic tissue before the nutrient-rich liquid digest is consumed. When such flies colonise the wound of a living human or animal (myiasis) and conditions are conducive, then their gentle, selective, and highly efficient feeding behaviour brings about rapid debridement of the wound.

This therapeutic benefit of myiasis has been recognised since ancient times and adopted by tribal healers and later by modern medicine. In recent years, much progress has been made in understanding the therapeutic principles of maggot-assisted debridement. The digestive secretions of course play a critical role. Now the race is on to isolate and synthetically produce therapeutic compounds for wound care drug development. However, the use of pharmaceuticals derived from maggot products may have limitations. For example, the use of individual products for debridement will likely preclude the other benefits associated with treatment using live larvae such as disinfection and wound healing, and may therefore limit the effectiveness of the treatment. Additionally, considering that secretions consist of a complex mixture of enzymes [40], one can argue that the efficacy of maggot therapy relies on this complex mix of substances that are produced by the live larvae and then deposited into the wound. In other words, the substitution of this mix of substances for a single, cost-effective pharmaceutical, or even a combination of pharmaceuticals, may not be possible. How medicinal maggots control infection and bring about wound healing is discussed in Chapters 9 and 10 of this book [21, 41]. There has been some success in producing recombinant forms of maggot-derived digestive enzymes and incorporating them into a delivery device [33, 35, 39], but more work is needed to determine which enzymes are effective, how their efficacy compares against live larvae, and how they can be produced reliably at a large scale for a reasonable cost.

References

1. Fonder, M.A., et al., *Treating the Chronic Wound: A Practical Approach to the Care of Nonhealing Wounds and Wound Care Dressings*. Journal of the American Academy of Dermatology, 2008. 58(2): pp. 185–206, https://doi.org/10.1016/j.jaad.2007.08.048.

2. Eming, S.A., T. Krieg, and J.M. Davidson, *Inflammation in Wound Repair: Molecular and Cellular Mechanisms*. Journal of Investigative Dermatology, 2007. 127(3): pp. 514–525, https://doi.org/10.1038/sj.jid.5700701.

3. Zhao, R., et al., *Inflammation in Chronic Wounds*. International Journal of Molecular Sciences, 2016. 17(12): pp. 2085–2085, https://doi.org/10.3390/ijms17122085.

4. Wilcox, J.R., M.J. Carter, and S. Covington, *Frequency of Debridements and Time to Heal: A Retrospective Cohort Study of 312,744 wounds*. JAMA Dermatology, 2013. 149(9): pp. 1050–1058, https://doi.org/10.1001/jamadermatol.2013.4960.

5. Wolcott, R.D., J.P. Kennedy, and S.E. Dowd, *Regular Debridement is the Main Tool for Maintaining a Healthy Wound Bed in Most Chronic Wounds*. Journal of Wound Care, 2009. 18(2): pp. 54–56, https://doi.org/10.12968/jowc.2009.18.2.38743.

6. Harvey, M., *The Natural History of Medicinal Flies*, in *A Complete Guide to Maggot Therapy: Clinical Practice, Therapeutic Principles, Production,*

Distribution, and Ethics, F. Stadler (ed.). 2022, Cambridge: Open Book Publishers, pp. 121–142, https://doi.org/10.11647/OBP.0300.07.

7. Parizad, N., K. Hajimohammadi, and R. Goli, *Surgical Debridement, Maggot Therapy, Negative Pressure Wound Therapy, and Silver Foam Dressing Revive Hope for Patients with Diabetic Foot Ulcer: A Case Report.* International Journal of Surgery Case Reports, 2021. 82: p. 105931, https://doi.org/10.1016/j.ijscr.2021.105931.

8. Sun, X., et al., *A Systematic Review of Maggot Debridement Therapy for Chronically Infected Wounds and Ulcers.* International Journal of Infectious Diseases, 2014. 25: pp. 32–37, https://doi.org/10.1016/j.ijid.2014.03.1397.

9. Siribumrungwong, B., C. Wilasrusmee, and K. Rerkasem, *Maggot Therapy in Angiopathic Leg Ulcers: A Systematic Review and Meta-analysis.* The International Journal of Lower Extremity Wounds, 2018. 17(4): pp. 227–235, https://doi.org/10.1177/1534734618816882.

10. Hanski, I., *Carrion Fly Community Dynamics: Patchiness, Seasonality and Coexistence.* Ecological Entomology, 1987. 12(3): pp. 257–266, https://doi.org/10.1111/j.1365-2311.1987.tb01004.x.

11. Rivers, D.B., C. Thompson, and R. Brogan, *Physiological Trade-offs of Forming Maggot Masses by Necrophagous Flies on Vertebrate Carrion.* Bulletin of Entomological Research, 2011. 101(05): pp. 599–611, https://doi.org/10.1017/S0007485311000241.

12. von Zuben, C.J., F.J. von Zuben, and W.A.C. Godoy, *Larval Competition for Patchy Resources in Chrysomya Megacephala (Dipt., Calliphoridae): Implications of the Spatial Distribution of Immatures.* Journal of Applied Entomology, 2001. 125(9–10): pp. 537–541, https://doi.org/10.1046/j.1439-0418.2001.00586.x.

13. Hobson, R.P., *On an Enzyme from Blow-fly Larvae Lucilia sericata which Digests Collagen in Alkaline Solution.* Biochemical Journal, 1931. 25(5): pp. 1458–1463, https://doi.org/10.1042/bj0251458.

14. Brown, A., et al., *Blow Fly Lucilia sericata Nuclease Digests DNA Associated with Wound Slough/Eschar and with Pseudomonas aeruginosa Biofilm.* Medical and Veterinary Entomology, 2012. 26(4): pp. 432–439, https://doi.org/10.1111/j.1365-2915.2012.01029.x.

15. Chambers, L., et al., *Degradation of Extracellular Matrix Components by Defined Proteinases from the Greenbottle Larva Lucilia sericata Used for the Clinical Debridement of Non-healing Wounds.* British Journal of Dermatology, 2003. 148(1): pp. 14–23, https://doi.org/10.1046/j.1365-2133.2003.04935.x.

16. dos Reis, S.F., C.J. von Zuben, and W.A.C. Godoy, *Larval Aggregation and Competition for Food in Experimental Populations of Chrysomya Putoria (Wied.) and Cochliomyia Macellaria (F.) (Dipt., Calliphoridae).* Journal of Applied Entomology, 1999. 123(8): pp. 485–489, https://doi.org/10.1046/j.1439-0418.1999.00397.x.

17. Ireland, S. and B. Turner, *The Effects of Larval Crowding and Food Type on the Size and Development of the Blowfly, Calliphora Vomitoria*. Forensic Science International, 2006. 159(2–3): pp. 175–181, https://doi.org/10.1016/j.forsciint.2005.07.018.

18. Mumcuoglu, K.Y., et al., *Destruction of Bacteria in the Digestive Tract of the Maggot of Lucilia sericata (Diptera: Calliphoridae)*. Journal of Medical Entomology, 2001. 38(2): pp. 161–166, https://doi.org/10.1603/0022-2585-38.2.161.

19. Thomas, S., *Maggot Therapy*. 2010, Medetec: Cardiff. pp. 563–632.

20. Mumcuoglu, K.Y., et al., *Maggot Therapy for the Treatment of Intractable Wounds*. International Journal of Dermatology, 1999. 38(8): pp. 623–627, https://doi.org/10.1046/j.1365-4362.1999.00770.x.

21. Nigam, Y. and M.R. Wilson, *The Antimicrobial Activity of Medicinal Maggots*, in *A Complete Guide to Maggot Therapy: Clinical Practice, Therapeutic Principles, Production, Distribution, and Ethics*, F. Stadler (ed.). 2022, Cambridge: Open Book Publishers, pp. 153–174, https://doi.org/10.11647/OBP.0300.09.

22. Gailit, J. and R.A.F. Clark, *Wound Repair in the Context of Extracellular Matrix*. Current Opinion in Cell Biology, 1994. 6(5): pp. 717–725, https://doi.org/10.1016/0955-0674(94)90099-X.

23. Barnard, D.R., *Skeletal-muscular Mechanisms of the Larva of Lucilia sericata (Meigen) in Relation to Feeding Habit (Diptera: Calliphoridae)*. Pan-Pacific Entomologist, 1977. 53(3): pp. 223–229.

24. Thomas, S., et al., *The Effect of Containment on the Properties of Sterile Maggots*. British Journal of Nursing, 2002. 11(Sup2): pp. S21-S28, https://doi.org/10.12968/bjon.2002.11.Sup2.10294.

25. Sherman, R.A., et al., *Maggot Therapy*, in *Biotherapy — History, Principles and Practice*, M. Grassberger, et al. (eds). 2013, Springer: Dordrecht; New York. pp. 5–29.

26. Church, J.C.T., *Larva Therapy in Modern Wound Care: A Review*. Primary Intention, 1999. 7(2): pp. 63–68.

27. Schmidtchen, A., et al., *Detection of Serine Proteases Secreted by Lucilia sericata in vitro and during Treatment of a Chronic Leg Ulcer*. Acta Dermato-Venereologica, 2003. 83(4): pp. 310–311, https://doi.org/10.1080/00015550310016689.

28. Wilson, M.R., et al., *The Impacts of Larval Density and Protease Inhibition on Feeding in Medicinal Larvae of the Greenbottle Fly Lucilia sericata*. Medical and Veterinary Entomology, 2016. 30(1): pp. 1–7, https://doi.org/10.1111/mve.12138.

29. Burgess, E.P.J., L.A. Malone, and J.T. Christeller, *Effects of Two Proteinase Inhibitors on the Digestive Enzymes and Survival of Honey Bees Apis Mellifera*. Journal of Insect Physiology, 1996. 42(9): pp. 823–828, https://doi.org/10.1016/0022-1910(96)00045-5.

30. Franco, O.L., et al., *Effects of Soybean Kunitz Trypsin Inhibitor on the Cotton Boll Weevil Anthonomus Grandis*. Phytochemistry, 2004. 65(1): pp. 81–89, https://doi.org/10.1016/j.phytochem.2003.09.010.

31. Johnston, K.A., J.A. Gatehouse, and J.H. Anstee, *Effects of Soybean Protease Inhibitors on the Growth and Development of Larval Helicoverpa Armigera*. Journal of Insect Physiology, 1993. 39(8): pp. 657–664, https://doi.org/10.1016/0022-1910(93)90071-X.

32. McManus, M.T. and E.P.J. Burgess, *Effects of the Soybean (Kunitz) Trypsin Inhibitor on Growth and Digestive Proteases of Larvae of Spodoptera Litura*. Journal of Insect Physiology, 1995. 41(9): pp. 731–738, https://doi.org/10.1016/0022-1910(95)00043-T.

33. Britland, S., et al., *Recombinant <i>Lucilia sericata</i> Chymotrypsin in a Topical Hydrogel Formulation Degrades Human Wound Eschar ex vivo*. Biotechnology Progress, 2011. 27(3): pp. 870–874, https://doi.org/10.1002/btpr.587.

34. Pritchard, D.I. and A.P. Brown, *Degradation of MSCRAMM Target Macromolecules in VLU Slough by Lucilia sericata Chymotrypsin 1 (ISP) Persists in the Presence of Tissue Gelatinase Activity*. International Wound Journal, 2015. 12(4): pp. 414–421, https://doi.org/10.1111/iwj.12124.

35. Telford, G., et al., *Degradation of Eschar from Venous Leg Ulcers Using a Recombinant Chymotrypsin from Lucilia sericata*. British Journal of Dermatology, 2010. 163(3): pp. 523–531, https://doi.org/10.1111/j.1365-2133.2010.09854.x.

36. Telford, G., et al., *Maggot Chymotrypsin I from Lucilia sericata Is Resistant to Endogenous Wound Protease Inhibitors*. British Journal of Dermatology, 2011. 164(1): pp. 192–196, https://doi.org/10.1111/j.1365-2133.2010.10081.x.

37. Pritchard, D.I., et al., *TIME Management by Medicinal Larvae*. International Wound Journal, 2016. 13(4): pp. 475–484, https://doi.org/10.1111/iwj.12457.

38. Valachova, I., et al., *Identification and Characterisation of Different Proteases in Lucilia sericata Medicinal Maggots Involved in Maggot Debridement Therapy*. Journal of Applied Biomedicine, 2014. 12(3): pp. 171–177, https://doi.org/10.1016/j.jab.2014.01.001.

39. Pöppel, A., et al., *A Jonah-like Chymotrypsin from the Therapeutic Maggot Lucilia sericata Plays a Role in Wound Debridement and Coagulation*. Insect Biochemistry and Molecular Biology, 2016. 70: pp. 138–147, https://doi.org/10.1016/j.ibmb.2015.11.012.

40. Franta, Z., et al., *Next Generation Sequencing Identifies Five Major Classes of Potentially Therapeutic Enzymes Secreted by Lucilia sericata Medical Maggots*. BioMed Research International, 2016. 2016: pp. 1–27, https://doi.org/10.1155/2016/8285428.

41. Nigam, Y. and M.R. Wilson, *Maggot-assisted Wound Healing*, in *A Complete Guide to Maggot Therapy: Clinical Practice, Therapeutic Principles, Production, Distribution, and Ethics*, F. Stadler (ed.). 2022, Cambridge: Open Book Publishers, pp. 175–194, https://doi.org/10.11647/OBP.0300.10.

9. The Antimicrobial Activity of Medicinal Maggots

Yamni Nigam and Michael R. Wilson

Bacterial infection of wounds is a serious and growing issue and contributes to a delay in wound healing. Whilst debridement is often the primary motivation for the clinical use of maggot therapy, there is accumulating evidence that the therapy has other therapeutic properties. In particular, larvae have a significant antibacterial effect on the wound surface through the antimicrobial action of their excretions and secretions and the disruption of microbial biofilms that are common in chronic wounds. This chapter describes the principles and mechanisms that allow medicinal maggots to successfully shape and control the microbial environment of the chronic wound.

Introduction

Bacterial infection of wounds is a serious and growing issue and contributes to a delay in wound healing. Progression of healing is said to be dependent on both bacterial count and microbial species present [1], so disinfection of the wound-site is vital to enable the wound to heal. Whilst debridement is often the primary motivation for the clinical use of maggot therapy, there is accumulating evidence that the therapy has other therapeutic properties. In particular, larvae have a significant antibacterial effect on the wound surface, not only through the removal

https://doi.org/10.11647/OBP.0300.09

of infected tissue, but also through the antimicrobial action of their excretions and secretions. When the American military surgeon William S. Baer encountered seriously wounded soldiers colonised by wild maggots during WW1, he observed the remarkably good condition the men were in and the absence of sepsis [2]. He considered the action of maggots to be that of scavengers sucking up bacteria and consuming dead tissue. He also noted the presence of excretions and secretions in the wound and believed that "some biological reaction" was responsible for helping the wound to heal, though the nature of this biochemical substance was something that he was not able to uncover.

In their natural environment, blowfly larvae exploit decaying carrion, which is a microbe-rich food source. Thus, it is intrinsic to their survival that they adapt to this environment and evolve strategies to cope with and control microbes [3]. It was this ability to control infection that motivated William S. Baer to eventually pioneer maggot therapy in his own peace-time clinical practice for the treatment of patients with osteomyelitis [2]. This chapter explains how medicinal maggots control wound infection.

Historical Investigations into the Antimicrobial Activity of Maggots

It had long been suspected that larvae possessed an antimicrobial quality. In the 1920s it was theorised that larvae were capable of destroying bacteria taken into their gut after the "remarkable sterility" of the gut contents of certain fly species was noted [4]. This was later expanded on by Robinson and Norwood [5,6], who found that bacteria were destroyed as they passed through the digestive system of medicinal maggots. As well as examining the destruction of bacteria in the gut, early studies also investigated the antimicrobial properties of larval excretions and secretions. Examining these "elimination products", Simmons [7, 8] demonstrated the presence of a potent antibacterial entity within the biological material. He also found that the use of non-disinfected larvae (compared to the use of the same material from disinfected organisms) increased the potency of the antibacterial activity, with a 5- to 10-minute incubation sufficient to prevent the growth of *Staphylococcus aureus* [7, 8]. Further research also determined the presence of a heat-stable antibacterial agent which could be partially purified using paper chromatography [9].

Resurgent Interest in Antibacterial Bioactivity from Maggots

More recently, there has been particular interest in understanding and identifying the therapeutic antimicrobial properties of maggot excretions and secretions, the main drive of this being the use of larvae as a source of novel antibiotics and anti-infectives, especially with the rise of drug-resistant forms of pathogenic bacteria such as methicillin-resistant *Staphylococcus aureus* (MRSA) [10].

The accumulation of evidence for maggot antimicrobial activity has been slow. Most of the compelling evidence on the nature of the therapeutic antimicrobial effects has come from scientific laboratory findings using maggot excretions and secretions. There have been numerous investigations into the types of bacteria vulnerable to maggot excretions and secretions. In one of the first modern investigations into the antimicrobial activity of maggot excretions and secretions, Thomas and colleagues [11] described variable bactericidal activity against different species and strains of bacteria, with marked activity against Gram-positive strains such as *Streptococcus* (group A, and group B) and *S. aureus*. Less marked activity was seen against MRSA and the Gram-negative *Pseudomonas* species, with no evidence of inhibition against the Gram-negative *Escherichia coli* and *Proteus* species.

Several tests have served to reaffirm the notion that maggot excretions and secretions are effective in destroying a broad range of Gram-positive bacteria. However, there is less consistency in results regarding Gram-negative species. For example, in a turbidometric assay using excretions and secretions from disinfected larvae, Bexfield and colleagues [12] observed significant antibacterial activity against Gram-positive species *S. aureus* (including MRSA), and *Bacillus thuringiensis*. In contrast to Thomas and colleagues [11], however, significant activity was also observed against Gram-negative species including *E. coli*, *Pseudomonas aeruginosa*, and *Enterobacter cloacae*. Findings in other investigations have also been inconsistent, with reports of maggot activity against both Gram-positive and Gram-negative species [13, 14], or activity against only Gram-positive and not against Gram-negative species [15].

Other investigators, too, noted antimicrobial activity against both Gram-positive and Gram-negative species, but observed that perhaps the activity against Gram-negatives was less pronounced. Using a colony forming units bioassay, it was demonstrated that maggots exhibited antibacterial activity against both S. aureus and E. coli, though the effectiveness of the activity was markedly less against E. coli than S. aureus [16]. A similar finding was reported in a clinical study, which noted that maggot therapy was more effective for Gram-positive-infected wounds than it was for Gram-negative-infected wounds [17]. A further investigation into the interaction of larvae with P. aeruginosa, a potent Gram-negative bacterium, found that the bacterium was harmful to the larvae, leading to a reduction in maggot food intake and their movement away from areas of contamination [18]. The authors found that this negative effect was caused by the action of specific quorum-sensing molecules that are released by bacteria in order to communicate with each other—usually prior to forming a biofilm. No bactericidal effect was detected against P. aeruginosa in this case [18].

Interestingly, a study by a Dutch group of clinicians and researchers found no antibacterial activity of maggot excretions and secretions at all, against either Gram-positive or Gram-negative species. However, recognising the clinical successes with maggot therapy and their own contradictory results in comparison with other reports, the authors suggested that the method of maggot secretion collection may account for the difference in results, not only in their own study, but also in that of others. This was expanded on by Barnes *et al.* [19] who, recognising the variety of methods employed in previous investigations and the variation in results, advocated for the standardisation of liquid culture assays used to quantify the antibacterial effectiveness of maggot excretions and secretions. In their own test, the authors found that different concentrations of maggot excretions and secretions and the presence of additional nutrition influenced the growth of tested bacteria (*E. coli, S. aureus,* and *P. aeruginosa*), and therefore would have contributed to the variation in previously reported results. Addressing this issue, the authors noted that whilst it is important to use media sufficiently high in nutritional content to enable bacterial growth, it should also not be detrimental to the antibacterial activity exhibited by the maggot excretions and secretions. Incidentally, in this test, the antibacterial effectiveness of maggot excretions and secretions was most potent against *E. coli* and less so against *S. aureus* [19].

These studies indicate the presence of antibacterial activity in maggot excretions and secretions but also demonstrate that care must be taken with regard to the method by which the excretions and secretions are collected, the choice of the bioassay used to assess the activity, and the need to establish sufficient control experiments to generate valid results from such studies. Regardless of the inconsistency of results related to the activity against Gram-negative bacteria, it is now widely accepted that there is an antibacterial entity present in the excretions and secretions of *L. sericata*. Indeed, excretions and secretions from medicinal maggots are used as positive controls in the study of antibacterial compounds found in excretions and secretions from other organisms [20].

Evidence for the Antimicrobial Activity of Medicinal Maggots

Maggots Can Destroy Ingested Bacteria

As well as investigations into the antibacterial action of larval excretions and secretions, there has also been some interest regarding the destruction of ingested bacteria in the maggot gut. By feeding larvae with *E. coli* that produce a fluorescent green protein and tracking this protein's movement through the alimentary tract, an Israeli team tracked the fate of ingested bacteria [21]. They showed that the majority of bacteria were destroyed in the mid-gut, with the remainder being destroyed in the hindgut, so that maggot faeces were either sterile or contained only a greatly reduced number of viable bacteria. In contrast, a subsequent study found that after ingestion of Methicillin-sensitive *Staphylococcus aureus* (MSSA) and Methicillin-resistant *Staphylococcus aureus* (MRSA), the strains remained viable within the maggot and were excreted into the environment [13]. However, it was noted by the authors that the larvae were exposed to a very large quantity of bacteria, which would not necessarily correspond to the bioburden of a wound, and therefore the capability to destroy bacteria in the gut may have been overwhelmed in this instance.

Clinical Evidence of Antibacterial Activity from Maggots

Whilst most of the evidence for the antimicrobial efficacy of *L. sericata* larvae comes from *in vitro* investigations, a small number of tests have also been conducted *in vivo*. In one such study swabs were tested from the wounds of 16 patients before and after treatment with maggot therapy and the chance of culturing Gram-positive and/or Gram-negative bacteria was determined [17]. For example, if three wound cultures were taken and two showed the growth of Gram-positive bacteria, the chance of culturing Gram-positive bacteria was given as 0.66. The results showed a reduction (although statistically not significant; $p=0.07$) in the chance of culturing Gram-positive bacteria after treatment with maggot therapy and a significant increase in the chance of culturing Gram-negative bacteria. The authors argued that the results indicated lower antibacterial effectiveness of maggot therapy in Gram-negative-infected wounds and suggested that treatment with a larger number of larvae may be necessary when treating a wound infected with Gram-negative bacteria.

A subsequent investigation similarly monitored the bacterial diversity before and after treatment with maggot therapy in 30 patients. The study found vast reductions in the species of bacteria present, though some species, mainly Gram-negative, were unaffected or increased in numbers, particularly *Proteus* species. As a result, the authors concluded that maggot therapy would be most appropriate in treating wounds infected with Gram-positive bacteria and advocated the need for special precautions when treating Gram-negative infections [16]. Incidentally, *Proteus* species is a frequent and natural commensal of *L. sericata* and previous laboratory studies [12] have also shown that it is unaffected by the antimicrobial activities of maggot excretions and secretions.

Randomised Controlled Trials and Antimicrobial Effects of Maggot Therapy

Randomised controlled trials are believed to be the gold standard for clinical studies. A recent randomised controlled trial was carried out with 50 patients who had a diabetic foot ulcer [22]. Patients were randomly assigned to a 'control' group, which received a conventional treatment of surgical debridement, antibiotic therapy, and offloading, or to a 'treatment' group, which received maggot therapy in addition to the conventional therapy. A swab culture was collected before and after each maggot application and analysed for the presence of *S. aureus* and *P. aeruginosa*. In the treatment group, the number of patients whose wound was infected with *S. aureus* significantly reduced after 48 hours of treatment, with a further reduction after a second application of larvae. The number of patients whose wound was infected with *P. aeruginosa*, meanwhile, did not reduce significantly after a single 48-hour treatment, but did after a second treatment. In the control group without maggot therapy, no significant reduction in the number of patients with a wound infected with either species was observed [22].

Animal Models and Antimicrobial Effects of Maggot Therapy

Tests of the antibacterial capability of larvae have also been conducted using a rat model [23]. Wounds were created in the rats and contaminated with a mixed population of Gram-positive and Gram-negative bacteria. The rats were then placed in one of four groups: 1) non-treated control, 2) antibiotic-treated, 3) maggot-treated, and 4) combined treatment with antibiotic and maggots. Results revealed that maggot-treated wounds reduced bacterial bioburden significantly faster compared to the control and antibiotic-treated groups, allowing for faster wound contraction and healing. The results of treatment with only maggots and the combined maggot and antibiotic treatment were similar [23].

Together with the clinical evidence, these few studies give an indication of the antibacterial capability of maggot therapy *in vivo* and serve to verify the findings of previous investigations conducted *in vitro*. The clinical evidence is still limited, however, and further work into the antibacterial effectiveness of larvae in clinical practice would be useful. However, despite the relative lack of clinical evidence, the idea that effective antibacterial molecules are contained in the excretions and secretions of *L. sericata* larvae is, at this point, widely accepted [24].

The Antimicrobial Compounds in Maggot Excretions and Secretions

Constitutive versus Inducible Antibacterial Activity

One key issue regarding the antibacterial activity is whether bioactivity is constitutive or inducible. In other words, are the antibacterial properties produced by larvae at a constant level, or is production stimulated upon bacterial attack? This is a potential issue for maggot therapy as the use of disinfected or medical-grade larvae is essential for its implementation in modern medicine, in part to meet regulatory requirements and to eliminate the risk of introducing new pathogens into the wound. The inducible nature of larval antibacterial properties could therefore have ramifications for their effectiveness in wound treatment or during *in vitro* experimentation.

Early investigation into the antimicrobial properties of *L. sericata* larvae originally suggested that non-disinfected maggots appeared to produce more bioactive excretions and secretions [7, 8]. Subsequent data produced using whole body extracts and haemolymph noted a three- to six-fold increase in the comparable bioactivity seen when using maggots removed from chronic wounds compared to disinfected maggots [14]. The study also found haemolymph-related activity increased 16-fold when disinfected maggots were injured with a needle containing bacteria. An additional study found that certain genes within the *L. sericata* genome would be differently expressed in second-instar larvae in response to receiving a septic wound (punctuated dorsolaterally with a needle that was contaminated with a lipopolysaccharide solution containing 10 mg/mL crude preparation of *E. coli*). This included genes that encode for signalling proteins, proteinases, homeostasis proteins, and potential antimicrobial peptides, indicating that the production of these factors was induced by the infection event [25]. Further investigations showed that homogenised whole-body extracts of larvae incubated with a bacterial suspension had greater antibacterial activity than extracts from disinfected larvae [26], and that preincubation of third-instar larvae in concentrations of *P. aeruginosa* resulted in the production of excretions and secretions that were significantly more effective than those from disinfected larvae in preventing and degrading biofilm [27].

A separate study found that the level of bacterial contamination had no bearing on the antibacterial potency of larval excretions and secretions [28]. Although this seems to contradict the observations described earlier, the authors draw attention to the fact that their study tested excretions and secretions while the earlier-mentioned studies tested internal haemolymph [25] and/or whole-body extracts [14, 26]. This would suggest that antibacterial factors of excretions and secretions are produced constitutively, whilst antibacterial properties of haemolymph may only be expressed when induced by the presence of bacteria. This idea was further corroborated after finding that a large antimicrobial peptide, the *Lucilia* defensin lucifensin (see below), was produced in the salivary glands and fat body of larvae and that certain infectious environments increased expression in the fat body, but had no effect on its expression of excretion and secretion products [29]. Indeed, many previous studies reporting on the *in vitro* antibacterial activity of collected excretions and secretions did so with disinfected larvae [11, 12, 16, 30, 31], demonstrating that this insect is able to produce and secrete constitutive antibacterial factors without prior exposure to bacteria.

Identification of Maggot-derived Antimicrobial Compounds

With the knowledge that maggot excretions and secretions contain antibacterial properties came an interest in discovering the identities of the compounds responsible. A study by Kerridge and colleagues [15] noted the antibacterial properties of maggot excretions and secretions and found that when extracted they were highly stable as a freeze-dried preparation. They went on to suggest these extractions could be used as a source of novel antibiotic-like compounds, which could be used for infection control. Indeed, the potential for these compounds to be used in the development of novel treatments is driving considerable research into the identification and characterisation of individual antimicrobial compounds or molecules. A summary of this research is presented in this section along with a summary table listing activities, characteristics, and modes of action (Table 9.1 available at https://hdl. handle.net/20.500.12434/2f7d13xl).

Partial characterisation of some small molecular antibacterial compounds was completed by Bexfield and colleagues [12, 30].

Particular attention was paid to a <500 Da fraction that showed broad-spectrum antibacterial activity, including activity against a range of MRSA strains [30]. This fraction was later identified as $C_{10}H_{16}N_6O_9$ and it was registered as the antibiotic Seraticin [32, 33]. Work on uncovering the mode of action of Seraticin indicates it may be due to inhibition of septal formation and cell division (Nigam, unpublished data). Another report also identified low molecular weight compounds that exhibited antimicrobial activity, including phydroxybenzoic acid (138 Da), phydroxyphenylacetic acid (152 Da) and proline diketopiperazine (194 Da), all of which showed activity against *Micrococcus luteus* and/or *P. aeruginosa*, and even more pronounced effects when used in combination [34].

Čeřovský and colleagues [35] later extracted and purified a defensin from the body tissues of *L. sericata* larvae which they believed to be the key antimicrobial component of maggot excretions and secretions. The compound was named "*Lucilia* defensin" or "lucifensin". This defensin was found to show an antibacterial effect against a range of *Staphylococcus* and *Streptococcus* species, though no effect was shown against Gram-negative species [36]. Its mode of action was also described, and involves a process of oligomerisation within the bacterial membrane, forming channels that result in membrane permeabilisation resulting in cell leakage and death [37, 38].

Lucifensin was successfully sequenced and chemically synthesised. The synthetic defensin is active against Gram-positive bacteria, but not Gram-negative strains such as *E. coli*, corroborating previous findings [38]. Additionally, lucifensin is produced in the salivary glands and fat body and certain infectious environments increase expression in the fat body, but not in excretion and secretion products [29]. The structure and characteristics of lucifensin were later described [39], and the potential for manufacturing an antibiotic-like pharmaceutical using a synthesised lucifensin was explored [37]. An almost identical defensin, named "lucifensin II", has also been isolated and described from a closely related blowfly species, *Lucilia cuprina* [40].

Zhang and colleagues [41] described the isolation and purification by ultrafiltration of an antimicrobial protein which they named MAMP. The <10 kDa fraction showed antimicrobial activity against standard and antibiotic-resistant strains of *S. aureas in vitro* and *in vivo*. The authors described possible mechanisms of action by interaction with the bacterial cell membrane and destruction of the cell surface structure. Pöppel and colleagues [10] used RNA sequencing to characterise the transcriptomes of various organs that contribute to the synthesis of antimicrobial peptides and found larvae capable of producing a broad spectrum of antimicrobial peptides. The group identified 47 genes encoding putative antimicrobial peptides, of which 23 were produced as synthetic analogues. These displayed antimicrobial activity against a range of pathogens including *P. aeruginosa*, *Proteus vulgaris*, and *Enterococcus faecalis*, though they found mostly additive effects against *E. coli* and *M. luteus*.

A cecropin antimicrobial peptide named "Lucilin" was identified and partially characterised, and showed activity against a number of Gram-negative bacteria [42]. A variant was also identified in the species *Lucilia exiamia*, which displayed similar properties [43]. In addition, researchers characterised two cationic antimicrobial peptides from *L. sericata*, LA-sarcotoxin and LS-stomoxyn [44]. These showed selective activity against a range of Gram-negative species. Pharmacological profiling indicated no cytotoxicity or cardiotoxicity, and no acute toxicity in experiments with mice, making them lead candidates for the development of novel antibiotics. Having said that, pharmacokinetic properties need to be improved for oral and systemic administration [44].

Table 9.1 Overview of antibacterial molecules/compounds. Inspired by an overview table of maggot bioactivates by Yan and colleagues [45, Table 1]. https://hdl.handle.net/20.500.12434/2f7d13xl.

Mechanism of Maggot Action on Bacterial Biofilms

A bacterial biofilm is an assemblage of microbial cells embedded in a complex self-produced polymeric matrix, which adhere to each other and/or to a surface [46]. Chronic wounds are highly prone to developing biofilm as necrotic tissue allows for bacterial attachment and the wound may be susceptible to infection due to impaired immune response [47–49]. Free-living planktonic bacteria easily attach to the fibrin surface, switching to create a strong, slowly metabolising, walled environment. This results in the depletion of nutrients which in turn causes starvation-induced growth arrest, thought to be a key mechanism in producing antibiotic tolerance in biofilm-forming bacteria [50]. This resistant, stable biofilm then serves to keep the wound in a chronically infected, non-healing state [51, 52]. Biofilms pose a serious problem to wound healing as they are widely recognised as being highly resistant to antibiotics as well as host immune responses [53]. Maggots, however, can tackle bacteria in this more resistant form, and various studies have sought to determine the effect of maggot excretions and secretions both on the ability of bacteria to form biofilm communities, and as an agent to disrupt existing bacterial biofilms.

Initial investigations into the effect of maggot excretions and secretions against biofilm found that different species of bacteria were impacted to varying degrees. The formation of biofilms composed of *S. aureus* was blocked by freeze-dried maggot excretions and secretions, whilst the formation of biofilms by *P. aeruginosa* was initially enhanced by the addition of maggot excretions and secretions before the biofilm collapsed after 10 hours. Against preformed biofilms, excretions and secretions were able to degrade *S. aureus*, whilst ten-fold more was required to degrade *P. aeruginosa* which only began 10 hours after application [31]. This difference in activity against different species was also observed in a subsequent investigation. Maggot excretions and secretions significantly reduced biofilm formation by *S. aureus* and *E. cloacae*, while growth of *P. mirabilis* was unaffected and even stimulated [54]. These results suggest that maggot ES may act selectively against different strains, rather than combatting a broad spectrum of bacteria.

Maggot excretions and secretions were also observed to disrupt biofilm formation of two different strains of *Staphylococcus epidermidis* (1457 and 5179-r1) that exhibit different mechanisms of bacterial adhesion and subsequent biofilm formation, thus corroborating the idea that more than one bioactive entity or mechanism present in maggot excretions and secretions may be involved in the prevention of biofilm formation [55]. The authors provided further support for this theory when they demonstrated differing effects of an *L. sericata*-derived recombinant chymotrypsin on bacterial adhesion of multiple *Staphylococcus* strains. They concluded that chymotrypsin was unlikely to represent a standalone agent. Rather, maggots secrete a variety of bioactive antibiofilm agents, of which chymotrypsin is only one component [56].

In a separate investigation which examined biofilm formation on surfaces commonly used in a medical setting, maggot excretions and secretions were found to prevent biofilm formation and disrupt existing biofilms of *P. aeruginosa*, with more effective excretions and secretions being produced by third-instar maggots than first-instar maggots. In a subsequent study, the research group also observed antibiofilm activity against *S. aureus* and *S. epidermidis* [57]. An *in vitro* experiment on dermal pig skin explants found that maggots were effective in combatting biofilms of *S. aureus* and *P. aeruginosa* [58]. Interestingly, results from an investigation into the effect of incubating maggots with *P. aeruginosa* bacteria, and then washing and collecting excretions and secretions from these bacteria pre-treated maggots, suggested that excretions and secretions from maggots previously exposed to *P. aeruginosa* were more effective in degrading biofilm of that species than those from disinfected maggots [27]. Additionally, fatty acid extract from dried *L. sericata* larvae was found to prevent biofilm formation of *S. aureus* and *Streptococcus pneumonia* and to eradicate preformed biofilms of these bacteria [59].

As well as whole extracts of larvae, isolated molecules derived from maggot excretions and secretions have also been found to display antibiofilm properties. The recombinant Chymotrypsin 1, a serine proteinase, was found to be effective in degrading macromolecules containing microbial surface components that recognise adhesive matrix molecules (MSCRAMMs). MSCRAMMs play an important role in the initial attachment of bacteria prior to biofilm formation and by degrading these molecules, Chymotrypsin 1 may work to impede colonisation and subsequent biofilm formation [60]. Further work corroborated this notion, finding that the recombinant Chymotrypsin can interfere with bacterial adhesion and disrupt protein-dependent bacterial biofilm-formation mechanisms [56]. Additionally, another molecule, a purified DNAse isolated from maggot excretions and secretions was found to degrade extracellular bacterial DNA in *Pseudomonas* biofilms [61]. Bacteria need to acquire extracellular DNA (either from host tissue itself or from their own bacterial sources) in order to help construct a biofilm, but maggot DNAse appeared capable of digesting all extracellular and bacterial sources of DNA, and thus inhibited the ability of bacteria to form a biofilm [61].

A common observation from biofilm investigations is that whilst maggot excretions and secretions are able to degrade and break down the biofilm of various species, the bacteria which are released from these biofilms are not destroyed [27, 31, 54, 55]. This was explored further by a group of researchers who noted that biofilms resisted antibiotics alone, but found that combining a treatment of maggot secretion and antibiotics (vancomycin, daptomycin or clindamycin) resulted in both the break-down of *S. aureus* biofilm and the elimination of the resulting bacteria [62]. This introduces a promising approach to the treatment of biofilm-infected chronic wounds, whereby use of a combination of maggot excretions and secretions and antibiotics could result in a more successful treatment than the use of a single method alone. Other findings also support this idea. A study investigating the combined use of maggot excretions and secretions with ciprofloxacin showed enhanced antimicrobial activity compared to the use of either individually [63]. Two other commonly used antibiotics, gentamicin and flucloxacillin, also showed enhanced synergistic antibacterial activity with maggot excretions and secretions [64].

Antifungal Activity of Maggot Excretions and Secretions

Within the scope of investigating antimicrobial activity of *L. sericata* larvae, research has primarily focussed on antibacterial compounds. The study of selective antifungal agents, meanwhile, has received much less attention. In an initial report, *L. sericata* larvae were found to be able to ingest yeasts, and ES collected from these maggots showed moderate antifungal activity against *Trichophyton terreste* mycelium [65]. This suggested the possibility of using maggot therapy in the treatment of wounds with fungal infections and superficial fungal infections. The authors went on to suggest that alkaline compounds in maggot excretions and secretions (such as ammonium carbonate, allantoin, and urea), may be partially responsible for this antifungal activity. Subsequent separate investigations also noted the potent antifungal activity of maggot excretions and secretions against *Candida*, *Aspergillus*, *Geotricum*, and *Saccharomyces* species [66, 67]. The antifungal component was characterised and found to be heat-stable and resistant to freeze-drying. Following ultrafiltration of maggot excretions and secretions into three main fractions (>10, 10–0.5, and <0.5 kDa), it was revealed that the greatest level of anti-*Candida* activity was observed in the <500 Da fraction, suggesting that maggots were capable of producing a very small, but very active, antifungal molecule [67]. In addition, a larger antibacterial molecule, Lucifensin, also showed slight antifungal activity against *Candida albicans* [38].

Characterisation of one of the maggot antifungal compounds was also achieved in a 2014 study which managed to produce a recombinant form of the discovered peptide. Named "Lucimycin", the novel antifungal peptide showed activity against a range of phyla including Ascomycota, Basidiomycota, and Zygomycota, as well as the oomycete plant pathogen *Phytophtora parasitica* [68]. This shows potential for the use of antifungal peptides isolated from *L. sericata* not only in human medicine for the treatment of fungal infections, but also in agriculture for crop protection. The possibility of producing transgenic plants capable of expressing lucimycin is also postulated [68].

Additionally, maggot therapy has been used successfully in the treatment of wounds with mycotic infection. In one described case study, maggots in biobags were used for the treatment of a complex hand injury that was infected with *Absidia corymbifera* [69]. Significant improvement in wound condition was reported after just two 72-hour applications of maggots. Maggots effectively removed necrotic tissue and the mycotic infection was successfully eradicated [69].

Summary

Dating back to the 1920s, the antimicrobial potential of medical maggots has been recognised and explored. In more recent years, the interest in understanding and identifying the antimicrobial properties of maggot excretions and secretions has been driven by the potential to use medical maggots as a source of novel antibiotics and anti-infectives. This is particularly relevant at this time considering the rise of drug-resistant forms of pathogenic bacteria such as MRSA.

There is mounting evidence for the antimicrobial activity of maggot ES against a range of bacteria and fungi. This includes efficacy against antibiotic-resistant bacterial strains, with greater activity generally observed against Gram-positive species and less so against Gram-negative bacteria. However, some studies have shown contradictory results in this regard, which may be a result of differing methods that have been used to test the antimicrobial effects of maggot excretions and secretions. Consequently, a greater consensus in testing methodology may be useful to produce more consistent and comparable results. Evidence has also shown action of maggot excretions and secretions against biofilms, to which chronic wounds can be prone, and which pose a significant problem to wound healing due to their resistance to antibiotics. This is therefore an important and promising area of investigation. Much of the evidence relating to the antimicrobial properties of maggots has relied on investigations conducted *in vitro*. A small number of clinical reports and case studies have been described, but their scope and scale has generally been limited, so the clinical evidence is still lacking. Further investigations would be useful to more conclusively demonstrate the antimicrobial properties of maggot therapy clinically.

As well as understanding the properties of maggot excretions and secretions, there is also great interest in identifying the compounds responsible with a view to developing new treatments. So far, a number of antibacterial molecules have been identified with varying structures, mechanisms, and activities against Gram-positive and Gram-negative bacteria, and susceptible and resistant strains. Some antibiofilm and antifungal molecules have also been described. The various research and discoveries in this area highlight the versatility of larval excretions and secretions as sources of effective antimicrobial molecules. It is anticipated that ongoing efforts in this field will advance our understanding of maggot therapy and its therapeutic principles and that this will lead to the development of new therapies. Many of these secreted factors are currently being isolated and investigated for the development of new antimicrobial drugs and treatments. However, when whole maggots are placed on a chronic and infected wound, they excrete not just a single antimicrobial compound, but a cocktail of such compounds thus providing an effective and unique antimicrobial environment. It is therefore unclear whether it will ever be possible to match the multiple therapeutic benefits conveyed by whole-organism maggot therapy with drugs based on individual active compounds of maggot excretions and secretions.

References

1. Edwards, R. and K.G. Harding, *Bacteria and Wound Healing*. Current Opinion in Infectious Diseases, 2004. 17(2): pp. 91–96, https://doi.org/10.1097/00001432-200404000-00004.

2. Baer, W.S., *The Treatment of Chronic Osteomyelitis with the Maggot (Larva of the Blow Fly)*. The Journal of Bone & Joint Surgery, 1931. 13(3): pp. 438–475, https://doi.org/10.1007/s11999-010-1416-3.

3. Harvey, M., *The Natural History of Medicinal Flies*, in *A Complete Guide to Maggot Therapy: Clinical Practice, Therapeutic Principles, Production, Distribution, and Ethics*, F. Stadler (ed.). 2022, Cambridge: Open Book Publishers, pp. 121–142, https://doi.org/10.11647/OBP.0300.07.

4. Duncan, J.T., *On a Bactericidal Principle Present in the Alimentary Canal of Insects and Arachnids*. Parasitology, 1926. 18(2): pp. 238–252, https://dx.doi.org/10.1017/S0031182000005205.

5. Robinson, W. and V.H. Norwood, *The Role of Surgical Maggots in the Disinfection of Osteomyelitis and Other Infected Wounds*. The Journal of Bone & Joint Surgery, 1933. 15(2): pp. 409–412.

6. Robinson, W. and V.H. Norwood, *Destruction of Pyogenic Bacteria in the Alimentary Tract of Surgical Maggots Implanted in Infected Wounds*. Journal of Laboratory and Clinical Medicine, 1934. 19(6): pp. 581–586.

7. Simmons, S.W., *A Bactericidal Principle in Excretions of Surgical Maggots Which Destroys Important Etiological Agents of Pyogenic Infections*. Journal of Bacteriology, 1935. 30(3): pp. 253–267, https://doi.org/10.1128/jb.30.3.253-267.1935.

8. Simmons, S.W., *The Bactericidal Properties of Excretions of the Maggot of Lucilia sericata*. Bulletin of Entomological Research, 1935. 26(4): pp. 559–563, https://doi.org/10.1017/S0007485300036907.

9. Pavillard, E.R. and E.A. Wright, *An Antibiotic from Maggots*. Nature, 1957. 180: pp. 916–917, https://doi.org/10.1038/180916b0.

10. Pöppel, A., et al., *Antimicrobial Peptides Expressed in Medicinal Maggots of the Blow Fly Lucilia sericata Show Combinatorial Activity against Bacteria*. Antimicrobial Agents and Chemotherapy, 2015. 59(5): pp. 2508–2514, https://doi.org/10.1128/AAC.05180-14.

11. Thomas, S., et al., *The Anti-microbial Activity of Maggot Secretions: Results of a Preliminary Study*. Journal of Tissue Viability, 1999. 9(4): pp. 127–132, https://doi.org/10.1016/S0965-206X(99)80032-1.

12. Bexfield, A., et al., *Detection and Partial Characterisation of Two Antibacterial Factors from the Excretions/Secretions of the Medicinal Maggot Lucilia sericata and Their Activity against Methicillin-resistant Staphylococcus aureus*

(*MRSA*). Microbes and Infection, 2004. 6(14): pp. 1297–1304, https://doi.org/10.1016/j.micinf.2004.08.011.

13.   Daeschlein, G., et al., *In vitro Antibacterial Activity of Lucilia sericata Maggot Secretions.* Skin Pharmacology and Physiology, 2007. 20(2): pp. 112–115, https://doi.org/10.1159/000097983.

14.   Huberman, L., et al., *Antibacterial Properties of Whole Body Extracts and Haemolymph of Lucilia sericata Maggots.* Journal of Wound Care, 2007. 16(3): pp. 123–127, https://doi.org/10.12968/jowc.2007.16.3.27011.

15.   Kerridge, A., H. Lappin-Scott, and J.R. Stevens, *Antibacterial Properties of Larval Secretions of the Blowfly, Lucilia sericata.* Medical and Veterinary Entomology, 2005. 19(3): pp. 333–337, https://doi.org/10.1111/j.1365-2915.2005.00577.x.

16.   Jaklič, D., et al., *Selective Antimicrobial Activity of Maggots against Pathogenic Bacteria.* Journal of Medical Microbiology, 2008. 57(5): pp. 617–625, https://doi.org/10.1099/jmm.0.47515-0.

17.   Steenvoorde, P. and G.N. Jukema, *The Antimicrobial Activity of Maggots: In-vivo Results.* Journal of Tissue Viability, 2004. 14(3): pp. 97–101, https://doi.org/10.1016/S0965-206X(04)43005-8.

18.   Andersen, A.S., et al., *Quorum-sensing-regulated Virulence Factors in Pseudomonas aeruginosa Are Toxic to Lucilia sericata Maggots.* Microbiology, 2010. 156(2): pp. 400–407, https://doi.org/10.1099/mic.0.032730-0.

19.   Barnes, K.M., R.A. Dixon, and D.E. Gennard, *The Antibacterial Potency of the Medicinal Maggot, Lucilia sericata (Meigen): Variation in Laboratory Evaluation.* Journal of Microbiological Methods, 2010. 82(3): pp. 234–237, https://doi.org/10.1016/j.mimet.2010.06.005.

20.   Barnes, K.M., D.E. Gennard, and R.A. Dixon, *An Assessment of the Antibacterial Activity in Larval Excretion/Secretion of Four Species of Insects Recorded in Association with Corpses, Using Lucilia sericata Meigen as the Marker Species.* Bulletin of Entomological Research, 2010. 100(6): pp. 635–640, https://doi.org/10.1017/S000748530999071X.

21.   Mumcuoglu, K.Y., et al., *Destruction of Bacteria in the Digestive Tract of the Maggot of Lucilia sericata (Diptera: Calliphoridae).* Journal of Medical Entomology, 2001. 38(2): pp. 161–166, https://doi.org/10.1603/0022-2585-38.2.161.

22.   Malekian, A., et al., *Efficacy of Maggot Therapy on Staphylococcus aureus and Pseudomonas aeruginosa in Diabetic Foot Ulcers.* Journal of Wound, Ostomy and Continence Nursing, 2019. 46(1): pp. 25–29, https://doi.org/10.1097/WON.0000000000000496.

23.   Borkataki, S., et al., *Therapeutic Use of Lucilia sericata Maggot in Controlling Bacterial Bio-burden in Rat Wound Model.* Tropical Biomedicine, 2018. 35(3): pp. 627–638.

24.   Cazander, G., et al., *Multiple Actions of Lucilia sericata Larvae in Hard-to-heal Wounds: Larval Secretions Contain Molecules that Accelerate Wound Healing,*

Reduce Chronic Inflammation and Inhibit Bacterial Infection. BioEssays, 2013. 35(12): pp. 1083–1092, https://doi.org/10.1002/bies.201300071.

25. Altincicek, B. and A. Vilcinskas, *Septic Injury-inducible Genes in Medicinal Maggots of the Green Blow Fly Lucilia sericata.* Insect Molecular Biology, 2009. 18(1): pp. 119–125, https://doi.org/10.1111/j.1365-2583.2008.00856.x.

26. Kawabata, T., et al., *Induction of Antibacterial Activity in Larvae of the Blowfly Lucilia sericata by an Infected Environment.* Medical and Veterinary Entomology, 2010. 24(4): pp. 375–381, https://doi.org/10.1111/j.1365-2915.2010.00902.x.

27. Jiang, K.C., et al., *Excretions/Secretions from Bacteria-pretreated Maggot Are More Effective against Pseudomonas aeruginosa Biofilms.* PloS ONE, 2012. 7(11): pp. e49815-e49815, https://doi.org/10.1371/journal.pone.0049815.

28. Barnes, K.M. and D.E. Gennard, *The Effect of Bacterially-dense Environments on the Development and Immune Defences of the Blowfly Lucilia sericata.* Physiological Entomology, 2011. 36(1): pp. 96–100, https://doi.org/10.1111/j.1365-3032.2010.00759.x.

29. Valachová, I., et al., *Expression of Lucifensin in Lucilia sericata Medicinal Maggots in Infected Environments.* Cell and Tissue Research, 2013. 353(1): pp. 165–171, https://doi.org/10.1007/s00441-013-1626-6.

30. Bexfield, A., et al., *The Antibacterial Activity against MRSA Strains and Other Bacteria of a <500 Da Fraction from Maggot Excretions/Secretions of Lucilia sericata (Diptera: Calliphoridae).* Microbes and Infection, 2008. 10(4): pp. 325–333, https://doi.org/10.1016/j.micinf.2007.12.011.

31. van der Plas, M.J.A., et al., *Maggot Excretions/Secretions Are Differentially Effective against Biofilms of Staphylococcus aureus and Pseudomonas aeruginosa.* Journal of Antimicrobial Chemotherapy, 2008. 61(1): pp. 117–122, https://doi.org/10.1093/jac/dkm407.

32. Bexfield, A., et al. *Antimicrobial Composition and a Method of Controlling Contamination and Infection Using Said Composition.* 2010. https://patents.google.com/patent/US20100215765.

33. Nigam, Y., et al., *The Physiology of Wound Healing by the Medicinal Maggot, Lucilia sericata*, S.J. Simpson, Editor. 2010, Elsevier: London. pp. 39–81.

34. Huberman, L., et al., *Antibacterial Substances of Low Molecular Weight Isolated from the Blowfly, Lucilia sericata.* Medical and Veterinary Entomology, 2007. 21(2): pp. 127–131, https://doi.org/10.1111/j.1365-2915.2007.00668.x.

35. Čeřovský, V., et al., *Lucifensin, the Long-sought Antimicrobial Factor of Medicinal Maggots of the Blowfly Lucilia sericata.* Cellular and Molecular Life Sciences, 2010. 67(3): pp. 455–466, https://doi.org/10.1007/s00018-009-0194-0.

36. Andersen, A.S., et al., *A Novel Approach to the Antimicrobial Activity of Maggot Debridement Therapy.* Journal of Antimicrobial Chemotherapy, 2010. 65(8): pp. 1646–1654, https://doi.org/10.1093/jac/dkq165.

37. Čeřovský, V. and R. Bém, *Lucifensins, the Insect Defensins of Biomedical Importance: The Story behind Maggot Therapy.* Pharmaceuticals, 2014. 7(3): pp. 251–264, https://doi.org/10.3390/ph7030251.

38. Čeřovský, V., et al., *Lucifensin, a Novel Insect Defensin of Medicinal Maggots: Synthesis and Structural Study.* ChemBioChem, 2011. 12(9): pp. 1352–1361, https://doi.org/10.1002/cbic.201100066.

39. Nygaard, M.K.E., et al., *The Insect Defensin Lucifensin from Lucilia sericata.* Journal of Biomolecular NMR, 2012. 52(3): pp. 277–282, https://doi.org/10.1007/s10858-012-9608-7.

40. El Shazely, B., et al., *Lucifensin II, a Defensin of Medicinal Maggots of the Blowfly Lucilia cuprina (Diptera: Calliphoridae).* Journal of Medical Entomology, 2013. 50(3): pp. 571–578, https://doi.org/10.1603/ME12208.

41. Zhang, Z., et al., *Activity of Antibacterial Protein from Maggots against Staphylococcus aureus in vitro and in vivo.* International Journal of Molecular Medicine, 2013. 31(5): pp. 1159–1165, https://doi.org/10.3892/ijmm.2013.1291.

42. Téllez, G.A. and J.C. Castaño-Osorio, *Expression and Purification of an Active Cecropin-like Recombinant Protein against Multidrug Resistance Escherichia coli.* Protein Expression and Purification, 2014. 100: pp. 48–53, https://doi.org/10.1016/j.pep.2014.05.004.

43. Téllez, G.A., et al., *Identification, Characterization, Immunolocalization, and Biological Activity of Lucilin Peptide.* Acta Tropica, 2018. 185: pp. 318–326, https://doi.org/10.1016/j.actatropica.2018.06.003.

44. Hirsch, R., et al., *Profiling Antimicrobial Peptides from the Medical Maggot Lucilia sericata as Potential Antibiotics for MDR Gram-negative Bacteria.* Journal of Antimicrobial Chemotherapy, 2019. 74(1): pp. 96–107, https://doi.org/10.1093/jac/dky386.

45. Yan, L., et al., *Pharmacological Properties of the Medical Maggot: A Novel Therapy Overview.* Evidence-Based Complementary and Alternative Medicine, 2018. 2018: pp. 1–11, https://doi.org/10.1155/2018/4934890.

46. Donlan, R.M., *Biofilms: Microbial Life on Surfaces.* 2002, Centers for Disease Control and Prevention (CDC), pp. 881–890.

47. Wolcott, R.D., D.D. Rhoads, and S.E. Dowd, *Biofilms and Chronic Wound Inflammation.* 2008, MA Healthcare London, pp. 333–341.

48. Siddiqui, A.R. and J.M. Bernstein, *Chronic Wound Infection: Facts and Controversies.* Clinics in Dermatology, 2010. 28(5): pp. 519–526, https://doi.org/10.1016/j.clindermatol.2010.03.009.

49. Zhao, G., et al., *Biofilms and Inflammation in Chronic Wounds.* Advances in Wound Care, 2013. 2(7): pp. 389–399, https://doi.org/10.1089/wound.2012.0381.

50. Nguyen, D., et al., *Active Starvation Responses Mediate Antibiotic Tolerance in Biofilms and Nutrient-limited Bacteria.* Science, 2011. 334(6058): pp. 982–986, https://doi.org/10.1126/science.1211037.

51. Harrison-Balestra, C., et al., *A Wound-isolated Pseudomonas aeruginosa Grows a Biofilm in vitro within 10 Hours and Is Visualized by Light Microscopy.* Dermatologic Surgery, 2003. 29(6): pp. 631–635, https://doi.org/10.1046/j.1524-4725.2003.29146.x.

52. Pritchard, D.I. and Y. Nigam, *Maximising the Secondary Beneficial Effects of Larval Debridement Therapy.* Journal of Wound Care, 2013. 22(11): pp. 610–616, https://doi.org/10.12968/jowc.2013.22.11.610.

53. Høiby, N., et al., *Antibiotic Resistance of Bacterial Biofilms.* International Journal of Antimicrobial Agents, 2010. 35(4): pp. 322–332, https://doi.org/10.1016/j.ijantimicag.2009.12.011.

54. Bohova, J., et al., *Selective Antibiofilm Effects of Lucilia sericata Larvae Secretions/Excretions against Wound Pathogens.* Evidence-Based Complementary and Alternative Medicine, 2014. 2014: pp. 1–9, https://doi.org/10.1155/2014/857360.

55. Harris, L.G., et al., *Disruption of Staphylococcus Epidermidis Biofilms by Medicinal Maggot Lucilia sericata Excretions/Secretions.* International Journal of Artificial Organs, 2009. 32(9): pp. 555–564, https://doi.org/10.1177/039139880903200904.

56. Harris, L.G., et al., *Lucilia sericata Chymotrypsin Disrupts Protein Adhesin-mediated Staphylococcal Biofilm Formation.* Applied and Environmental Microbiology, 2013. 79(4): pp. 1393–1395, http://dx.doi.org/10.1128/AEM.03689-12.

57. Cazander, G., et al., *Maggot Excretions Inhibit Biofilm Formation on Biomaterials.* Clinical Orthopaedics and Related Research, 2010. 468(10): pp. 2789–2796, https://doi.org/10.1007/s11999-010-1309-5.

58. Cowan, L.J., et al., *Chronic Wounds, Biofilms and Use of Medicinal Larvae.* Ulcers, 2013. 2013(Article ID 487024): pp. 1–7, https://doi.org/10.1155/2013/487024.

59. Liu, J., et al., *Antibacterial and Anti-biofilm Effects of Fatty Acids Extract of Dried Lucilia sericata Larvae against Staphylococcus aureus and Streptococcus pneumoniae in vitro.* Natural Product Research, 2019. https://doi.org/10.1080/14786419.2019.1627353.

60. Pritchard, D.I. and A.P. Brown, *Degradation of MSCRAMM Target Macromolecules in VLU Slough by Lucilia sericata Chymotrypsin 1 (ISP) Persists in the Presence of Tissue Gelatinase Activity.* International Wound Journal, 2015. 12(4): pp. 414–421, https://doi.org/10.1111/iwj.12124.

61. Brown, A., et al., *Blow Fly Lucilia sericata Nuclease Digests DNA Associated with Wound Slough/Eschar and with Pseudomonas aeruginosa Biofilm.*

Medical and Veterinary Entomology, 2012. 26(4): pp. 432–439, https://doi.org/10.1111/j.1365-2915.2012.01029.x.

62. van der Plas, M.J.A., et al., *Combinations of Maggot Excretions/Secretions and Antibiotics Are Effective against Staphylococcus aureus Biofilms and the Bacteria Derived Therefrom.* The Journal of Antimicrobial Chemotherapy, 2010. 65(5): pp. 917–923, https://doi.org/10.1093/jac/dkq042.

63. Arora, S., C. Baptista, and C.S. Lim, *Maggot Metabolites and Their Combinatory Effects with Antibiotic on Staphylococcus aureus.* Annals of Clinical Microbiology and Antimicrobials, 2011. 10(6): pp. 1–8, https://doi.org/10.1186/1476-0711-10-6.

64. Cazander, G., et al., *Synergism between Maggot Excretions and Antibiotics.* Wound Repair and Regeneration, 2010. 18(6): pp. 637–642, https://doi.org/10.1111/j.1524-475X.2010.00625.x.

65. Alnaimat, S.M., M. Wainwright, and S.H. Aladaileh, *An Initial in vitro Investigation into the Potential Therapeutic Use of Lucilia sericata Maggot to Control Superficial Fungal Infections.* Jordan Journal of Biological Sciences, 2013. 6(2): pp. 137–142, https://doi.org/10.12816/0000271.

66. Amer, M.S., et al., *Antimicrobial and Antiviral Activity of Maggots Extracts of Lucilia sericata (Diptera: Calliphoridae).* Egyptian Journal of Aquatic Biology and Fisheries, 2019. 23(4): pp. 51–64, https://doi.org/10.21608/ejabf.2019.52173.

67. Evans, R., E. Dudley, and Y. Nigam, *Detection and Partial Characterization of Antifungal Bioactivity from the Secretions of the Medicinal Maggot, Lucilia sericata.* Wound Repair and Regeneration, 2015. 23(3): pp. 361–368, https://doi.org/10.1111/wrr.12287.

68. Pöppel, A., et al., *Lucimycin, an Antifungal Peptide from the Therapeutic Maggot of the Common Green Bottle Fly Lucilia sericata.* Biological Chemistry, 2014. 395(6): pp. 649–656, https://doi.org/10.1515/hsz-2013-0263.

69. Bohac, M., et al., *Maggot Therapy in Treatment of a Complex Hand Injury Complicated by Mycotic Infection.* Bratislava Medical Journal, 2015. 116(11): pp. 671–673, https://doi.org/10.4149/BLL_2015_128.

10. Maggot-assisted Wound Healing

Yamni Nigam and Michael R. Wilson

Unlike any other wound care device or pharmaceutical, medicinal maggots convey multiple therapeutic benefits at the same time when applied to chronic and/or infected wounds. In addition to providing an ideal healing environment through debridement and infection control, maggot excretions and secretions actively promote wound healing through a wide range of specific physiological mechanisms and pathways. After a brief review of early studies into the healing properties of medicinal maggots, and what is known from randomised clinical trials, the chapter explains in detail the biochemical and physiological principles of maggot-mediated wound healing.

Introduction

For years there have been anecdotal reports from clinicians suggesting that wounds treated with maggots have better outcomes and heal faster compared to non-maggot treated wounds. It is only in recent years, however, that these reports have been further investigated. The evidence supporting maggot-induced promotion of healing comes from randomised controlled trials, clinical studies, and scientific laboratory investigations.

A wound typically goes through three major phases on its way to complete healing [1]. These are the phases of inflammation (including haemostasis), proliferation and maturation (or remodelling). The

https://doi.org/10.11647/OBP.0300.10

inflammatory phase serves to immediately protect the body, and results in the active recruitment of phagocytic and destructive white blood cells (leucocytes) [1]. These cells debride injured and non-viable tissue, and substantially diminish the bioburden of the wound, enabling it to progress to the next phase of healing. Wounds will only progress to healing if the debridement and disinfection processes have been successful [2].

Once the wound has entered the proliferative phase, several physiological events occur. This includes the process of granulation, which involves the laying down of new foundation tissue in the wound base. Specialised cells called fibroblasts migrate inwards from the wound margins and begin to generate and assemble collagen, the major component of wound connective tissue. Fibroblasts are stimulated by chemical activators and messengers, known as cytokines, which are mostly released by macrophages (the dominant leucocyte towards the end of the inflammatory phase). Fibroblasts themselves secrete a variety of cytokines (e.g. platelet-derived growth factor (PDGF) and tissue growth factor beta (TGFb)), allowing other vital cells such as endothelial cells and angiocytes to proliferate and grow new blood vessels [3]. New blood vessels provide much-needed oxygen and nutrients that help to facilitate the growth and proliferation of new tissue filling the wound.

Early Studies on Maggot-led Healing

One of the first reports to explore the exact mechanisms involved in wound healing by maggots was a study which examined the outcomes of pressure ulcers in spinal cord injury patients, some of which were treated conventionally, and some with maggots. Not only did debridement occur more rapidly in patients treated with maggot therapy, but also the wound surface area decreased and wound healing was faster [4]. A later, larger-scale study discovered that pressure ulcers treated with maggots were found to contain twice the amount of granulation tissue compared to wounds not treated with maggot therapy. A set of 31 wounds was observed, at first receiving conventional treatment and then the very same wounds were treated with maggot therapy. While conventional treatment resulted in a 1.2 cm^2 per week increase in wound area, subsequent maggot therapy resulted in a 1.2

cm² decrease in wound surface area [5]. In a further study examining changes to necrotic tissue and total surface area of non-healing wounds following maggot therapy, the size and shape of diabetic foot ulcers was calculated, including other measures such as coverage of granulation tissue and time to healing. Maggot-treated wounds were associated with hastened growth of granulation tissue and greater healing rates. After 4 weeks of maggot therapy and 1 to 2 treatment cycles per week, on average 56% of the wound base was covered with healthy granulation tissue. However, in conventionally treated wounds granulation tissue covered only on average 15% of the wound base after 4 weeks [6].

The findings from Sherman and colleagues encouraged other researchers to undertake clinical investigations on maggot-assisted wound healing. For example, in a study of 30 patients with chronic leg ulcers who were treated with maggots over 4 days, investigators measured several parameters after removal of the larvae [7]. These included a wound score on a sliding scale from 0 to 15, with higher scores indicating poorer wound condition. The score accounted for various characteristics including slough coverage, exudation, inflammation, and malodour. Wound scores dramatically improved after only a single application of maggots, from 13.5 to 6.3, with a particularly remarkable improvement in granulation. The investigators also used remittance spectroscopy to monitor the optical characteristics of the wound area in the visible and near-infra-red spectral range. Before maggot therapy, wounds were necrotic, fibrin-covered, and without granulation tissue. Typical spectra in these wounds showed a high remittance. However, after maggot therapy, the remittance spectra changed. The authors observed a marked decrease in remittance because of the large absorption of the fresh granulation tissue. The findings suggested an increase in local blood flow and a decrease in oedema, which were responsible for red granulation tissue formation and an improvement in wound healing following treatment with maggots [7].

A separate clinical study assessing the healing of diabetic foot ulcers in non-ambulatory patients, found that time to healing was significantly shorter in the group treated with maggot therapy (18.5 weeks) compared to the control group (22.4 weeks), and patients in the control group were also three times more likely to require an amputation [8].

Randomised Controlled Trials on Wound Healing Using Maggots

There have also been various clinical trials including randomised controlled trials (RCTs) that have investigated the effectiveness of maggot therapy. More recently, meta-analyses of these studies have been conducted that have sought to collate and review the evidence. The first such meta-analysis consisted of 7 trials conducted from 1995–2009, including three randomised controlled trials and four non-randomised trials [9]. This analysis suggested that whilst larvae were effective in debridement, there was not enough evidence to say that maggot therapy resulted in faster healing. This was primarily due to the sub-optimal design of some of the studies with the authors citing problems concerning small sample sizes, unclear inclusion and exclusion criteria, lack of blinding of outcome assessors, and lack of randomisation resulting in poor-quality data. It was concluded that better designed investigations were required in this area in order to form more concrete conclusions about the efficacy of maggot therapy compared to conventional treatments [9].

A later meta-analysis considered 12 comparative studies, including six randomised controlled trials, from 2000–2014. Based on the analysis of these twelve studies, the authors concluded that larval therapy was both more effective and more efficient in the debridement of chronic ulcers when compared with conventional treatments, but it was also associated with quicker healing rates of chronic wounds. They noted a shortened time to healing in ulcers, a longer antibiotic-free time period, and a decreased amputation risk compared with conventional therapies [10]. A more recent review of clinical studies of maggot therapy from 2000–2015 showed a significantly higher rate of successful debridement compared with conventional treatment, but also that time to healing was significantly (3.1 weeks) shorter than the conventional strand [11]. It was, however, suggested that the shorter time to healing may be aided by more successful debridement using maggot therapy, or a combination of this with some other enhanced-healing mechanism. Such reports highlight the need for larger, well-designed RCTs to scientifically investigate and evaluate maggot-enhanced healing. Unfortunately, the relative paucity of such gold-standard trials for maggot therapy means that some researchers, practitioners, and regulators remain sceptical about the benefits of the therapy. Chapter 11 also discusses the need for randomised controlled trials as a necessary step toward the establishment of new medicinal fly species in clinical practice [12].

Scientific Mechanisms by Which Maggots Promote Wound Healing

Ever since early scientific reports of maggot therapy and the discovery of their effectiveness in wound treatment, there have been theories on how maggots stimulate the healing process. Initially, it was suspected that wound healing was somehow stimulated by the physical action of the larvae crawling over the wound surface [13, 14]. Early research suggested that stimulation of tissue growth was due to the action of allantoin or ammonia bicarbonate, both of which are present in maggot excretions, and both of which were found to promote wound healing [15, 16]. In recent years, research has focussed on the notion that wound healing effects are primarily due to the action of maggot secretions which can aid wound healing by a number of different mechanisms. As such, several *in vitro* studies provide convincing molecular evidence to support the hypothesis that maggots promote wound healing through mechanisms other than debridement.

Effect of Maggots on the Inflammatory Phase of Wound Healing

Chronic wounds are, by definition, non-healing and are unable to progress rapidly through the three main stages of wound healing (inflammation, proliferation and maturation), often remaining in the inflammatory phase [17]. Various investigations have found that maggot secretions may play a role in inhibiting the mechanisms and processes that perpetuate this chronic state of inflammation, and thereby help the wound to heal. Neutrophils are the first line of defence against infection. Upon phagocytosis of a pathogen, a respiratory burst occurs which causes the reduction of oxygen to form superoxide, hydrogen peroxide (H_2O_2), and the hydroxyl radical. These reactive oxygen species, along with other oxygen-derived molecules, participate in the elimination of the pathogen [18].

Several studies suggest that the beneficial effects of maggots may lie in their ability to reduce these levels of pro-inflammatory factors. For example, a study investigating the effect of *L. sericata* salivary gland extract on the activity of human neutrophils (stimulated with opsonised zymosan) found that exposure to high concentrations of the extract resulted in a significant reduction in both the level of superoxide and the release of myeloperoxidase, a pro-inflammatory molecule [19]. Just prior to this, a study had also looked at the effect of maggot secretions on human neutrophil pro-inflammatory responses [20]. Neutrophils from healthy donors were stimulated with either formyl-MetLeu-Phe (fMLP) or phorbol-12-myristate-13-acetate (PMA) and incubated with increasing concentrations of secretions ranging from 0.5–100 µg/mL. Hydrogen peroxide production via fMLP-stimulated neutrophils was inhibited by as little as 5 µg/mL of secretions, whilst PMA-induced hydrogen peroxide production was inhibited in a dose-dependent manner. Incubation with maggot secretions also reduced fMLP-stimulated expression of CD11b/CD18, a protein involved in the innate immune system which mediates inflammation, and inhibited fMLP-induced neutrophil migration. The authors concluded that maggot secretions inhibited the production and expression of pro-inflammatory mediators such as reactive oxygen species and components of the complement system, and prevented the movement of neutrophils to the wound area. Therefore, maggot secretion may contribute to the healing of chronic wounds via the inhibition of ongoing inflammation and tissue breakdown [20].

Monocytes are white blood cell precursors to macrophages. Along with neutrophils they are involved in the innate immune system and engulf apoptotic cells and pathogens as well as controlling the inflammatory process by secreting cytokines and growth factors, which in turn recruit more inflammatory cells [21]. Monocytes and macrophages are considered to be the two most vital leukocytes for wound healing [22]. Once monocytes infiltrate an area of inflamed tissue, they differentiate into either pro-inflammatory or anti-inflammatory/pro-angiogenic macrophages under the influence of cytokines and growth factors present in the wound. In a chronic wound, the balance between pro-inflammatory and anti-inflammatory macrophages is upset, in favour of pro-inflammatory cells. Anti-inflammatory macrophages produce high levels of IL-10, which is a cytokine with potent anti-inflammatory properties, as well as growth factors such as basic fibroblast growth factor (bFGF) and vascular endothelial growth factor (VEGF). In addition, they are involved in many cellular activities including proliferation of fibroblasts and epidermal cells, and the formation of new blood vessels [23]. The effect of maggot secretions on the release of pro-inflammatory mediators from human monocytes has been investigated using mononuclear cells obtained from healthy donors incubated with a range of maggot secretions in the presence or absence of lipopolysaccharides or lipoteichoic acid [21]. Maggot secretions inhibited the production of the pro-inflammatory cytokines TNF-a, IL-12, and macrophage migration inhibitory factor while increasing the production of the anti-inflammatory cytokine IL-10, all via elevated levels of cyclic AMP [21]. The same authors also conducted a study to investigate the effects of maggot secretions on the differentiation of monocytes into pro-inflammatory and anti-inflammatory/pro-angiogenic macrophages [23]. Peripheral blood mononuclear cells from healthy donors were stimulated with or without lipopolysaccharides, in the presence of maggot secretions. The results showed that maggot secretions steered monocyte differentiation towards a pro-angiogenic macrophage type with a decreased production of the pro-inflammatory cytokines [23].

In addition, the human complement system, a cascade of potent serum enzymes which form part of the innate immune system, plays an important role in regulating this inflammatory response. Activation of the complement system plays a critical role in the innate immune response to tissue injury and is necessary for normal physiological healing [24]. However, an inappropriate activation system can cause prolonged inflammation, thus maintaining tissue damage and impeding wound healing [22, 24, 25]. Cazander and colleagues [26] hypothesised that the wound healing effect of maggot therapy may be due to the maggot secretions exerting an effect on the complement system. Using sera from healthy and post-operative patients in an *in vitro* study, maggot secretions were found to reduce complement activation in both cohorts of patients in a dose-dependent manner. The authors concluded that this was most likely through the degradation of complement components C3 and C4 in the enzymatic cascade [26].

Thus, it would appear from *in vitro* investigations to date that maggot secretions may aid wound healing by reducing pro-inflammatory mediators and breaking down components of the complement system. It has been suggested that suppressing the complement system could be evolutionarily advantageous to the larvae in surviving on live hosts. Whilst medicinal maggots of the species *L. sericata* and *L. cuprina* do not harm the living tissue of humans, they are a common pest of other animals, especially sheep, in which harmful myiasis by larvae can be fatal if left untreated. It is suggested that the maggots may have evolved this trait as a means of suppressing the immune response of their hosts to enable their continued feeding [26]. This has an unintended benefit on non-healing human wounds, as suppression of the inflammatory response can help in the progression of wound healing.

Effects of Maggots on Fibroblasts

A healing wound will show the growth and appearance of healthy extracellular matrix (ECM) or granulation tissue, a collagen-rich connective tissue which forms on the surface of a healing wound. Fibroblasts are the cells that synthesise ECM and collagen, so it is critical that these cells can migrate into the wound bed once debridement and disinfection of the wound is complete. The growth stimulating effects of maggots on human dermal fibroblasts have been extensively investigated.

In one of the first investigations of this kind, human fibroblasts were cultured *in vitro* and treated either with larval haemolymph, larval alimentary secretions, or the insect hormone 20-hydroxyecdysone (EC). Human fibroblasts showed a significant increase in cell numbers under all three treatment conditions when compared to untreated cells. High concentrations of EC can be found in *L. sericata* haemolymph leading the authors to conclude that insect growth-stimulating molecules (such as EC and others) present in the maggot extracts could be secreted into the host wound, where they stimulate human wound tissue. Therefore, this is another mechanism by which maggot therapy promotes wound healing [27].

When tissues are injured, fibroblasts in the local vicinity also differentiate into myo-fibroblasts, which are highly contractile and aid wound contraction [28]. Fibroblasts also secrete proteases, which play a key role in the wound healing process (the main proteases being matrix metalloproteinases and serine proteases) by breaking down damaged proteins that constitute the ECM, resulting in new tissue formation and closure of the wound [29, 30]. In 2003, a study identified the predominant proteolytic enzymes secreted from *L. sericata* larvae as serine proteases (trypsin-like and chymotrypsin-like) and a metalloproteinase, and showed that maggot secretions could solubilise fibrin clots and degrade laminin, collagen types I and III, and fibronectin [31]. The authors concluded that the proteolytic activity of maggot secretions may promote wound healing by remodelling components of the ECM [31].

Fibroblasts not only synthesise components of ECM but interact with it via integrins and are modified/modulated by growth factors and cytokines that reside within the ECM to increase proliferation and change morphology [31]. In order to investigate this further, the same authors developed a three-dimensional model to observe fibroblast migration and morphology in response to maggot secretions [32]. This novel model more closely mimicked the microenvironment *in vivo* and provided a better understanding of the interactions between the ECM, resident cells, and maggot secretions in the wound healing process. Both 2D and 3D studies conducted demonstrated that fibroblasts seeded onto fibronectin- or collagen-coated plates and incubated with maggot secretions showed reduced cell-ECM adhesion and filopodia inhibition, thus preventing cell spreading along with degradation of fibrin [29, 32, 33]. In addition, the authors showed that maggot secretions could enhance the migration of fibroblasts across fibronectin-coated surfaces, which correlated with the degradation of fibronectin by serine proteinases (which they had previously identified in maggot secretions) [33]. Therefore, maggot secretions may aid in wound healing by increasing fibroblast cell motility, releasing bioactive compounds from the ECM, and enhancing interactions between fibroblasts and the ECM.

The effect of maggot secretions on fibroblast motility was also corroborated later by researchers [34], who found that maggot secretion markedly accelerated the migration of fibroblasts and epidermal keratinocytes during wound closure without any significant mitogenic effect. In support of the above study, subsequent findings [35] showed that when fibroblasts were cultured with extracts from maggot salivary glands (over 5–10 days), the cells exhibited a phenotype typical of cells with an increased metabolism (e.g. voluminous nuclear membrane, large reticular nuclei, distinct Golgi apparatus etc.) leading the authors to conclude that maggot salivary gland extracts increased cell metabolism and protein production, which correlated with the formation of microfibrillar nets required for fibroblast cell migration and production of ECM. The same effect was also noted when incorporating larval secretions into a hydrogel which was then applied to a laboratory wound model, raising the possibility that larval secretions or isolated active compounds could be successfully incorporated into pharmaceutical products for wound healing [32].

Finally, the effects of maggot secretions on haemostatic processes have also been investigated. During haemostasis, blood platelets are activated, which results in the initiation and formation of a platelet plug. In conjunction with this is the coagulation cascade which causes soluble fibrinogen to be converted into a network of insoluble fibrin fibres. This process prevents excessive bleeding and provides a matrix to aid future cell migration [36]. This fibrin network or clot is then broken down by the fibrinolytic system. Fibrinolysis is activated by the serine proteases, urokinase-type plasminogen activator (Urokinase or uPA) or tissue-type plasminogen activator, which converts plasminogen to plasmin which, in turn, degrades the fibrin mesh [37]. However, in chronic wounds, fibrinolysis may be impaired due to increased levels of the fibrinolysis inhibitor (plasminogen activator inhibitor-150), potentially leading to the formation of necrotic tissue and fibrin slough that can act as a nutrient-rich source for bacteria [38]. These, in turn, may increase the inflammatory response and prevent wound closure [39].

Interestingly, it was reported in a 2014 *in vitro* study that the serine protease sericase, present in maggot secretions, augmented plasminogen activator-induced fibrinolysis via the degradation of plasminogen into an activated form which could, in turn, lyse clots and fibrin cuffs to potentially allow cells at the wound edge to migrate through the ECM to form granulation tissue, and thus aid in the closure of a wound [39].

Effects of Maggots on Angiogenesis and Tissue Reperfusion

Maggots may also play a vital role in tissue reperfusion, with larval activity found to combat a number of actions which impair blood-flow to the wound site [20, 23, 39]. Angiogenesis is the formation of new blood vessels from pre-existing vessels, and it is a vital process for wound healing, relying on the interplay between endothelial cells, fibroblasts, macrophages and the surrounding ECM. Macrophages produce growth factors to stimulate angiogenesis and the ECM also provides a reservoir of pro-angiogenic factors which are released during its degradation. In 2014, a finding of considerable clinical significance was reported by a team of Japanese surgeons, who showed a quantifiable improvement in tissue perfusion (amount of oxygen reaching the wound site) after the application of maggots [40]. They did this by measuring the skin perfusion pressure (the amount of oxygen getting to the tissue) surrounding a post-amputation chronic wound of a patient with critical limb ischaemia, before and after maggot therapy. Following treatment, skin perfusion pressure increased dramatically, from 12 to 54 mmHg on the dorsal aspect of the foot, and from 17 to 44 mmHg on the plantar aspect. The authors surmised that maggot therapy had somehow contributed to the increase in blood supply to the ischaemic wound [40].

In parallel with clinical observations and studies, there is a growing body of *in vitro* work that elucidates how larval secretions help to stimulate angiogenesis and encourage the development of new blood vessels. Research from our own group supports the notion that maggot secretions promote angiogenesis. We identified the amino acids L-histidine, 3-guanidinopropionic acid, and L-valinol in maggot secretions and demonstrated, *in vitro*, that these isolated components specifically enhanced the proliferation of human endothelial cells, whilst having no effect on fibroblasts, with the amino acid valinol eliciting the greatest increase in endothelial cell proliferation [41]. In another investigation, Zhang and colleagues [42] investigated the effect of dried *L. sericata* extracts on full thickness dorsal-skin excision wounds of male Sprague Dawley rats. After 3 days of treatment, a significant increase in wound capillary density, vascular endothelial growth factor A (*VEGFA*) mRNA expression, and VEGF-A protein expression were detected in rat wounds treated with *L. sericata* fatty acid extracts compared to treatment with the Chinese wound medicine, JingWanHong (positive control). Wound contraction was also significantly increased compared to treatment with a negative control (Vaseline). Thus, the observed wound healing properties of maggot secretions may be due in part to pro-angiogenic properties via the up-regulation of vascular endothelial growth factor (VEGF) expression. Additionally, van der Plas and colleagues [23] showed that in addition to reducing the production of pro-inflammatory cytokines, maggot secretions also increased the production of pro-angiogenic growth factors, basic fibroblast growth factor (bFGF) and VEGF in anti-inflammatory macrophages. These findings suggest that secretions from maggots may assist in the correction of the macrophage balance within a chronic wound via the promotion of angiogenic growth factors.

The migration of resident epidermal keratinocytes and dermal cells, including fibroblasts and dermal microvascular cells, from the wound margins into the wound bed, is a crucial step during the proliferative phase of wound healing. The most widely studied protein kinase pathways known to regulate cell migration during wound healing are the PI3K:AKT1 and MEK1/2:ERK1/2 pathways. PI3K is activated by many pro-angiogenic factors, including VEGF and bFGF. Activation of PI3K in turn recruits and activates AKT1, which then alters the activity or abundance of specific transcription factors for cell migration and viability. The involvement of both pathways in maggot secretion-induced cell migration was investigated by Wang and colleagues [43]. Human microvascular epidermal cells were utilised for a wound healing assay. Cells were grown to confluency in 6-well culture dishes and were then exposed to maggot secretions (10μg/mL) or a control treatment (phosphate buffered saline solution). It was observed that maggot secretions significantly increased microvascular epidermal cell migration when compared with the control group. To assess the effect of maggot secretions on the PI3K:AKT1 and MEK1/2:ERK1/2 pathways specific inhibitors for the protein kinases, AKT1 and ERK1/2, were added to the culture medium. The inhibitor to PI3K:AKT1 partially blocked maggot secretion-enhanced cell migration. However, there was no change in cell migration following treatment with the MEK1/2:ERK1/2 inhibitor. Protein analysis confirmed that maggot secretions activated AKT1 but no ERK1/2. Thus, it was concluded that maggot secretions could be exerting their angiogenic wound healing effects, in part by the activation of the key signalling protein, AKT1 [43].

Recent studies have shed further light on the role of maggots in enhancing wound healing through angiogenesis. In one experiment, researchers incubated endothelial cells (cells which give rise to new capillaries) with maggot secretions [44]. They showed significantly higher proliferation of endothelial cells and the formation of capillary tubes compared with cells that were incubated with a control. The same researchers also monitored levels of two glycoproteins (CD34 and CD68) which up-regulate endothelial cell activity and are markers of angiogenesis and proliferation. The researchers found that wound tissue obtained from patients after maggot therapy had more of these proteins than they had before. These raised levels of glycoproteins enabled better endothelial cell activity and promoted enhanced angiogenesis [44].

A recent thorough and convincing study exploring the molecule micro-RNA (miR-126), both *in vitro* and *in vivo*, further increased our understanding of how maggots support angiogenesis [45]. MiR-126 is expressed by endothelial cells and is responsible for many positive functions, including angiogenesis, whilst low levels of this RNA are associated with vascular disease and poor angiogenesis. The researchers cultured human umbilical vein endothelial cells in the presence of larval secretions and saw a significant rise in expression of miR-126. Next, the investigators turned their attention to patients and examined miR-126 levels in peripheral blood. The patients examined were grouped: 79 patients with normal blood glucose; 93 patients with type II diabetes, but with no diabetic foot ulcers (DFU), and 90 patients with type II diabetes and the existence of one or more DFU. The researchers discovered that the 79 patients with normal blood glucose exhibited normal miR-126 levels; the 93 patients with type II diabetes, but no DFU had low miR-126 levels, and the 90 patients with type II diabetes and DFU had very low miR-126 levels. The 90 patients with DFU were then divided into two groups, with 47 being treated with maggots, and 43 untreated (control). The investigators discovered that miR-126 levels in all 47 patients increased and were significantly higher following treatment with maggots. They concluded that maggot therapy increased the expression of a key molecule involved in capillary formation and wound healing. Thus, mounting scientific evidence suggests that maggots stimulate blood capillary formation, resulting in more oxygen to the wound [45]. These findings may also explain the clinical results of the Japanese skin perfusion pressure study mentioned earlier [40].

Growth Factor Effects of Maggot Secretions

Endogenous hepatocyte growth factor (HGF) is important for cutaneous wound healing. In a recent study blood samples from patients treated with maggots showed a significant increase in HGF after just a single application [46]. The authors attributed the increased levels of HGF to proteases within the secretions, leading to the promotion of healthy granulation tissue. The expression of this factor was also found to increase in proportion to the protein concentration of the maggot secretions. The authors went on to suggest that formation of healthy granulation tissue observed during maggot therapy resulted from the increased presence of HGF, and that maggot secretions promoted HGF production via a positive feedback loop involving HGF and the STAT3 signalling pathway [46]. The STAT3 signalling pathway was also confirmed in a recent study in which the authors detected five signalling pathways that are involved in wound healing, and suggested that two of these were activated in the presence of maggot whole-body extracts and accompanied by their downstream gene expression [47].

Wound healing is regulated and controlled by a number of key human growth factors (e.g. VEGF or platelet-derived growth factor (PDGF)), and larvae produce their own array of insect hormones and factors which control their growth as they develop [48]. A recent laboratory study explored the homology of factors in maggot secretions and human growth factors that are known to be pivotal to wound healing. Although this was a preliminary study, Western blots with maggot secretions demonstrated the presence of proteins homologous to the human growth factors VEGF and PDGF, among others [49]. It is therefore likely that these homologous maggot proteins support accelerated wound healing in maggot therapy.

Summary

Unlike any other wound care device or pharmaceutical, medicinal maggots convey multiple therapeutic benefits at the same time when applied to chronic and/or infected wounds. As discussed in previous chapters, maggots are highly efficient and precise when it comes to debridement of dead or devitalised tissue [50, 51]. Cadavers, the primary breeding substrate for flies that are suitable for maggot therapy, are microbe- and pathogen-rich environments. Therefore, maggots had to evolve strategies to control infection [52, 53], which they bring to the chronic wound environment, either on their own in the case of beneficial myiasis, or when applied therapeutically by clinicians for maggot therapy [53, 54]. Finally, this chapter presents the evidence for maggot-assisted wound healing. Of course, debridement and infection control are important enablers of wound healing, but it is now clear that medicinal maggots have a far more active role in wound healing. The maggots' excretions and secretions actively promote wound healing through a wide range of specific physiological mechanisms and pathways. Consequently, there is good reason to believe that the wound healing benefits of maggot therapy may be maximised by repeated reapplication of medicinal maggots onto an already clean and debrided wound-bed [55]. Of course, it is tempting to identify for this purpose active compounds from maggot excretions and secretions that may be developed into pharmaceuticals. However, as mentioned in the previous two chapters [50, 53] on the therapeutic principles of maggot therapy, such a reductionist approach to the complex chronic wound may be more convenient to the patient and practitioner but whether it is as efficacious and affordable as whole-organism maggot therapy is uncertain and may depend greatly on the nature of the wound and its stage along the healing trajectory.

References

1.   Komi, D.E.A., K. Khomtchouk, and P.L. Santa Maria, *A Review of the Contribution of Mast Cells in Wound Healing: Involved Molecular and Cellular Mechanisms.* Clinical Reviews in Allergy & Immunology, 2020. 58(3): pp. 298–312, https://doi.org/10.1007/s12016-019-08729-w.

2. Bazaliński, D., et al., *Effectiveness of Chronic Wound Debridement with the Use of Larvae of Lucilia Sericata*. Journal of Clinical Medicine, 2019. 8(11): pp. 1845–1845, https://doi.org/10.3390/jcm8111845.

3. Creager, M.D., et al., *3.18 Immunohistochemistry*. 2017, Elsevier. pp. 387–405.

4. Sherman, R.A., F. Wyle, and M. Vulpe, *Maggot Therapy for Treating Pressure Ulcers in Spinal Cord Injury Patients*. The Journal of Spinal Cord Medicine, 1995. 18(2): pp. 71–74, https://doi.org/10.1080/10790268.1995.11719382.

5. Sherman, R.A., *Maggot versus Conservative Debridement Therapy for the Treatment of Pressure Ulcers*. Wound Repair and Regeneration, 2002. 10(4): pp. 208–214, https://doi.org/10.1046/j.1524-475X.2002.10403.x.

6. Sherman, R.A., *Maggot Therapy for Treating Diabetic Foot Ulcers Unresponsive to Conventional Therapy*. Diabetes Care, 2003. 26(2): pp. 446–451, https://doi.org/10.2337/diacare.26.2.446.

7. Wollina, U., et al., *Biosurgery Supports Granulation and Debridement in Chronic Wounds — Clinical Data and Remittance Spectroscopy Measurement*. International Journal of Dermatology, 2002. 41(10): pp. 635–639, https://doi.org/10.1046/j.1365-4362.2002.01354.x.

8. Armstrong, D.G., et al., *Maggot Therapy in "Lower-extremity Hospice" Wound Care: Fewer Amputations and More Antibiotic-free Days*. Journal of the American Podiatric Medical Association, 2005. 95(3): pp. 254–257, https://doi.org/10.7547/0950254.

9. Zarchi, K. and G.B.E. Jemec, *The Efficacy of Maggot Debridement Therapy — A Review of Comparative Clinical Trials*. International Wound Journal, 2012. 9(5): pp. 469–477, https://doi.org/10.1111/j.1742-481X.2011.00919.x.

10. Sun, X., et al., *A Systematic Review of Maggot Debridement Therapy for Chronically Infected Wounds and Ulcers*. International Journal of Infectious Diseases, 2014. 25: pp. 32–37, https://doi.org/10.1016/j.ijid.2014.03.1397.

11. Siribumrungwong, B., C. Wilasrusmee, and K. Rerkasem, *Maggot Therapy in Angiopathic Leg Ulcers: A Systematic Review and Meta-analysis*. The International Journal of Lower Extremity Wounds, 2018. 17(4): pp. 227–235, https://doi.org/10.1177/1534734618816882.

12. Thyssen, P.J. and F.S. Masiero, *Bioprospecting and Testing of New Fly Species for Maggot Therapy*, in *A Complete Guide to Maggot Therapy: Clinical Practice, Therapeutic Principles, Production, Distribution, and Ethics*, F. Stadler (ed.). 2022, Cambridge: Open Book Publishers, pp. 195–234, https://doi.org/10.11647/OBP.0300.11.

13. Buchman, J., *The Rationale of the Treatment of Chronic Osteomyelitis with Special Reference to Maggot Therapy*. Annals of Surgery, 1934. 99(2): pp. 251–259, https://doi.org/10.1097/00000658-193402000-00003.

14. Buchman, J. and J.E. Blair, *Maggots and Their Use in the Treatment of Chronic Osteomyelitis*. Surgery, Gynecology and Obstetrics, 1932. 55: pp. 177–190.

15. Robinson, W., *Stimulation of Healing in Non-healing Wounds by Allantoin Occurring in Maggot Secretions and of Wide Biological Distribution*. The Journal of Bone & Joint Surgery, 1935. 17(2): pp. 267–271.

16. Robinson, W., *Ammonium Bicarbonate Secreted by Surgical Maggots Stimulates Healing in Purulent Wounds*. The American Journal of Surgery, 1940. 47(1): pp. 111–115, https://doi.org/10.1016/S0002-9610(40)90125-8.

17. Frykberg, R.G. and J. Banks, *Challenges in the Treatment of Chronic Wounds*. Advances in Wound Care, 2015. 4(9): pp. 560–582, https://doi.org/10.1089/wound.2015.0635.

18. Uhlinger, D.J., et al., *The Respiratory Burst Oxidase of Human Neutrophils. Guanine Nucleotides and Arachidonate Regulate the Assembly of a Multicomponent Complex in a Semirecombinant Cell-free System*. The Journal of Biological Chemistry, 1993. 268(12): pp. 8624–8631, https://doi.org/10.1016/0891-5849(90)90668-9.

19. Pecivova, J., et al., *Effect of the Extract from Salivary Glands of Lucilia sericata on Human Neutrophils*. Neuro Endocrinology Letters, 2008. 29(5): pp. 794–797.

20. van der Plas, M.J.A., et al., *Maggot Excretions/Secretions Inhibit Multiple Neutrophil Pro-inflammatory Responses*. Microbes and Infection, 2007. 9(4): pp. 507–514, https://doi.org/10.1016/j.micinf.2007.01.008.

21. van der Plas, M.J.A., et al., *Maggot Secretions Suppress Pro-inflammatory Responses of Human Monocytes through Elevation of Cyclic AMP*. Diabetologia, 2009. 52(9): pp. 1962–1970, https://doi.org/10.1007/s00125-009-1432-6.

22. Bryant, R.A. and D.P. Nix, *Acute and Chronic Wounds: Current Management Concepts*. 2007, Mosby, Missouri.

23. van der Plas, M.J.A., J.T. van Dissel, and P.H. Nibbering, *Maggot Secretions Skew Monocyte-macrophage Differentiation away from a Pro-inflammatory to a Pro-angiogenic Type*. PLoS ONE, 2009. 4(11), https://doi.org/10.1371/journal.pone.0008071.

24. Cazander, G., G.N. Jukema, and P.H. Nibbering, *Complement Activation and Inhibition in Wound Healing*. Clinical and Developmental Immunology, 2012. 2012: pp. 1–14, https://doi.org/10.1155/2012/534291.

25. Makrides, S.C., *Therapeutic Inhibition of the Complement System*. Pharmacological Reviews, 1998. 50(1): pp. 59–87.

26. Cazander, G., et al., *Maggot Excretions Affect the Human Complement System*. Wound Repair and Regeneration, 2012. 20(6): pp. 879–886, https://doi.org/10.1111/j.1524-475X.2012.00850.x.

27. Prete, P.E., *Growth Effects of Phaenicia sericata Larval Extracts on Fibroblasts: Mechanism for Wound Healing by Maggot Therapy*. Life Sciences, 1997. 60(8): pp. 505–510, https://doi.org/10.1016/S0024-3205(96)00688-1.

28. Li, B. and J.H. Wang, *Fibroblasts and Myofibroblasts in Wound Healing: Force Generation and Measurement.* Journal of Tissue Viability, 2011. 20(4): pp. 108–120, https://doi.org/10.1016/j.jtv.2009.11.004.

29. Horobin, A.J., et al., *Maggots and Wound Healing: An Investigation of the Effects of Secretions from Lucilia sericata Larvae upon Interactions between Human Dermal Fibroblasts and Extracellular Matrix Components.* British Journal of Dermatology, 2003. 148(5): pp. 923–933, https://doi.org/10.1046/j.1365-2133.2003.05314.x.

30. International, C., *The Role of Proteases in Wound Diagnostics. An Expert Working Group Review.* London: Wounds International, 2011.

31. Chambers, L., et al., *Degradation of Extracellular Matrix Components by Defined Proteinases from the Greenbottle Larva Lucilia sericata Used for the Clinical Debridement of Non-healing Wounds.* British Journal of Dermatology, 2003. 148(1): pp. 14–23, https://doi.org/10.1046/j.1365-2133.2003.04935.x.

32. Horobin, A.J., K.M. Shakesheff, and D.I. Pritchard, *Promotion of Human Dermal Fibroblast Migration, Matrix Remodelling and Modification of Fibroblast Morphology within a Novel 3D Model by Lucilia sericata Larval Secretions.* The Journal of Investigative Dermatology, 2006. 126(6): pp. 1410–1418, https://doi.org/10.1038/sj.jid.5700256.

33. Horobin, A.J., K.M. Shakesheff, and D.I. Pritchard, *Maggots and Wound Healing: An Investigation of the Effects of Secretions from Lucilia sericata Larvae upon the Migration of Human Dermal Fibroblasts over a Fibronectin-coated Surface.* Wound Repair and Regeneration, 2005. 13(4): pp. 422–433, https://doi.org/10.1111/j.1067-1927.2005.130410.x.

34. Smith, A.G., et al., *Greenbottle (Lucilia sericata) Larval Secretions Delivered from a Prototype Hydrogel Wound Dressing Accelerate the Closure of Model Wounds.* Biotechnology Progress, 2006. 22(6): pp. 1690–1696, https://doi.org/10.1021/bp0601600.

35. Polakovičova, S., et al., *The Effect of Salivary Gland Extract of Lucilia sericata Maggots on Human Dermal Fibroblast Proliferation within Collagen/Hyaluronan Membrane in vitro: Transmission Electron Microscopy Study.* Advances in Skin & Wound Care, 2015. 28(5): pp. 221–226, https://doi.org/10.1097/01.ASW.0000461260.03630.a0.

36. Laurens, N., P. Koolwijk, and M.P.M. De Maat, *Fibrin Structure and Wound Healing.* Journal of Thrombosis and Haemostasis, 2006. 4(5): pp. 932–939, https://doi.org/10.1111/j.1538-7836.2006.01861.x.

37. van Meijer, M. and H. Pannekoek, *Structure of Plasminogen Activator Inhibitor 1 (PAI-1) and Its Function in Fibrinolysis: An Update.* Fibrinolysis, 1995. 9(5): pp. 263–276, https://doi.org/10.1016/S0268-9499(95)80015-8.

38. Wysocki, A.B., et al., *Temporal Expression of Urokinase Plasminogen Activator, Plasminogen Activator Inhibitor and Gelatinase-B in Chronic Wound Fluid Switches from a Chronic to Acute Wound Profile with Progression to Healing.*

Wound Repair and Regeneration, 1999. 7(3): pp. 154–165, https://doi.org/10.1046/j.1524-475X.1999.00154.x.

39. van der Plas, M.J.A., et al., *A Novel Serine Protease Secreted by Medicinal Maggots Enhances Plasminogen Activator-induced Fibrinolysis*. PloS ONE, 2014. 9(3): pp. e92096-e92096, https://doi.org/10.1371/journal.pone.0092096.

40. Maeda, T.M., et al., *Increase in Skin Perfusion Pressure after Maggot Debridement Therapy for Critical Limb Ischaemia*. Clinical and Experimental Dermatology, 2014. 39(8): pp. 911–914, https://doi.org/10.1111/ced.12454.

41. Bexfield, A., et al., *Amino Acid Derivatives from Lucilia sericata Excretions/ Secretions May Contribute to the Beneficial Effects of Maggot Therapy via Increased Angiogenesis*. British Journal of Dermatology, 2010. 162(3): pp. 554–562, https://doi.org/10.1111/j.1365-2133.2009.09530.x.

42. Zhang, Z., et al., *Fatty Acid Extracts from Lucilia sericata Larvae Promote Murine Cutaneous Wound Healing by Angiogenic Activity*. Lipids in Health and Disease, 2010. 9(1): p. 24, https://doi.org/10.1186/1476-511X-9-24.

43. Wang, S., et al., *Maggot Excretions/Secretions Induces Human Microvascular Endothelial Cell Migration through AKT1*. Molecular Biology Reports, 2010. 37(6): pp. 2719–2725, https://doi.org/10.1007/s11033-009-9806-x.

44. Sun, X., et al., *Maggot Debridement Therapy Promotes Diabetic Foot Wound Healing by Up-regulating Endothelial Cell Activity*. Journal of Diabetes and its Complications, 2016. 30(2): pp. 318–322, https://doi.org/10.1016/j.jdiacomp.2015.11.009.

45. Zhang, J., et al., *Increasing the miR-126 Expression in the Peripheral Blood of Patients with Diabetic Foot Ulcers Treated with Maggot Debridement Therapy*. Journal of Diabetes and its Complications, 2017. 31(1): pp. 241–244, https://doi.org/10.1016/j.jdiacomp.2016.07.026.

46. Honda, K., et al., *A Novel Mechanism in Maggot Debridement Therapy: Protease in Excretion/Secretion Promotes Hepatocyte Growth Factor Production*. American Journal of Physiology. Cell Physiology, 2011. 301(6): pp. C1423-C1430, https://doi.org/10.1152/ajpcell.00065.2011.

47. Li, P.N., et al., *Molecular Events Underlying Maggot Extract Promoted Rat in vivo and Human in vitro Skin Wound Healing*. Wound Repair and Regeneration, 2015. 23(1): pp. 65–73, https://doi.org/10.1111/wrr.12243.

48. Nijhout, H.F., et al., *The Developmental Control of Size in Insects*. Wiley Interdisciplinary Reviews: Developmental Biology, 2014. 3(1): pp. 113–134, https://doi.org/10.1002/wdev.124.

49. Evans, R., et al., *Human Growth Factor Homologues, Detected in Externalised Secretions of Medicinal Larvae, Could Be Responsible for Maggot-induced Wound Healing*. International Journal of Research in Pharmacy and Biosciences, 2019. 6(5): pp. 1–10.

50. Nigam, Y. and M.R. Wilson, *Maggot Debridement*, in *A Complete Guide to Maggot Therapy: Clinical Practice, Therapeutic Principles, Production, Distribution, and Ethics*, F. Stadler (ed.). 2022, Cambridge: Open Book Publishers, pp. 143–152, https://doi.org/10.11647/OBP.0300.08.

51. Sherman, R. and F. Stadler, *Wound Aetiologies, Patient Characteristics, and Healthcare Settings Amenable to Maggot Therapy*, in *A Complete Guide to Maggot Therapy: Clinical Practice, Therapeutic Principles, Production, Distribution, and Ethics*, F. Stadler (ed.). 2022, Cambridge: Open Book Publishers, pp. 39–62, https://doi.org/10.11647/OBP.0300.03.

52. Harvey, M., *The Natural History of Medicinal Flies*, in *A Complete Guide to Maggot Therapy: Clinical Practice, Therapeutic Principles, Production, Distribution, and Ethics*, F. Stadler (ed.). 2022, Cambridge: Open Book Publishers, pp. 121–142, https://doi.org/10.11647/OBP.0300.07.

53. Nigam, Y. and M.R. Wilson, *The Antimicrobial Activity of Medicinal Maggots*, in *A Complete Guide to Maggot Therapy: Clinical Practice, Therapeutic Principles, Production, Distribution, and Ethics*, F. Stadler (ed.). 2022, Cambridge: Open Book Publishers, pp. 153–174, https://doi.org/10.11647/OBP.0300.09.

54. Sherman, R., *Medicinal Maggot Application and Maggot Therapy Dressing Technology*, in *A Complete Guide to Maggot Therapy: Clinical Practice, Therapeutic Principles, Production, Distribution, and Ethics*, F. Stadler (ed.). 2022, Cambridge: Open Book Publishers, pp. 79–96, https://doi.org/10.11647/OBP.0300.05.

55. Pritchard, D.I. and Y. Nigam, *Maximising the Secondary Beneficial Effects of Larval Debridement Therapy*. Journal of Wound Care, 2013. 22(11): pp. 610–616, https://doi.org/10.12968/jowc.2013.22.11.610.

11. Bioprospecting and Testing of New Fly Species for Maggot Therapy

Patricia J. Thyssen, Franciéle S. Masiero and

Frank Stadler

Lucilia sericata, the green bottle blowfly, has a long history of clinical use and an excellent safety record which makes it safe for therapeutic clinical use. In regions where it is naturally absent, maggot therapy cannot be offered to patients with chronic wounds unless an alternative local species is found. This chapter explains how new species are identified and tested for their therapeutic efficacy and clinical safety. The process involves the bioprospecting for candidate fly species, pre-clinical *in vitro* and animal studies to make sure they are therapeutically active and safe, and clinical trials of maggot therapy with human patients.

Introduction

The Diptera is one of the most taxonomically diverse insect orders. The flies also stand out with regard to the diversity of their feeding habits, including parasitism, saprophagy, predation, and omnivory. Flies can be found all over the planet, although many species may have only limited distribution due to physiological adaptations to survive in a certain biogeoclimatic region. For a detailed discussion of the natural history of medicinal flies, please refer to Chapter 7 of this book [1].

https://doi.org/10.11647/OBP.0300.11

Lucilia sericata (Meigen), the green bottle blowfly, has a long history of clinical use and an excellent safety record which makes it safe for therapeutic clinical use. In regions where it is absent, maggot therapy cannot be offered to patients with chronic wounds unless an alternative local species is found. This is because in most countries there are quarantine regulations in place for the introduction of living organisms, for whatever purposes, which is a necessary precaution to protect agricultural production and the environment from pests and diseases. How to establish laboratory colonies for medicinal maggot production and how to identify suitable species that have been previously used for maggot therapy is explained in Chapter 13 of this book [2]. Given that there are more than 1,500 blowfly species (Calliphoridae) known to date [3], it may seem that the identification of additional species for use in maggot therapy would be something simple, but this is not the case.

This chapter explains how new medicinal fly species are identified and tested for their therapeutic efficacy and clinical safety, so that maggot therapy is made possible in regions where *L. sericata* is not present. The process begins with bioprospecting which is the search for candidate fly species that possess the key characteristics required for clinical application. However, before shortlisted species can be tested on humans, they must first be subjected to pre-clinical trials to make sure they are therapeutically active and safe. Once there is evidence showing a good safety profile and at least effective debridement, which is a prerequisite for infection control and wound healing, clinical trials can be conducted to treat patients under controlled conditions with medicinal maggots from a new species. Such clinical trials are a prerequisite for the approval of maggot therapy in a country or block of countries with the same regulatory framework. After the efficacy and safety of maggot therapy have been demonstrated and the approval as a therapeutic good is obtained, medicinal maggots must be produced on a reliable basis, in line with good manufacturing practice, and at scale for country-wide delivery of maggot therapy services. Please refer to Chapters 12 to 18 of this book for guidance on the production and supply of medicinal maggots [2, 4–9].

Bioprospecting for Medicinal Fly Species

Bioprospecting is the process of searching for organisms with characteristics or properties that make them useful to humans as new foods, new materials, new engineering applications, or new medicines. Fortunately, it is not all that difficult to prospect for potential new medicinal fly species. Eating habits such as necrophagy or parasitism can be discovered from observation in nature or at clinics that treat cases of myiasis in humans or domestic animals. Myiasis is the unintentional colonisation of a wound with fly maggots. Unless the species involved is parasitic and consumes living tissue, as is the case for both the New World screwworm *Cochliomyia hominivorax* (Coquerel) and the Old World screwworm *Chrysomya bezziana* (Villeneuve) [10], there is a good chance that the maggots found are therapeutically efficacious. Additionally, there are a large number of reports in the literature that can be useful to screen for and identify the appropriate feeding habit of a fly species, i.e., taking into account that the species must be obligatorily necrophagous, which means they must only feed on dead tissue. As is recommended for other scientific literature-based investigations, only data published in reputable, peer-reviewed and indexed scientific journals should be considered. In addition, public- or animal-health information held in regional public databases may also be useful in the search for new medicinal fly species.

A pre-selection of information in the literature can be very convenient to save time and to plan future research more effectively, but it should never be the only way to choose a fly species as a natural candidate for maggot therapy. There are a number of problems that are usually not evident at the time of screening. In most countries, reporting of a myiasis infestation in either animals or humans is not mandatory. For this reason, larvae of myiasis-causing flies are invariably removed and discarded, rather than properly diagnosed by specialists [11, 12]. An accurate diagnosis of the agent responsible for myiasis is necessary to gain more information about this disease presentation and to avoid misinformation. Flies that ingest the living tissue of their hosts (classified as causing obligatory myiasis, i.e., are parasites) should not be used for the treatment of wounds, since there is a risk that the damage caused will be greater than the benefit [13].

What about a species that is in transition from parasitism to necrophagy? *Lucilia eximia* (Wiedemann), known as carrion-breeding fly [14], is a good example of a parasitic transition phenomenon, since it has occasionally been incriminated as a facultative myiasis-causing fly (i.e., a fly with larvae that normally develop in carrion but can opportunistically parasitise and exploit living tissue or ingest devitalised tissues from living hosts) in domestic and wild animals in the New World [15–17]. Another intriguing species is *Lucilia cuprina* (Wiedemann), which causes obligatory myiasis, predominantly in sheep, in Australia and New Zealand [18]. Stevens and Wall [19] studied the genetics of this species from specimens collected in Africa, Europe, Australasia, North America and the islands of Hawaii. The results supported the existence of an intraspecific genetic variation in *L. cuprina*, possibly related to geographic isolation [20] and strong climatic influence, which are factors that *a priori* determined which "species" would become predominant in different regions of the world [20]. Thus, in an independent evolution of the parasitic habit [21], one of the strains, *L. cuprina cuprina*, distributed in the Neotropical, Eastern and Southern regions of the Nearctic, would be responsible for facultative myiasis (therefore natural candidates for maggot therapy), while the other strain, *L. cuprina dorsalis*, present in the Australasian and Afrotropical regions, became an obligatory myiasis agent. Consequently, being able to correctly identify species is as important as knowing their biology. In Egypt, for example, *L. cuprina* larvae were accidentally used in two people to treat their wounds, but the initial intention was that *L. sericata* larvae were used [22]; the authors mentioned, without identifying the strain, that the treatment was safe and successful, but the outcome could have been unfavourable.

Competition between maggots from the same or different fly species in the same wound is another factor worth considering. *Chrysomya albiceps* (Wiedemann) is a calliphorid fly species originally from Africa and widely distributed in Asia, southern Europe, and several countries in South America. It is one of the species of great forensic relevance due to the frequency with which it colonises corpses [23] and it is known that its larvae are voracious predators of other fly larvae [24, 25]. While *Ch. albiceps* is not a parasitic species, its eligibility for maggot therapy is questionable considering that under adverse conditions (such as under temporary starvation during transport, for example) the larvae of this species could opt for cannibalism [24, 26], which would result in a reduction in the number of larvae placed in the wound and would consequently impair the evolution of the treatment.

Other characteristics that deserve to be highlighted when selecting a candidate species for maggot therapy are associated with (i) its distribution, (ii) ease of breeding and maintenance, and (iii) the development cycle. The wound temperature is around 32°C [27–29], but in very warm climates this temperature may increase. Thus, it would be advisable to use local, warm-adapted species for treatment, since they may cope with these very high temperatures better than cold-climate species. Maggot therapy at scale will only be possible if the flies used can be easily mass-reared and maintained in the insectary. Mass rearing and efficient production, with a minimum of work and cost, is further supported by species that have a short development cycle of under four weeks from egg to egg.

Pre-clinical Trials to Assess Nutritional Strategy, Safety, and Therapeutic Efficacy of Medicinal Maggots

Assessing the nutritional strategy is the first step to making sure that a 'new' species of fly considered for maggot therapy can be used safely. After all, it would not be desirable to use fly species that are parasitic and consume living flesh. Such pre-clinical trials should be done using *in vitro* experimentation and *in vivo* with laboratory animals and real wounds. *In vitro* experimentation without laboratory animals has the advantage that (i) it does not involve vertebrate animals and therefore does not require animal ethics approval, (ii) with some exceptions, it is inexpensive regarding inputs and infrastructure, (iii) fewer people are involved in its execution, (iv) it allows for a greater number of replicates, and (v) the results can be obtained in a relatively short time.

The first pre-clinical trial that should be conducted is the *in vitro* testing to evaluate both the nutritional strategy of fly larvae and their debridement rate. The latter is determined by the amount of tissue that one larva is able to ingest per time spent on the wound.

Possible cytotoxic properties and mechanisms by which the larvae promote healing and control infection can be investigated through a series of *in vitro* tests using human or animal cell cultures from rats, mice, and monkeys (Vero cells, T lymphocytes, macrophages), or by the cultivation of microorganisms (multi-drug resistant bacteria, fungi that cause mycoses, or protozoa that cause cutaneous diseases such as leishmaniasis). In tests with cell cultures, larvae should not be used because their vigorous activity may disturb or damage the cell culture. The larvae may also struggle to survive due to the lack of food and inappropriate environmental conditions (temperature, amount of oxygen and light). Instead, larval excretions and secretions rich in low- and medium-molecular weight proteins such as proteases and antimicrobial peptides are routinely extracted for this purpose. It is somewhat limiting, though, that for each hypothesis to be investigated, a separate test must be conducted to obtain the desired response (Table 11.1). Moreover, such testing can require special equipment and technical expertise with cell culture and experimental design. Inadequate setup of experimental groups, for example, can generate data with high bias and little scientific benefit.

Table 11.1 List of some *in vitro* tests performed to (i) characterise the antimicrobial factors and investigate the activities of larvae and their products against bacteria, fungi and parasites; (ii) to evaluate the mechanisms of action that contribute to wound healing; and (iii) to investigate how to improve aspects related to production, survival and disinfection of immature (eggs and maggots).

In vitro tests performed to observe:	Target Species*
Characterisation of antimicrobial factors (peptides)	*Calliphora vicina* (Robineau-Desvoidy) (alloferon 1 and 2) [30], *Lucilia cuprina* (lucifensin II) [31], *L. eximia* (lucilin)[32], *L. sericata* (lucifensin, lucimycin)[33, 34], *Protophormia terraenovae* (Robineau-Desvoidy) (phormia A and B) [35], *Sarconesiopsis magellanica* (Le Guillou) (sarconesin, sarconesin II) [36, 37]
Antibacterial, antifungal and/or antileishmania activities of larval excretions/secretions, specific peptides, fat body or hemolymph extracts	*Ca. vicina* [30, 38, 39] *Chrysomya albiceps* [40], *Chrysomya megacephala* (Fabricius) [40, 41], *Chrysomya putoria* (Wiedemann) [40], *Chrysomya rufifacies* (Macquart) [42], *Co. macellaria* [42, 43], *L. cuprina* [31, 44–46], *L. eximia* [32], *L. sericata* [33, 34, 39, 47–49], *Musca domestica* Linnaeus [50], *P. terraenovae* [35], *S. magellanica* [35, 37, 39, 49, 51, 52]
Action against bacterial biofilm	*Ca. vicina* [53], *L. sericata* [54–57]
Synergism between larval excretions/secretions and antibiotics	*L. cuprina* [45], *L. sericata* [56, 58]

In vitro tests performed to observe:	Target Species*
Combined use of larvae and topical agents	*Co. macellaria* [59]
ES stimulus on fibroblast migration and components of the extracellular matrix	*L. eximia* [32], *L. sericata* [60]
ES and their ability to inhibit pro-inflammatory responses	*L. eximia* [32], *L. sericata* [61]
Angiogenesis stimulus	*L. sericata* [62, 63]
Transgenic larvae and their ability to express and secrete human platelet-derived growth factor	*L. sericata* [64]
Larval growth, survival, and debridement efficacy	*Co. macellaria* [59], *L. sericata* [65, 66]
Survival of embryos by cryopreservation	*L. sericata* [67]
Efficiency of egg disinfection	*Ch. megacephala* [68, 69], *Ch. putoria* [69], *Ch. rufifacies* [68], *Ca. vicina* [70], *Co. macellaria* [68, 69], *L. cuprina* [68, 71, 72], *L. Sericata* [68]

The most important question to be answered in pre-clinical trials is whether the larvae of the chosen species feed only on devitalised tissue or also feed on living flesh. This question must be answered using *in vivo* animal models, because *in vitro* tests cannot reproduce the complexity of biological, physiological, and immunological interactions between maggots and hosts. The evaluation of cytotoxicity in response to the products produced by the larvae is also of critical importance, but as seen previously, it can be appropriately observed through *in vitro* tests. If both results are promising, then it is demonstrated that maggot therapy is safe and development can enter the clinical trial phase.

In vivo tests can also be performed to help identify safety or even efficacy for treatments of wounds with specific aetiology, such as cutaneous parasitic infections, or those where the individual has some type of comorbidity such as diabetes (Table 11.2). In maggot therapy the animal models that have been most used are mice, rats, and rabbits. However, *in vivo* experiments should only be conducted when necessary because (i) they are expensive, with experimental animals raised in specialised laboratory animal facilities costing approximately USD10.00

and USD15.00 per pathogen-free (SPF) mouse and rat, respectively; and (ii) there are added training and animal welfare requirements for researchers to consider. The study design must be approved by a recognised ethics committee and experiments should be carried out with the fewest possible replicates (animals) to prevent the unnecessary sacrifice of laboratory animals.

Table 11.2 List of some *in vivo* tests performed (i) to assess the nutritional strategy and safety of larvae, (ii) to investigate the activities of larvae and their products against bacteria, viruses, and parasites, (iii) to investigate the capacity to enhance antitumoural activity, and (iv) to assess the mechanisms of action and effectiveness of different therapeutic approaches in wound healing.

In vivo tests performed for/to:	Target Species*
assess the nutritional strategy and the safe use of a "new species" for maggot therapy	*Co. macellaria* [73]
assess the capacity to enhance antitumoural activity	*Ca. vicina* [30]
assess the antibacterial, antiviral and/ or antileishmania activities of larval excretions/secretions or peptides	*Ca. vicina* [30, 39], *M. domestica* [74], *L. sericata* [39, 75–77], *S. magellanica* [75].
assess the effectiveness of maggot therapy and/or larval products in wound healing in animals with or without diabetes	*Co. macellaria* [78, 79], *L. cuprina* [41, 80, 81], *L. sericata* [82–84], *S. magellanica* [82, 85]
compare the effectiveness between maggot therapy and conventional treatments for wound healing	*Co. macellaria* [79]
assess the effectiveness of maggot therapy between different fly species	*L. sericata* [82], *S. magellanica* [82]

From an animal ethics point of view and to avoid unnecessary sacrifice of experimental animals, it would be helpful to use animals, for example pets or farm animals, that have been accidentally injured. However, it is very difficult to ensure the homogeneity in species, age, sex, wound type, aetiology and other factors required for unbiased planning of the experiment and the analysis of results. Although, it is not impossible to plan a prospective-style trial with such animals, but the time it would take to accumulate a meaningful case number of sufficiently homogeneous nature is probably impractical, unless the researchers have access to a regular supply of injured animals such as from large-scale farming activities or veterinary practice.

While small individual immunogenic differences may exist, when wounds are artificially induced within the same group of laboratory animals, the samples are still sufficiently homogeneous. There are several ways to induce wounds in anaesthetised laboratory animals, ranging from scarification of the skin [76, 81, 83, 84] to chemical burns [73]. Wounds may also be induced with wound-causing parasites [39]. Wounds may or may not be inoculated with pathogenic bacteria [52, 82]. For a comparative evaluation of the therapeutic action of fly larvae it is important to take into consideration how the wound was induced. Any initial variations in size and depth of the wound, in infection status, or microbe/parasite load must be accounted for in the analysis in order not to distort results and lead to wrong conclusions.

Before starting an *in vivo* test, it is mandatory to submit to an institutional ethics committee an application to conduct an experiment with animals, together with a very detailed design of the study. This application will be assessed by the committee against the guidelines of regional or international associations for guarantee animal welfare (e.g., World Organization for Animal Health (OIE), World Veterinary Association (WVA), United States Department of Agriculture (USDA)). These assessments can take time, particularly when the experimental design and methodologies lack detail and are poorly researched.

Preclinical Research Protocols

The following three protocols explain (i) how to conduct an *in vitro* test to assess the nutritional strategy and debridement efficacy of medicinal maggots, (ii) how to assess the antimicrobial action of larval excretions and secretions (ES) against bacteria, and (iii) how to conduct *in vivo* experiments to assess the therapeutic safety and efficacy of fly species after preliminary *in vitro* testing. Each protocol is accompanied by a schematic summary of the process (Figures 11.1 to 11.3)

How to Conduct an In Vitro Test to Assess the Nutritional Strategy and Debridement Efficacy of Medicinal Maggots

1. Establish fly colonies as described in Chapter 13 [2] of this book. For guidance on colony maintenance in the insectary, please refer to Chapter 14 [7].

2. Harvest eggs from established colonies with some raw minced liver.

3. Remove eggs from the liver bait and disinfect by washing them for 3 min with 1% sodium hypochlorite (NaOCl) [69].

4. Place disinfected eggs on filter paper into a Petri dish and incubate them at 25°C until the larvae hatch.

5. Prepare the *in vitro* wound model: place a 20 g portion of raw minced pork muscle (this meat should be used for the wound model because it resembles closely human tissue and results in larval growth very similar to that of human tissue [87, 88]) and a few drops of artificial blood (250 g portion of fresh bovine liver triturated in 50 mL of distilled water) into a small plastic container (approx. 145 mL—use inexpensive containers with a tightly fitting lid).

6. Introduce 30 newly hatched larvae to each wound model replicate (consider that maggots debride approximately 150 mg of necrotic tissue per day [27]). The maggots used should always be of the same age and developmental stage.

7. If performance at the point of care is to be simulated then maggots to be tested should be packaged as per regular shipment and left for 24 h (or the typical time it takes for delivery) before testing.

8. If the debridement efficiency of bagged maggots is to be tested then the bag is placed onto the meat and a tie should be applied to ensure close contact between the bag and the meat surface.

9. A piece of fine-weave chiffon fabric or other synthetic mesh fabric may be sandwiched between container and lid to confine maggots. The lid needs to be fitted with a hole about

4 cm², large enough to permit ventilation but small enough to prevent excessive moisture loss from the chamber.

10. Incubate at 33±1°C. This temperature range corresponds to the wound bed temperature range of 31–35°C [27, 28].

11. The incubation time to assess the nutritional strategy and/ or debridement activity will depend on whether free-range or bagged application is simulated. Free-range application is much faster, necessitating removal of maggots after 24, 48 or 72 h of application (the duration of each experiment corresponds to common maggot therapy treatment times [89–91]. Bagged application is less efficient and bags may remain on the wound for up to 96 h [92, 93].

12. After the incubation period, debridement efficacy can be established with the measurement of the: (i) weight of the remaining meat (measured to the nearest mg); (ii) number of surviving maggots; (iii) developmental stage (instar) of surviving maggots; (iv) weight or length of maggots (since weight and size are correlated it will not be necessary to measure both). In both cases, measurements should be taken after maggots have been quickly euthanised by rapid immersion in near boiling water (approximately 70°C)—it is important to consistently stick to one method for comparability of results over time.

13. With adequate replication (there should be at least three replicates for each experimental group), the data generated will allow descriptive statistical analysis and also analysis of variance between assay runs. This can reveal whether debridement efficacy is maintained, increases or declines over time.

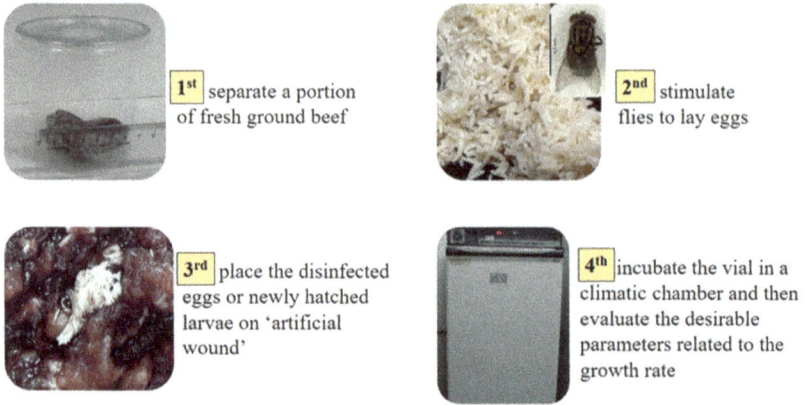

Figure 11.1 Summary model and protocol of an *in vitro* test to assess the nutritional strategy and debridement activity of medicinal larvae (adapted from Masiero and colleagues [59]).

How to Assess the Antimicrobial Action of Larval Excretions/ Secretions (ES) against Bacteria

1. Establish fly colonies as described in Chapter 13 [2] of this book. For guidance on colony maintenance in the insectary, please refer to Chapter 14 [7].

2. Harvest eggs from established colonies with some raw minced liver.

3. Remove eggs from the liver bait and disinfect by washing them for 3 min with 1% sodium hypochlorite (NaOCl) [69].

4. Place disinfected eggs on filter paper and incubate them at 25°C until the larvae hatch.

5. Transfer newly hatched larvae to a container with minced beef at a dose of 1 larva per gram of beef.

6. Allow larvae to feed for 72 h.

7. Remove larvae from the meat and wash them 3 times in sterile distilled water.

8. Add 25 live larvae to 800 µL of sterile distilled water, held in a 1.5 mL microtube. Incubate for 1 h in the dark at 37±2°C.

9. Remove larvae from the microtube, discard them and centrifuge the resultant liquid at 4000 x g at 4°C for 15 min.

10. Sterilise the liquid, i.e., the excretions/secretions (ES) by passing them through a 0.45 μm filter.

11. Refrigerate ES at 10±2°C for up to 24 h.

Agar plate test:

1. Different concentrations of ES and bacteria can be tested on agar plates with results measured in colony-forming unit (CFU). Experimental groups may be divided into: (i) ES; (ii) ES + bacterial inoculum; (iii) bacterial inoculum; and (iv) control, i.e., bacterial inoculum plus an antimicrobial agent for which efficacy is known.

2. Seeding and reading of the plates: aliquots of 25 μL of each experimental group should be plated by spreading onto Petri dishes containing BHI agar (Brain Heart Infusion) with three replicates for each treatment. Seedings are done at 0 h, 1 h, 2 h, 4 h and 12 h after the extraction of ES.

3. Petri dishes are incubated at 37°C, according to the reading period set.

4. Count CFU using a colony counter. Plates presenting more than 300 CFUs are considered uncountable.

Microtiter plate and optical density test:

1. Reading by OD: dose a 96-well microtiter plate so that each vertical well row represents one treatment (ES, ES + bacterial inoculum, bacterial inoculum, bacterial inoculum + control antibiotic, and sterile Luria-Bertani broth.

2. The experimental groups are tested at least in triplicate. A total volume of 200 μL (1:1 in ES + bacterial inoculum and bacterial inoculum + control antibiotic groups) is introduced into each well.

3. Incubate the microplate at 37°C.

4. Measure changes in the OD at 540 nm (wavelength) with a microplate reader spectrometer. Measure every 1 h (for up to 6 h) and then after 24 h at 540 nm.

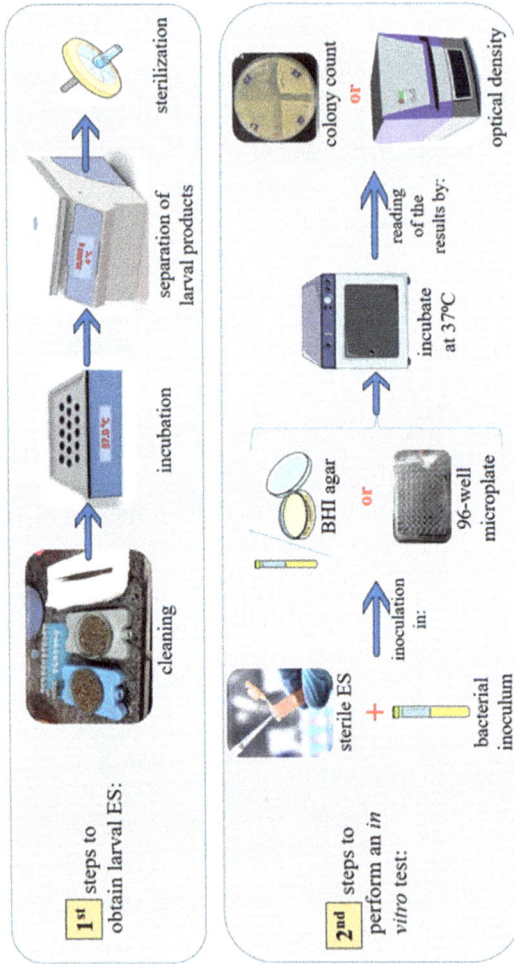

Figure 11.2 Summary model of *in vitro* test to assess the antimicrobial action of larval excretions/secretions of medicinal blowfly larvae against bacteria (adapted from Masiero and colleagues [43]).

How to Conduct In Vivo Experiments to Assess Therapeutic Safety and Efficacy of Fly Species after Preliminary In Vitro Testing

1. Establish fly colonies as described in Chapter 13 [2] of this book. For guidance on colony maintenance in the insectary, please refer to Chapter 14 [7].

2. Harvest eggs from established colonies with some raw minced liver.

3. Remove eggs from the liver bait and disinfect by washing them for 3 min with 1% sodium hypochlorite (NaOCl) [69].

4. Place disinfected eggs on filter paper and incubate them at 25°C until the larvae hatch.

5. Transfer new hatched larvae to a container containing 1 g sterile diet [94] or blood agar per transferred larva.

6. Allow larvae to feed on diet for 12 h before depositing them on the wound.

7. Obtain around 13 male (or female) 12-week-old Wistar rats (*Rattus norvegicus alvinus*, Rodentia, Mammalia), weighing approximately 350 g.

8. Keep the rats in individual cages at a temperature of 22±2°C and a 12-h photoperiod.

9. Before lesions are induced, administer anaesthesia and analgesia with ketamine hydrochloride (75 mg/kg) and xylazine (10 mg/kg) both intraperitoneal.

10. Shave the dorsal region and administer 0.2 mL of a 1:4 solution of hydrochloric acid and distilled water subcutaneously.

11. Lesions will open on their own within three days. Analgesic medicine should be given systematically to control discomfort.

12. Randomly divide animals into at least two groups (N= 6 in each group)

13. Treat one group with maggot therapy (5 larvae/cm²) and the other, being the control group, with a treatment for which efficacy is known and supported by strong evidence. During

treatment, the lesions must be covered with a confinement dressing made of polyurethane dressing, sterile gauze, and tape to prevent escape and suffocation of larvae [79].

14. Administer treatments for 48–72 h.

15. Evaluate lesions daily, from the beginning of the application of the treatments until the end of the experiment or complete healing. Possible assessment metrics include:

    a. Healing progress, wound shape, wound edge characteristics, wound depth, quantity of necrotic tissue, type and quantity of exudate, and amount of granulation tissue.

    b. The wounds can also be evaluated according to Pressure Ulcer Scale for Healing (PUSH) (National Pressure Ulcer Advisory Panel, 1998). Particular attention (and a more detailed examination) should be paid on the initial day of treatment (day 0) and on days 3, 7, and 12 after treatment, to capture significant changes in the lesions [73].

    c. Additionally, photographic records before, during, and after each treatment are recommended in order to document the results and to assess the ratio of wound healing (RWH). RWH represents the reduction percentage of the wound in relation to its size before the beginning of the treatment [95]. It is calculated by the following formula, where: A(i) = wound area at day zero, i.e., prior to treatment; A(f) = wound area on the day of evaluation. Areas can be calculated using any software suitable for this purpose.

$$RWH = \frac{A(i) - A(f)}{A(i)} \times 100$$

    d. Collect histopathological samples at 0 h (before application of any therapeutic treatment) and at 3, 7, and 12 days after administration of treatments.

e. On day 0, euthanise the one animal not assigned to a treatment group and obtain tissue samples. At days 3, 7, and 12, euthanise two randomly selected animals from each group for tissue sampling. Use a scalpel to excise a 5mm tick section of wound extending 5mm beyond the wound margin to include normal skin tissue.

f. Fix the samples for 24 h in 10% paraformaldehyde and dehydrate in 70% ethanol.

g. Then embed samples in paraffin and cut 5 μm sections.

h. Stain sections with hematoxylin-eosin (HE), and examine under an optical microscope for signs of inflammation, epithelial regeneration, and blood vessel formation.

Clinical Trials

Any investigative procedure performed with human subjects with the aim of providing information on the safety and efficacy of drugs and other medical therapies is called a clinical trial. As illustrated in Figure 11.4, these trials are generally divided into three phases starting with a small number of participants (phase I) where aspects related to safety are evaluated, followed by studies with a larger number of participants (phase II), which often compare the 'new' product or protocol with a currently prescribed treatment. Once favourable safety and efficacy data are gathered, the phase III trials are conducted, covering a much larger number of participants. Phase IV clinical trials follow the approval of a medical product or therapy by a regulatory agency (or health authority) and once placed on the market. In this phase, the long-term safety and efficacy of the therapy is being investigated using thousands of participants. It is important to remember that all clinical trials irrespective of the phase can only be carried out with the approval of the relevant ethics committee and respective local health authorities, because the trial involves either human or animal subjects (for veterinary therapies).

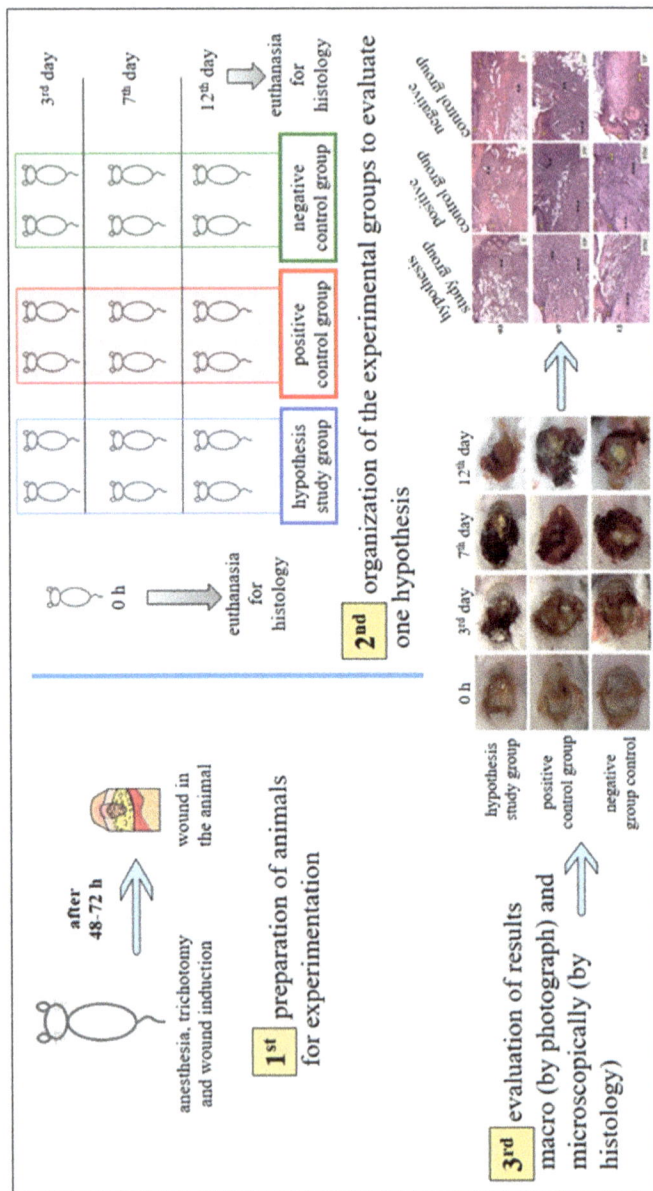

Figure 11.3 Summary model for *in vivo* experimentation to assess the safety and efficacy of blowfly species after preliminary *in vivo* experimentation and pre-selection for maggot therapy (adapted from Nassu and Thyssen [73] and Masiero and colleagues [95]).

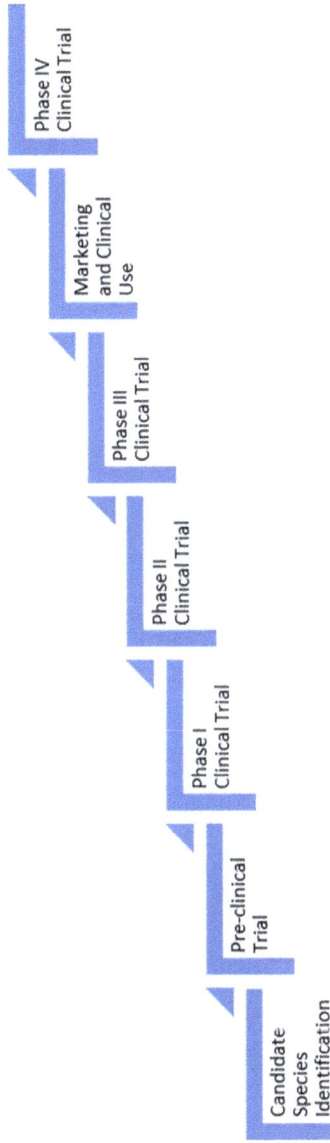

Figure 11.4 Step-wise process for the evaluation of a fly species for maggot therapy from bioprospecting to clinical use and beyond.

There are other relevant issues to consider when planning a clinical trial. They may be carried out in a single centre (usually phase I and II trials) or in several (multicentre trials). The latter are commonly phase III trials because of the number of participants involved. As for the methodology for acquiring sample data, the trials can be classified as blind, double-blind, randomised controlled, retrospective, or prospective. In a blind study, neither the study subject nor the examiner knows what treatment (response variable) is administered at any stage. It is commonly seen as one of the most effective and efficient mechanisms to guarantee the quality, reliability, integrity and consistency of the results obtained. For somewhat obvious reasons, trials with maggot therapy cannot be properly blinded because there is no way to "eliminate" the sensation of larvae moving in the wound, which is likely to be perceived by the patient, even if maggots are applied in biobags. As for the visual appearance of the dressing, practitioners will invariably notice even young maggots during application of biobags or free-range maggots on gauze pads. At the end of treatment during dressing removal, there is no hiding which wound received medicinal maggots. Consequently, blind maggot therapy trials are only possible if participating patients commit to secrecy and do not reveal what treatment they have received. Moreover, the researchers evaluating the therapeutic outcome must remain ignorant with regard to the treatment and do not witness dressing application and removal. The randomised controlled clinical trial (better known as RCT) is often used to test the effectiveness of a product or therapeutic approach in a given population compared to a control treatment, i.e., a product/approach with known effects. Randomisation with regard to which patient gets what treatment is a strategy used to increase the validity of the results obtained. The term control indicates that the participants will not receive a single intervention factor, otherwise it would be a descriptive study of effects with limited scientific value. It is the author's opinion that RCTs would be the preferred way to validate the use of maggot therapy. In Brazil, for example, the national health authority does not authorise the wide-scale use of a medical product or therapy like maggot therapy without consistent results from a RCT.

As mentioned above, studies can also be retrospective (in which the researcher studies participants based on an outcome) or prospective (when the outcome has not yet occurred). The type of study or experimental design must be chosen to minimise the chance of researcher bias. If retro- or prospective studies are undertaken then researchers must be careful to not only search for evidence that is consistent with their hypothesis but also to disregard those that may actually be more relevant [96]. In addition, Hanson [97] provides step-by-step guidance on how to design, conduct and report clinical research, including helpful tables and checklists.

The global burden of chronic and difficult-to-heal wounds is steadily growing. Most patients receiving maggot therapy are diabetics due to the frequency with which they are affected by difficult-to-heal wounds and the high number of unsuccessful treatments that often lead to infections, amputation of extremities, or death. It is estimated that the number of people with diabetes worldwide affected by complications of the lower limb is between 40 and 60 million [98]! Maggot therapy is very promising both in terms of its efficacy and affordability, particularly in austere environments [99, 100]. However, there appear to be only few large and well-designed clinical trials developed or under way that seek to assess the efficacy of maggot therapy in terms of its ability to debride wounds, control infections, and promote wound healing, although these therapeutic benefits have long been observed in practice and in the laboratory. Some of the most significant studies and clinical trials conducted to date (where the number of participants is equal to or > 10), including nonrandomised retrospective studies, nonrandomised prospective studies, RCTs (multicenter or blind) and meta-analysis, are shown in Table 11.3.

Table 11.3 Examples of some of the most significant studies and clinical trials conducted to assess the efficacy of maggot therapy taking into account the main objectives to be achieved and the target species of blowflies used for maggot therapy. Those with sample size less than ten have been excluded.

Type of study/ clinical trial design	Main goal	Country and Reference
Nonrandomised retrospective study	To compare the healing rate between wounds treated with maggot therapy (*L. sericata*) (n = 14) and conventional treatment (n = 6).	USA [101]
	To compare the treatment of infected wounds with maggot therapy (the fly species used was not mentioned, but was most likely *L. sericata*) and antibiotics.	USA [102]
	To compare time and healing rate in the treatment of infected pressure ulcers or diabetic foot ulcers (n = 23) with maggot therapy (*L. sericata*) and conventional treatment (n = 20).	China [103]
	To assess the healing evolution in decubitus (pressure) ulcers in the sacral region (n = 36). No control group was included.	Turkey [47]
Multicentre retrospective study	To assess the healing rate in the treatment of wounds (n = 723) with maggot therapy (*L. sericata*) by loose or bagged larvae.	Israel [104]
Nonrandomised prospective study	To compare the treatment of infected chronic diabetic foot ulcers in individuals aged 18–80 years with maggot therapy (*L. sericata*) and antibiotics. No control group was included.	UK [105]
	To compare the healing rate between wounds treated with maggot therapy (*L. cuprina*) (n = 29) and conventional debridement (n = 30).	Malaysia [106]
	To assess the treatment of chronic ulcers of distinct aetiologies in individuals aged 32–87 years with maggot therapy (*L. eximia*). No control group was included.	Colombia [91]
	To compare the treatment of infected lower limb wounds with maggot therapy (*L. sericata*) (n = 80)—in this case, considering two aspects: the treated area (legs or feet) and number of applied larvae (5 or 10 larvae/cm2)—and ozone therapy (n = 49).	Poland [107]

Type of study/ clinical trial design	Main goal	Country and Reference
Meta-analysis	To assess the outcomes and median costs of diabetic ulcer treatments with either maggot therapy or conventional treatment by pooling four previous cohort studies.	Thailand [108]
	To assess the time and healing rate in the treatment of wounds with mixed aetiologies. Twelve studies were included in the meta-analysis.	China [109]
RCT	To compare the median percentage area reduction of venous leg ulcers treated with four-layer compression bandaging (group I, n = 20) or four-layer compression bandaging + larvae (*L. sericata*) (group II, n = 20).	UK [110]
	To compare the treatment of infected (by *Staphylococcus aureus* or *Pseudomonas aeruginosa*) diabetic foot ulcers (n = 50) with maggot therapy (*L. sericata*) and conventional treatment (antibiotic therapy, debridement, and offloading).	Iran [111]
Three-arm RCT	To compare cost-effectiveness, time, and healing rate in the treatment of venous ulcers in which participants (n = 267) were assigned to one of three treatment groups: 1) loose larvae (*L. sericata*), 2) bagged larvae (*L. sericata*), and 3) hydrogel.	UK [112, 113]
Blinded RCT	To compare debridement rate and reduce the bacterial load and wound area in venous ulcers treated with maggot therapy (*L. sericata*) or surgical debridement followed by one topical application of silver sulfadiazine per week (for four weeks). It was mentioned that the statistician was not aware of the origin of the data that was received for analysis.	Mexico [114]

Type of study/ clinical trial design	Main goal	Country and Reference
Multicentre blinded RCT	To compare the debridement rate of venous ulcers, with 40 cm2 (or smaller) and > 2 cm deep (n= 119), treated with maggot therapy (bagged *L. sericata* larvae) and conventional treatment (surgical debridement + dressing of hydrogel or alginate) in individuals during a two-week hospital stay.	France [115]
	To compare the debridement speed of venous or arterial/venous ulcers (n = 64) treated with maggot therapy (*L. sericata*) or hydrogel.	UK [116]

Regulatory Approval

Unfortunately, in most countries (particularly those in the southern hemisphere) the use of maggot therapy is still limited to clinical research studies which prevent the treatment of a large number of wound patients who would benefit from maggot therapy (Table 11.3). The reasons for this include:

- MT is subject to regulatory and bureaucratic limitations before it reaches the patient. Under such circumstances, a very detailed research proposal must be presented to a local ethics committee, which will authorise its execution, provided the wellbeing and safety of patients are assured.

- In addition, it is also necessary to obtain the consent of every patient participating in the study. The human ethics of maggot therapy is discussed in detail in Chapter 19 of this book [117].

- A single or even multiple treatment centres may not have a large number of patients with wounds that are amenable to maggot therapy.

- Likewise, the treatment centres may lack appropriate infrastructure to cater for a large number of patients within the timeframe of a clinical trial.

To market and use medicinal maggots or wound care products derived from medicinal maggots on a routine basis, the medical product must be approved for use by the relevant ministries of health or their regulatory agencies. Health regulatory agencies are usually independent statutory bodies under the law with the main objective to regulate and inspect products or activities to protect healthcare consumers. Some of the best-known regulatory bodies and agencies are, for example, the Food and Drug Administration in the United States, the Medicines and Healthcare products Regulatory Agency in the United Kingdom, and the European Medicines Agency.

Obtaining authorisation for the use of a medical product or therapy can be quite challenging, because stringent safety and efficacy criteria must be met [118]. Such requirements are necessary as an additional measure that protects not only patients but also their treating physicians from harm and liability. In recent decades, medicine has advocated evidence-based practice [119], i.e., clinical decision making based on data obtained from systematic reviews of primary research as conducted by Cochrane [120]. Another mechanism to assess the overall quality of evidence for clinical decision making is GRADE which stands for Grading of Recommendations, Assessment, Development and Evaluations [96]. It is the most widely adopted tool for grading the quality of evidence and for making recommendations, endorsed by over 100 organisations worldwide. GRADE classifies the evidence as very low, low, moderate or high considering the following criteria: limitation of study design, imprecision, inconsistency, indirectness and bias of publication. As can be seen in Table 11.3, most studies conducted to evaluate the therapeutic efficacy of maggot therapy do not meet such high standards. The main reasons why most maggot therapy studies are not eligible for inclusion in systematic reviews or meta-analyses include: non-random allocation, non-blind evaluation of results, absence or poor description of the control group, simultaneous intervention, lack of clarity or non-follow-up of the outcome, studies with inadequate sample sizes, heterogeneity of the treated groups, and the lack of standardisation in the use of maggot therapy. For example, in the latest systematic review of the Cochrane Database on the debridement of diabetic foot ulcers to assess the rate of healing [121], only one RCT with maggot therapy was eligible for inclusion in the analysis.

Having said this, the existing substantive body of evidence [108, 109, 111, 116] and clinical experience leaves maggot therapy practitioners and patients with little doubt that maggot-assisted wound care is highly efficacious. It is therefore important that future clinical trials are designed according to best practice. To that end, researchers planning such studies are encouraged to consider the recommendations on clinical data collection, prepared by the European Wound Management Association's Patient Outcome Group [122], that describe criteria for producing rigorous outcomes in both RCTs and clinical studies, and describe how to ensure studies are consistent and reproducible. Another helpful read is a protocol proposed by Fan and colleagues [123] on how to conduct a systematic review and meta-analysis, which draws attention to particularly topical issues, such as the choice of participants for a given clinical trial (the inclusion of very heterogeneous wounds has been common) and poorly standardised practice in relation to the use of maggot therapy. For example, there may be significant differences in the effect of debridement with variations only in these two parameters.

We do not provide detailed guidance on how to apply for authorisation to use maggot therapy from regulatory agencies, as the list of documents and their order of presentation tend to vary significantly from country to country. In Brazil, as in other jurisdictions, specialised consultants can be hired to initiate this process at the Brazilian National Health Surveillance Agency (ANVISA), and we have observed that this action avoids delays in the evaluation of requests.

Clinical Use and Commercial Production

In the 1930s and '40s after William S. Baer introduced maggot therapy to modern medicine, medicinal maggots were produced in US, Canadian, and European hospitals for in-house use and Lederle Laboratories (Pearl River, NY) supplied medicinal maggots commercially. However, with the advent of antibiotics, maggot therapy fell out of favour [124]. However, since the late 1980s and early '90s, interest in maggot therapy has been steadily growing again. Today, two examples of successful commercialisation of *L. sericata* larvae for therapeutic purposes stand out. In Europe, BioMonde is the main supplier of medicinal maggots with origins dating back to 1994. In Europe, medicinal maggots are produced in accordance with current European Good Manufacturing Practice requirements. Until December 2020, BioMonde offered two products, loose (free-range) larvae and BioBag™ dressings. Due to regulatory and supply restrictions, as well as commercial unfeasibility, BioMonde discontinued the supply of free-range maggots in January 2021. In the US, medicinal maggots have been commercially produced and supplied by MonarchLabs since 2005. As far as regulatory approval is concerned, the Food and Drug Administration considers medicinal maggots a medical device [125].

It is important to note that in both cases the enterprises that commercialised medicinal maggots were spin-offs from research programmes at prestigious universities [126–128]. This is not a surprise because it is a long and costly research process until medicinal maggots can be commercially produced, marketed and applied in the clinical setting, especially for new medicinal fly species (but also for *L. sericata* in jurisdictions where maggot therapy is not yet approved). Unfortunately, partnerships between universities and the commercial sector in low- and middle-income countries are impractical for a number of reasons, including low institutional productivity and inadequate professional qualification. The absence of reliable, fast, and affordable delivery services for highly perishable maggots is also a barrier to commercialisation in low- and middle-income countries. Recent efforts by MedMagLabs [129] to locate medicinal maggot production at the point of care to avoid supply chain interruptions are promising. Regardless, these barriers to maggot therapy may explain why there has been little progress as far as maggot therapy in developing countries is concerned [130], despite the fact that highly efficacious maggot therapy is generally cheaper than other treatments for hard-to-heal wounds, especially in the low- and middle-income country context [113, 131].

In the US and Europe educational resources and training activities are offered by maggot therapy producers [132], researchers [133], professional bodies [134], and foundations [135]. The positive impact on patients' quality of life through qualitative studies of patient perceptions and experiences is still little explored but the few studies report favourable outcomes. For example, positive experiences among patients who used maggot therapy were reported by Kithching [136] and Silva and colleagues [137]. The latter study was carried out in South

America using *Ch. megacephala*, a newly selected medicinal fly species [90]. The patients who received the treatment perceived maggot therapy as the most successful treatment yet on their journey to wound healing.

Summary

It is highly desirable that a number of fly species representing all major biogeographic regions are available for maggot therapy [2]. This will ensure that maggot therapy can be implemented globally. This is because national quarantine authorities will be reluctant to permit the importation of non-native fly species, especially if they are considered agricultural pests. Moreover, it is conceivable that this bioprospecting will result in new fly species with superior or different therapeutic properties compared to those found in *L. sericata*.

The selection of a new fly species for maggot therapy must take into account the life-cycle of the species, which should be short so it facilitates mass rearing. The environmental requirements and the species' adaptability to maintenance in the insectary must also be considered. Any new target species with favourable characteristics must be assessed, either *in vitro* or in animal models, for their safety and efficacy. For example, they must not consume living tissue and pre-clinical testing must indicate likely therapeutic benefit to the patient. When development proceeds to clinical trials, it is important that these are planned and executed according to best practice to ensure that the data generated is acceptable to the medical regulators and demonstrates clearly the benefits and safety of maggot therapy with the species under investigation.

References

1.   Harvey, M., *The Natural History of Medicinal Flies*, in *A Complete Guide to Maggot Therapy: Clinical Practice, Therapeutic Principles, Production, Distribution, and Ethics*, F. Stadler (ed.). 2022, Cambridge: Open Book Publishers, pp. 121–142, https://doi.org/10.11647/OBP.0300.07.

2.   Stadler, F., et al., *Fly Colony Establishment*, in *A Complete Guide to Maggot Therapy: Clinical Practice, Therapeutic Principles, Production, Distribution, and Ethics*, F. Stadler (ed.). 2022, Cambridge: Open Book Publishers, pp. 257–288 (p. 269), https://doi.org/10.11647/OBP.0300.13.

3. Courtney, G.W., et al., *Biodiversity of Diptera*, in *Insect Biodiversity: Science and Society*, R.G. Foottit and P.H. Adler (eds). 2017, Wiley-Blackwell: New Jersey, USA, pp. 229–278.

4. Stadler, F., *Laboratory and Insectary Infrastructure and Equipment*, in *A Complete Guide to Maggot Therapy: Clinical Practice, Therapeutic Principles, Production, Distribution, and Ethics*, F. Stadler (ed.). 2022, Cambridge: Open Book Publishers, pp. 237–256, https://doi.org/10.11647/OBP.0300.12.

5. Stadler, F., *Packaging Technology*, in *A Complete Guide to Maggot Therapy: Clinical Practice, Therapeutic Principles, Production, Distribution, and Ethics*, F. Stadler (ed.). 2022, Cambridge: Open Book Publishers, pp. 349–362, https://doi.org/10.11647/OBP.0300.16.

6. Stadler, F., *Distribution Logistics*, in *A Complete Guide to Maggot Therapy: Clinical Practice, Therapeutic Principles, Production, Distribution, and Ethics*, F. Stadler (ed.). 2022, Cambridge: Open Book Publishers, pp. 363–382, https://doi.org/10.11647/OBP.0300.17.

7. Stadler, F. and P. Takáč, *Medicinal Maggot Production*, in *A Complete Guide to Maggot Therapy: Clinical Practice, Therapeutic Principles, Production, Distribution, and Ethics*, F. Stadler (ed.). 2022, Cambridge: Open Book Publishers, pp. 289–330, https://doi.org/10.11647/OBP.0300.14.

8. Stadler, F. and P. Tatham, *Drone-assisted Medicinal Maggot Distribution in Compromised Healthcare Settings*, in *A Complete Guide to Maggot Therapy: Clinical Practice, Therapeutic Principles, Production, Distribution, and Ethics*, F. Stadler (ed.). 2022, Cambridge: Open Book Publishers, pp. 383–402, https://doi.org/10.11647/OBP.0300.18.

9. Takáč, P., et al., and F. Stadler, *Establishment of a Medicinal Maggot Production Facility and Treatment Programme in Kenya*, in *A Complete Guide to Maggot Therapy: Clinical Practice, Therapeutic Principles, Production, Distribution, and Ethics*, F. Stadler (ed.). 2022, Cambridge: Open Book Publishers, pp. 289–330, https://doi.org/10.11647/OBP.0300.14.

10. Bernhardt, V., et al., *Myiasis in Humans-A Global Case Report Evaluation and Literature Analysis*. Parasitology Research, 2019. 118(2): pp. 389–397, https://doi.org/10.1007/s00436-018-6145-7.

11. Loureiro, J.F., et al., [*Colon Myiasis*]. Revista da Associacao Medica Brasileira, 2010. 56(6): p. 638, https://doi.org/10.1590/s0104-42302010000600008.

12. Marcondes, C.B., *Dermatobia Hominis (Diptera: Cuterebridae) in Africa and the Need for Caution in its Taxonomy*. Journal of Infection and Public Health, 2014. 7(1): pp. 73–74, https://doi.org/10.1016/j.jiph.2013.07.007.

13. Osorio, J.H., *Diagnostic Mistake and Wrong Treatment of Cutaneous Myiasis by Cochliomyia Hominivorax (Coquerel) (Diptera: Calliphoridae)*. Brazilian Journal of Biological Sciences, 2016. 3(5): pp. 231–239.

14. Carvalho, L.M.L., et al. *Observations on the Succession Patterns of Necrophagous Insects on a Pig Carcass in an Urban Area of Southeastern Brazil*. Anil Aggrawals Internet Journal of Forensic Medicine and Toxicology 2004 5(1) ; pp. 33–39.

15. Azeredo-Espin, A.M. and N.G. Madeira, *Primary Myiasis in Dog Caused by Phaenicia Eximia (Diptera:Calliphoridae) and Preliminary Mitochondrial DNA Analysis of the Species in Brazil*. J Med Entomol, 1996. 33(5): pp. 839–843, https://doi.org/10.1093/jmedent/33.5.839.

16. Cansi, E.R., et al., *Myiasis by Screw Worm Cochliomyia Hominivorax (Coquerel) (Diptera: Calliphoridae) in a Wild Maned Wolf Chrysocyon Brachyurus (Mammalia: Canidae), in Brasília, Brazil*. Neotropical Entomology, 2011. 40(1): pp. 150–151, https://doi.org/10.1590/s1519-566x2011000100025.

17. Moretti, T.C. and P.J. Thyssen, *Miíase primária em coelho doméstico causada por Lucilia eximia (Diptera: Calliphoridae) no Brasil: relato de caso*. Arquivo Brasileiro de Medicina Veterinaria e Zootecnia, 2006. 58(1): pp. 28–30, https://doi.org/10.1590/S0102-09352006000100005.

18. Hall, M. and R. Wall, *Myiasis of Humans and Domestic Animals*. Advances in Parasitololgy, 1995. 35: pp. 257–334, https://doi.org/10.1016/s0065-308x(08)60073-1.

19. Stevens, J. and R. Wall, *Species, Sub-species and Hybrid Populations of the Blowflies Lucilia cuprina and Lucilia sericata (Diptera:Calliphoridae)*. Proceedings Biological Sciences, 1996. 263(1375): pp. 1335–1341, https://doi.org/10.1098/rspb.1996.0196.

20. Stevens, J. and R. Wall, *The Evolution of Ectoparasitism in the Genus Lucilia (Diptera:Calliphoridae)*. International Journal for Parasitology, 1997. 27(1): pp. 51–59, https://doi.org/10.1016/s0020-7519(96)00155-5.

21. Stevens, J. and R. Wall, *Genetic Variation in Populations of the Blowflies Lucilia cuprina and Lucilia sericata (Diptera: Calliphoridae). Random Amplified Polymorphic DNA Analysis and Mitochondrial DNA Sequences*. Biochemical Systematics and Ecology, 1997. 25(2): pp. 81–97, https://doi.org/10.1016/S0305-1978(96)00038-5.

22. Tantawi, T.I., K.A. Williams, and M.H. Villet, *An Accidental but Safe and Effective Use of Lucilia cuprina (Diptera: Calliphoridae) in Maggot Debridement Therapy in Alexandria, Egypt*. Journal of Medical Entomology, 2010. 47(3): pp. 491–494, https://doi.org/10.1093/jmedent/47.3.491.

23. Thyssen, P.J., et al., *Implications of Entomological Evidence during the Investigation of Five Cases of Violent Death in Southern Brazil*. Journal of Forensic Science and Research, 2018. 2: pp. 001–008, https://doi.org/10.29328/journal.jfsr.1001013.

24. Faria, L.D.B., L.A. Trinca, and W.A.C. Godoy, *Cannibalistic Behavior and Functional Response in Chysomya Albiceps (Diptera: Calliphoridae)*. Journal of Insect Behavior, 2004. 17: pp. 251–261, https://dx.doi.org/10.1023/B:JOIR.0000028574.91062.18.

25. Spindola, A.F., et al., *Attraction and Oviposition of Lucilia eximia (Diptera: Calliphoridae) to Resources Colonized by the Invasive Competitor Chrysomya albiceps (Diptera: Calliphoridae)*. Journal of Medical Entomology, 2017. 54(2): pp. 321–328, https://doi.org/10.1093/jme/tjw170.

26. Rosa, G.S., et al., *The Dynamics of Intraguild Predation in Chrysomya albiceps Wied. (Diptera: Calliphoridae): Interactions between Instars and Species under Different Abundances of Food*. Neotropical Entomology, 2006. 35(6): p. 775–780, https://doi.org/10.1590/s1519-566x2006000600009.

27. Blake, F.A., et al., *The Biosurgical Wound Debridement: Experimental Investigation of Efficiency and Practicability*. Wound Repair and Regeneration, 2007. 15(5): pp. 756–761, https://doi.org/10.1111/j.1524-475X.2007.00298.x.

28. Dini, V., et al., *Correlation Between Wound Temperature Obtained With an Infrared Camera and Clinical Wound Bed Score in Venous Leg Ulcers*. Wounds, 2015. 27(10): pp. 274–278 http://www.woundsresearch.com/article/correlation-between-wound-temperature-obtained-infrared-camera-and-clinical-wound-bed-score.

29. McGuiness, W., E. Vella, and D. Harrison, *Influence of Dressing Changes on Wound Temperature*. Journal of Wound Care, 2004. 13(9): pp. 383–385, https://doi.org/10.12968/jowc.2004.13.9.26702.

30. Chernysh, S., et al., *Antiviral and Antitumor Peptides from Insects*. Procedings of the National Academie of Science of the Unites States of America, 2002. 99(20): pp. 12628–12632, https://doi.org/10.1073/pnas.192301899.

31. El Shazely, B., et al., *Lucifensin II, a Defensin of Medicinal Maggots of the Blowfly Lucilia cuprina (Diptera: Calliphoridae)*. Journal of Medical Entomology, 2013. 50(3): pp. 571–578, https://doi.org/10.1603/me12208.

32. Téllez, G.A., et al., *Identification, Characterization, Immunolocalization, and Biological Activity of Lucilin Peptide*. Acta Tropica, 2018. 185: pp. 318–326, https://doi.org/10.1016/j.actatropica.2018.06.003.

33. Ceřovský, V., et al., *Lucifensin, a Novel Insect Defensin of Medicinal Maggots: Synthesis and Structural Study*. ChemBioChem, 2011. 12(9): pp. 1352–1361, https://doi.org/10.1002/cbic.201100066.

34. Pöppel, A.K., et al., *Lucimycin, an Antifungal Peptide from the Therapeutic Maggot of the Common Green Bottle Fly Lucilia sericata*. Biological Chemistry, 2014. 395(6): pp. 649–656, https://doi.org/10.1515/hsz-2013-0263.

35. Lambert, J., et al., *Insect Immunity: Isolation from Immune Blood of the Dipteran Phormia Terranovae of Two Insect Antibacterial Peptides with Sequence Homology to Rabbit Lung Macrophage Bactericidal Peptides*. Proceedings of the National Academie of the United States of America, 1989. 86(1): pp. 262–266, https://doi.org/10.1073/pnas.86.1.262.

36. Díaz-Roa, A., et al., *Sarconesin II, a New Antimicrobial Peptide Isolated from Sarconesiopsis magellanica Excretions and Secretions*. Molecules, 2019. 24(11), https://doi.org/10.3390/molecules24112077.

37. Díaz-Roa, A., et al., *Sarconesin: Sarconesiopsis magellanica Blowfly Larval Excretions and Secretions with Antibacterial Properties*. Frontiers in Microbiology, 2018. 9(2249): pp. 1–13, https://doi.org/10.3389/fmicb.2018.02249.

38. Dallavecchia, D.L., et al., *Antibacterial and Antifungal Activity of Excretions and Secretions of Calliphora Vicina*. Medical and Veterinary Entomology, 2021. 35(2): pp. 225–229, https://doi.org/10.1111/mve.12486.

39. Sanei-Dehkordi, A., et al., *Anti Leishmania Activity of Lucilia sericata and Calliphora vicina Maggots in Laboratory Models*. Experimental Parasitology, 2016. 170: p. 59–65, https://doi.org/10.1016/j.exppara.2016.08.007.

40. Ratcliffe, N.A., et al., *Detection and Preliminary Physico-chemical Properties of Antimicrobial Components in the Native Excretions/Secretions of Three Species of Chrysomya (Diptera, Calliphoridae) in Brazil*. Acta Tropica, 2015. 147: pp. 6–11, https://doi.org/10.1016/j.actatropica.2015.03.021.

41. Mohamed, N.T., *Fractionation and Purification of Bioactive Peptides in Excretory/Secretory Products of Third Instar Larvae of Chrysomya Megacephala (Calliphoridae: Diptera)*. Bulletin of Envrionment, Pharmacy and Life Sciences, 2015. 4(10): pp. 69–74.

42. Fonseca-Muñoz, A., et al., *Bactericidal Activity of Chrysomya rufifacies and Cochliomyia macellaria (Diptera: Calliphoridae) Larval Excretions-Secretions Against Staphylococcus aureus (Bacillales: Staphylococcaceae)*. Journal of Medical Entomology, 2019. 56(6): pp. 1598–1604, https://doi.org/10.1093/jme/tjz109.

43. Masiero, F.S., et al., *First Record of Larval Secretions of Cochliomyia macellaria (Fabricius, 1775) (Diptera: Calliphoridae) Inhibiting the Growth of Staphylococcus aureus and Pseudomonas aeruginosa*. Neotropical Entomology, 2017. 46(1): pp. 125–129, https://doi.org/10.1007/s13744-016-0444-4.

44. Abdel-Samad, M.R.K., *Antiviral and Virucidal Activities of Lucilia cuprina Maggots' Excretion/Secretion (Diptera: Calliphoridae): First Work*. Heliyon, 2019. 5(11): e02791, https://doi.org/10.1016/j.heliyon.2019.e02791.

45. Arora, S., C. Baptista, and C.S. Lim, *Maggot Metabolites and Their Combinatory Effects with Antibiotic on Staphylococcus aureus*. Annals of Clinical Microbiology and Antimicrobials, 2011. 10(6): pp. 1–8, https://doi.org/10.1186/1476-0711-10-6.

46. Teh, C.H., et al., *In vitro Antibacterial Activity and Physicochemical Properties of a Crude Methanol Extract of the Larvae of the Blow Fly Lucilia cuprina*. Medical and Veterinary Entomology, 2013. 27(4): pp. 414–420, https://doi.org/10.1111/mve.12012.

47. Polat, E., et al., *Treatment of Pressure Ulcers with Larvae of Lucilia sericata*. Türkiye Fiziksel Tıp ve Rehabilitasyon Dergisi, 2017. 63(4): pp. 307–312, https://doi.org/10.5606/tftrd.2017.851.

48. Thomas, S., et al., *The Anti-microbial Activity of Maggot Secretions: Results of a Preliminary Study.* Journal of Tissue Viability, 1999. 9(4): pp. 127–132, https://doi.org/10.1016/s0965-206x(99)80032-1.

49. Laverde-Paz, M.J., et al., *Evaluating the Anti-leishmania Activity of Lucilia sericata and Sarconesiopsis magellanica Blowfly Larval Excretions/Secretions in an in vitro Model.* Acta Tropica, 2018. 177: pp. 44–50, https://doi.org/10.1016/j.actatropica.2017.09.033.

50. Fu, P., J. Wu, and G. Guo, *Purification and Molecular Identification of an Antifungal Peptide from the Hemolymph of Musca domestica (Housefly).* Cellular & Molecular Immunology, 2009. 6(4): pp. 245–251, https://doi.org/10.1038/cmi.2009.33.

51. Díaz-Roa, A., et al., *Sarconesiopsis magellanica (Diptera: Calliphoridae) Excretions and Secretions Have Potent Antibacterial Activity.* Acta Tropica, 2014. 136: pp. 37–43, https://doi.org/10.1016/j.actatropica.2014.04.018.

52. Góngora, J., et al., *Evaluación de la actividad antibacterial de los extractos de cuerpos grasos y hemolinfa derivados de la mosca Sarconesiopsis magellanica (Diptera: Calliphoridae).* Infectio, 2015. 19(1): pp. 3–9, https://doi.org/10.1016/j.infect.2014.09.003.

53. Gordya, N., et al., *Natural Antimicrobial Peptide Complexes in the Fighting of Antibiotic Resistant Biofilms: Calliphora vicina Medicinal Maggots.* PLoS ONE, 2017. 12(3): e0173559, https://doi.org/10.1371/journal.pone.0173559.

54. Harris, L.G., et al., *Disruption of Staphylococcus epidermidis Biofilms by Medicinal Maggot Lucilia sericata Excretions/Secretions.* International Journal of Artificial Organs, 2009. 32(9): pp. 555–564, https://doi.org/10.1177/039139880903200904.

55. Jiang, K.C., et al., *Excretions/Secretions from Bacteria-pretreated Maggot Are More Effective against Pseudomonas aeruginosa Biofilms.* PLoS ONE, 2012. 7(11): e49815, https://doi.org/10.1371/journal.pone.0049815.

56. van der Plas, M.J., et al., *Combinations of Maggot Excretions/Secretions and Antibiotics Are Effective against Staphylococcus aureus Biofilms and the Bacteria Derived Therefrom.* Journal of Antimicrobial Chemotherapy, 2010. 65(5): pp. 917–923, https://doi.org/10.1093/jac/dkq042.

57. van der Plas, M.J., et al., *Maggot Excretions/Secretions Are Differentially Effective against Biofilms of Staphylococcus aureus and Pseudomonas aeruginosa.* Journal of Antimicrobial Chemotherapy, 2008. 61(1): pp. 117–122, https://doi.org/10.1093/jac/dkm407.

58. Cazander, G., et al., *Synergism between Maggot Excretions and Antibiotics.* Wound Repair and Regeneration, 2010. 18(6): pp. 637–642, https://doi.org/10.1111/j.1524-475X.2010.00625.x.

59. Masiero, F.S., et al., *In vitro Evaluation of the Association of Medicinal Larvae (Insecta, Diptera, Calliphoridae) and Topical Agents Conventionally Used for*

the Treatment of Wounds. Acta Tropica, 2019. 190: pp. 68–72, https://doi. org/10.1016/j.actatropica.2018.10.015.

60. Horobin, A.J., K.M. Shakesheff, and D.I. Pritchard, *Promotion of Human Dermal Fibroblast Migration, Matrix Remodelling and Modification of Fibroblast Morphology within a Novel 3D Model by Lucilia sericata Larval Secretions*. The Journal of Investigative Dermatology, 2006. 126(6): pp. 1410–1408, https:// doi.org/10.1038/sj.jid.5700256.

61. van der Plas, M.J., et al., *Maggot Secretions Suppress Pro-inflammatory Responses of Human Monocytes through Elevation of Cyclic AMP*. Diabetologia, 2009. 52(9): pp. 1962–1970, https://doi.org/10.1007/s00125-009-1432-6.

62. Bexfield, A., et al., *Amino Acid Derivatives from Lucilia sericata Excretions/ Secretions May Contribute to the Beneficial Effects of Maggot Therapy via Increased Angiogenesis*. British Journal of Dermatology, 2010. 162(3): pp. 554–562, https://doi.org/10.1111/j.1365-2133.2009.09530.x.

63. Wang, S.Y., et al., *Maggot Excretions/Secretions Induces Human Microvascular Endothelial Cell Migration through AKT1*. Molecular Biology Reports, 2010. 37(6): pp. 2719–2725, https://doi.org/10.1007/s11033-009-9806-x.

64. Linger, R.J., et al., *Towards Next Generation Maggot Debridement Therapy: Transgenic Lucilia sericata Larvae that Produce and Secrete a Human Growth Factor*. BMC Biotechnology, 2016. 16(30): pp. 1–12, https://doi.org/10.1186/ s12896-016-0263-z.

65. Čičková, H., M. Kozánek, and P. Takáč, *Growth and Survival of Blowfly Lucilia sericata Larvae under Simulated Wound Conditions: Implications for Maggot Debridement Therapy*. Medical and Veterinary Entomology, 2015. 29(4): pp. 416–424, https://doi.org/10.1111/mve.12135.

66. Wilson, M.R., et al., *The Impacts of Larval Density and Protease Inhibition on Feeding in Medicinal Larvae of the Greenbottle Fly Lucilia sericata*. Med Vet Entomol, 2016. 30(1): pp. 1–7, https://doi.org/10.1111/mve.12138.

67. Rajamohan, A., J.P. Rinehart, and R.A. Leopold, *Cryopreservation of Embryos of Lucilia sericata (Diptera: Calliphoridae)*. Journal of Medical Entomology, 2014. 51(2): pp. 360–367, https://doi.org/10.1603/me13188.

68. Brundage, A.L., T.L. Crippen, and J.K. Tomberlin, *Methods for External Disinfection of Blow Fly (Diptera: Calliphoridae) Eggs prior to Use in Wound Debridement Therapy*. Wound Repair Regen, 2016. 24(2): pp. 384–393, https://doi.org/10.1111/wrr.12408.

69. Thyssen, P.J., et al., *Sterilization of Immature Blowflies (Calliphoridae) for Use in Larval Therapy*. Journal of Medicine and Medical Sciences, 2013. 4(10): pp. 405–409 https://www.interesjournals.org/articles/sterilization-of- immature-blowflies-calliphoridae-for-use-in-larval-therapy.pdf.

70. Dallavecchia, D.L., et al., *Efficacy of UV-C Ray Sterilization of Calliphora vicina (Diptera: Calliphoridae) Eggs for Use in Maggot Debridement Therapy*. Journal

of Medical Entomology, 2019. 56(1): pp. 40–44, https://doi.org/10.1093/jme/tjy140.

71.   Limsopatham, K., et al., *Sterilization of Blow Fly Eggs, Chrysomya megacephala and Lucilia cuprina, (Diptera: Calliphoridae) for Maggot Debridement Therapy Application.* Parasitology Research, 2017. 116(5): pp. 1581–1589, https://doi.org/10.1007/s00436-017-5435-9.

72.   Mohd Masri, S., et al., *Sterilisation of Lucilia cuprina Wiedemann Maggots Used in Therapy of Intractable Wounds.* Tropical Biomedicine, 2005. 22(2): pp. 185–189.

73.   Nassu, M.P. and P.J. Thyssen, *Evaluation of Larval Density Cochliomyia macellaria F. (Diptera: Calliphoridae) for Therapeutic Use in the Recovery of Tegumentar Injuries.* Parasitology Research, 2015. 114(9): pp. 3255–3260, https://doi.org/10.1007/s00436-015-4542-8.

74.   Parrado, A.E.R., et al., *Terapia Larval con Musca domestica en el tratamiento de la úlcera leishmánica en un modelo murino.* Acta Biológica Colombiana, 2020. 25(1): pp. 82–95, https://doi.org/10.15446/abc.v25n1.77177.

75.   Cruz-Saavedra, L., et al., *The Effect of Lucilia sericata- and Sarconesiopsis magellanica-derived Larval Therapy on Leishmania panamensis.* Acta Tropica, 2016. 164: pp. 280–289, https://doi.org/10.1016/j.actatropica.2016.09.020.

76.   Zhang, Z., et al., *Activity of Antibacterial Protein from Maggots against Staphylococcus aureus in vitro and in vivo.* International Journal of Molecular Medicine, 2013. 31(5): pp. 1159–1165, https://doi.org/10.3892/ijmm.2013.1291.

77.   Arrivillaga, J., J. Rodríguez, and M. Oviedo, [*Preliminary Evaluation of Maggot (Diptera: Calliphoridae) Therapy as a Potential Treatment for Leishmaniasis Ulcers*]. Biomédica, 2008. 28(2): pp. 305–310, https://dx.doi.org/10.7705/biomedica.v28i2.102.

78.   Masiero, F.S., et al., *Histological Patterns in Healing Chronic Wounds Using Cochliomyia macellaria (Diptera: Calliphoridae) Larvae and Other Therapeutic Measures.* Parasitology Research, 2015. 114(8): pp. 2865–2872, https://doi.org/10.1007/s00436-015-4487-y.

79.   Masiero, F.S. and P.J. Thyssen, *Evaluation of Conventional Therapeutic Methods versus Maggot Therapy in the Evolution of Healing of Tegumental Injuries in Wistar Rats with and without Diabetes mellitus.* Parasitology Research, 2016. 115(6): pp. 2403–2407, https://doi.org/10.1007/s00436-016-4991-8.

80.   Hassan, M.I., et al., *The Using of Lucilia cuprina Maggots in the Treatment of Diabetic Foot Wounds.* Journal of the Egyptian Society of Parasitology, 2014. 44(1): pp. 125–129, https://doi.org/10.12816/0006451.

81.   Li, P.N., et al., *Molecular Events Underlying Maggot Extract Promoted Rat in vivo and Human in vitro Skin Wound Healing.* Wound Repair and Regeneration, 2015. 23(1): pp. 65–73, https://doi.org/10.1111/wrr.12243.

82. Díaz-Roa, A., et al., *Evaluating Sarconesiopsis magellanica Blowfly-derived Larval Therapy and Comparing It to Lucilia sericata-derived Therapy in an Animal Model*. Acta Tropica, 2016. 154: pp. 34–41, https://doi.org/10.1016/j.actatropica.2015.10.024.

83. Tombulturk, F.K., et al., *Effects of Lucilia sericata on Wound Healing in Streptozotocin-induced Diabetic Rats and Analysis of Its Secretome at the Proteome Level*. Human & Experimental Toxicology, 2018. 37(5): pp. 508–520, https://doi.org/10.1177/0960327117714041.

84. Zhang, Z., et al., *Fatty Acid Extracts from Lucilia sericata Larvae Promote Murine Cutaneous Wound Healing by Angiogenic Activity*. Lipids in Health and Disease, 2010. 9(24): pp. 1–9, https://doi.org/10.1186/1476-511x-9-24.

85. Góngora, J., et al., *Evaluating the Effect of Sarconesiopsis magellanica (Diptera: Calliphoridae) Larvae-derived Haemolymph and Fat Body Extracts on Chronic Wounds in Diabetic Rabbits*. Journal of Diabetes Research, 2015. 2015: p. 270253, https://doi.org/10.1155/2015/270253.

86. Arora, S., L.C. Sing, and C. Baptista, *Antibacterial Activity of Lucilia cuprina Maggot Extracts and Its Extraction Techniques*. International Journal of Integrative Biology, 2010. 9(1): pp. 43–48.

87. Bernhardt, V., et al., *Of Pigs and Men-Comparing the Development of Calliphora vicina (Diptera: Calliphoridae) on Human and Porcine Tissue*. International Journal of Legal Medicine, 2017. 131(3): pp. 847–853, https://doi.org/10.1007/s00414-016-1487-0.

88. Clark, K., L. Evans, and R. Wall, *Growth Rates of the Blowfly, Lucilia sericata, on Different Body Tissues*. Forensic Science International, 2006. 156(2–3): pp. 145–149, https://doi.org/10.1016/j.forsciint.2004.12.025.

89. Figueroa, L., et al., *Experiencia de terapia larval en pacientes con úlceras crónicas*. Parasitología Latinoamericana, 2006. 61: pp. 160–164.

90. Pinheiro, M.A., et al., *Use of Maggot Therapy for Treating a Diabetic Foot Ulcer Colonized by Multidrug Resistant Bacteria in Brazil*. Indian Journal of Medical Research, 2015. 141(3): pp. 340–342 https://journals.lww.com/ijmr/Fulltext/2015/41030/Use_of_maggot_therapy_for_treating_a_diabetic_foot.13.aspx.

91. Wolff, M.I., et al., *Lucilia eximia (Diptera: Calliphoridae), una nueva alternativa para la terapia larval y reporte de casos en Colombia*. Iatreia, 2010. 23(2): pp. 107–116.

92. Steenvoorde, P., C.E. Jacobi, and J. Oskam, *Maggot Debridement Therapy: Free-range or Contained? An in-vivo Study*. Advances in Skin & Wound Care, 2005. 18(8): pp. 430–435, https://doi.org/10.1097/00129334-200510000-00010.

93. Thomas, S., et al., *The Effect of Containment on the Properties of Sterile Maggots*. British Journal of Nursing, 2002. 11(12 Suppl): pp. S21–22, S24, S26 passim, https://doi.org/10.12968/bjon.2002.11.Sup2.10294.

94. Estrada, D.A., et al., [*Chrysomya albiceps* (*Wiedemann*) (*Diptera: Calliphoridae*) *Developmental Rate on Artificial Diet with Animal Tissues for Forensic Purpose*]. Neotropical Entomology, 2009. 38(2): pp. 203–207, https://doi. org/10.1590/s1519-566x2009000200006.

95. Masiero, F.S., et al., *First Report on the Use of Larvae of Cochliomyia macellaria* (*Diptera: Calliphoridae*) *for Wound Treatment in Veterinary Practice*. Journal of Medical Entomology, 2020. 57(3): pp. 965–968, https://doi.org/10.1093/ jme/tjz238.

96. Guyatt, G.H., et al., *GRADE: An Emerging Consensus on Rating Quality of Evidence and Strength of Recommendations*. BMJ, 2008. 336(7650): pp. 924– 926, https://doi.org/10.1136/bmj.39489.470347.AD.

97. Hanson, B.P., *Designing, Conducting and Reporting Clinical Research. A Step by Step Approach*. Injury, 2006. 37(7): pp. 583–594, https://doi.org/10.1016/j. injury.2005.06.051.

98. IDF. *IDF Diabetes Atlas*. 2021. https://diabetesatlas.org/.

99. Sherman, R.A. and M.R. Hetzler, *Maggot Therapy for Wound Care in Austere Environments*. Journal of Special Operations Medicine, 2017. 17(2): pp. 154–162.

100. Stadler, F., R.Z. Shaban, and P. Tatham, *Maggot Debridement Therapy in Disaster Medicine*. Prehospital and Disaster Medicine, 2016. 31(1): pp. 79–84, https://doi.org/10.1017/s1049023x15005427.

101. Sherman, R.A., *Maggot Therapy for Treating Diabetic Foot Ulcers Unresponsive to Conventional Therapy*. Diabetes Care, 2003. 26(2): pp. 446–451, https:// doi.org/10.2337/diacare.26.2.446.

102. Armstrong, D.G., et al., *Maggot Therapy in "Lower-extremity Hospice" Wound Care: Fewer Amputations and More Antibiotic-free Days*. Journal of the American Podiatric Medical Association, 2005. 95(3): pp. 254–257, https:// doi.org/10.7547/0950254.

103. Wang, S.Y., et al., *Clinical Research on the Bio-debridement Effect of Maggot Therapy for Treatment of Chronically Infected Lesions*. Orthopaedic Surgery, 2010. 2(3): pp. 201–206, https://doi.org/10.1111/j.1757-7861.2010.00087.x.

104. Gilead, L., K.Y. Mumcuoglu, and A. Ingber, *The Use of Maggot Debridement Therapy in the Treatment of Chronic Wounds in Hospitalised and Ambulatory Patients.* Journal of Wound Care, 2012. 21(2): pp. 78, 80, 82–85, https://doi. org/10.12968/jowc.2012.21.2.78.

105. Bowling, F.L., E.V. Salgami, and A.J. Boulton, *Larval Therapy: A Novel Treatment in Eliminating Methicillin-resistant Staphylococcus aureus from Diabetic Foot Ulcers*. Diabetes Care, 2007. 30(2): pp. 370–371, https://doi. org/10.2337/dc06-2348.

106. Paul, A.G., et al., *Maggot Debridement Therapy with Lucilia cuprina: A Comparison with Conventional Debridement in Diabetic Foot Ulcers*.

International Wound Journal, 2009. 6(1): pp. 39–46, https://doi.org/10.1111/j.1742-481X.2008.00564.x.

107. Szczepanowski, Z., et al., *Microbiological Effects in Patients with Leg Ulcers and Diabetic Foot Treated with Lucilia sericata Larvae*. International Wound Journal, 2022. 19(1): pp. 135–143, https://doi.org/10.1111/iwj.13605.

108. Wilasrusmee, C., et al., *Maggot Therapy for Chronic Ulcer: A Retrospective Cohort and a Meta-analysis*. Asian Journal of Surgery, 2014. 37(3): pp. 138–147, https://doi.org/10.1016/j.asjsur.2013.09.005.

109. Sun, X., et al., *A Systematic Review of Maggot Debridement Therapy for Chronically Infected Wounds and Ulcers*. International Journal of Infectious Diseases, 2014. 25: pp. 32–37, https://doi.org/10.1016/j.ijid.2014.03.1397.

110. Davies, C.E., et al., *Maggots as a Wound Debridement Agent for Chronic Venous Leg Ulcers under Graduated Compression Bandages: A Randomised Controlled Trial*. Phlebology, 2015. 30(10): pp. 693–699, https://doi.org/10.1177/0268355514555386.

111. Malekian, A., et al., *Efficacy of Maggot Therapy on Staphylococcus aureus and Pseudomonas aeruginosa in Diabetic Foot Ulcers: A Randomized Controlled Trial*. Journal of Wound, Ostomy and Continence Nursing, 2019. 46(1): pp. 25–29, https://doi.org/10.1097/won.0000000000000496.

112. Dumville, J.C., et al., *Larval Therapy for Leg Ulcers (VenUS II): Randomised Controlled Trial*. BMJ, 2009. 338: p. b773, https://doi.org/10.1136/bmj.b773.

113. Soares, M.O., et al., *Cost Effectiveness Analysis of Larval Therapy for Leg Ulcers*. BMJ, 2009. 338: p. b825, https://doi.org/10.1136/bmj.b825.

114. Contreras-Ruiz, J., et al., [*Comparative Study of the Efficacy of Larva Therapy for Debridement and Control of Bacterial Burden Compared to Surgical Debridement and Topical Application of an Antimicrobial*]. Gaceta médica de México, 2016. 152(Suppl 2): pp. 78–87, http://www.anmm.org.mx/GMM/2016/s2/GMM_152_2016_S2_78-87.pdf.

115. Opletalová, K., et al., *Maggot Therapy for Wound Debridement: A Randomized Multicenter Trial*. Archives of Dermatology, 2012. 148(4): pp. 432–438, https://doi.org/10.1001/archdermatol.2011.1895.

116. Mudge, E., et al., *A Randomized Controlled Trial of Larval Therapy for the Debridement of Leg Uulcers: Results of a Multicenter, Randomized, Controlled, Open, Observer Blind, Parallel Group Study*. Wound Repair Regen, 2014. 22(1): pp. 43–51, https://doi.org/10.1111/wrr.12127.

117. Stadler, F., *The Ethics of Maggot Therapy*, in *A Complete Guide to Maggot Therapy: Clinical Practice, Therapeutic Principles, Production, Distribution, and Ethics*, F. Stadler (ed.). 2022, Cambridge: Open Book Publishers, pp. 405–430, https://doi.org/10.11647/OBP.0300.19.

118. Gottrup, F., *Evidence Is a Challenge in Wound Management*. The International Journal of Lower Extremity Wounds, 2006. 5(2): pp. 74–75, https://doi.org/10.1177/1534734606288412.

119. Sackett, D.L., et al., *Evidence Based Medicine: What It Is and What It Isn't*. BMJ, 1996. 312(7023): pp. 71–72, https://doi.org/10.1136/bmj.312.7023.71.

120. Cochrane. *About Us*. https://www.cochrane.org/about-us.

121. Edwards, J. and S. Stapley, *Debridement of Diabetic Foot Ulcers*. Cochrane Database of Systematic Reviews, 2010. 2010(1): Cd003556, https://doi.org/10.1002/14651858.CD003556.pub2.

122. Gottrup, F., J. Apelqvist, and P. Price, *Outcomes in Controlled and Comparative Studies on Non-healing Wounds: Recommendations to Improve the Quality of Evidence in Wound Management*. Journal of Wound Care, 2010. 19(6): pp. 237–268, https://doi.org/10.12968/jowc.2010.19.6.48471.

123. Fan, W., et al., *Safety and Efficacy of Larval Therapy on Treating Leg Ulcers: A Protocol for Systematic Review and Meta-analysis*. BMJ Open, 2020. 10(10): e039898, https://doi.org/10.1136/bmjopen-2020-039898.

124. Whitaker, I.S., et al., *Larval Therapy from Antiquity to the Present Day: Mechanisms of Action, Clinical Applications and Future Potential*. Postgraduate Medical Journal, 2007. 83(980): pp. 409–413, https://doi.org/10.1136/pgmj.2006.055905.

125. FDA. *510(k) Summary. Monarch Labs, LLC*. 2007. https://www.accessdata.fda.gov/cdrh_docs/pdf7/K072438.pdf.

126. Grassberger, M. and W. Fleischmann, *The Biobag — A New Device for the Application of Medicinal Maggots*. Dermatology, 2002. 204(4): p. 306, https://doi.org/10.1159/000063369.

127. Sherman, R.A., *A New Dressing Design for Use with Maggot Therapy*. Plastic and Reconstructive Surgery, 1997. 100(2): pp. 451–456, https://doi.org/10.1097/00006534-199708000-00029.

128. Sherman, R.A. and F.A. Wyle, *Low-cost, Low-maintenance Rearing of Maggots in Hospitals, Clinics, and Schools*. American Journal of Tropical Medicine and Hygiene, 1996. 54(1): pp. 38–41, https://doi.org/10.4269/ajtmh.1996.54.38.

129. MedMagLabs. *Creating Hope in Conflict: A Humanitarian Grand Challenge*. http://medmaglabs.com/creating-hope-in-conflict/.

130. Roy, D. and R. Sherman, *Commnetary: Why is Maggot Therapy Not More Commonly Practiced in India?* Medical Journal of Dr. D.Y. Patil University, 2014. 7(5): pp. 642–643.

131. Eamkong, S., S. Pongpanich, and C. Rojanaworarit, *Comparison of Curing Costs between Maggot and Conventional Therapies for Chronic Wound Care*. Journal of Health Research, 2010. 24(suppl 2): pp. 21–25.

132. BioMonde. *Larval Academy*. https://biomonde.com/en/hcp/elearning/larval-academy.

133. Nigam, Y. *Love A Maggot*. https://loveamaggot.com/about/.

134. Mexican Association for Wound Care and Healing. *Clinical Practice Guidelines for the Treatment of Acute and Chronic Wounds with Maggot Debridement Therapy*. 2010. https://s3.amazonaws.com/aawc-new/memberclicks/GPC_larvatherapy.pdf.

135. BTER. *BioTherapeutics, Education and Research Foundation*. https://www.bterfoundation.org/.

136. Kitching, M., *Patients' Perceptions and Experiences of Larval Therapy*. Journal of Wound Care, 2004. 13(1): pp. 25–29, https://doi.org/10.12968/jowc.2004.13.1.26560.

137. Silva, S.M., et al., *Terapia larval sob a ótica do paciente*. ESTIMA Brazilian Journal of Enterostomal Therapy, 2020. 18(e3020), https://doi.org/10.30886/estima.v18.963_IN.

PART 3

PRODUCTION OF MEDICINAL MAGGOTS

12. Laboratory and Insectary Infrastructure and Equipment

Frank Stadler

Medicinal maggot production laboratory infrastructure requirements depend on pre-existing infrastructure, the current research and/or production activities, and on the production objectives—whether medicinal maggots are to be produced for research, therapy, or a combination of both. This chapter provides a typology of production facilities and describes the physical insectary and laboratory infrastructure and equipment necessary to maintain medicinal fly colonies and prepare medicinal maggots for use in human and veterinary medicine. Importantly, reliable production of safe and high-quality medicinal maggots does not necessarily require sophisticated and expensive laboratories and equipment.

Introduction

This chapter is concerned with the physical insectary and laboratory infrastructure and equipment necessary to maintain medicinal fly colonies and prepare medicinal maggots for use in human and veterinary medicine. It focusses specifically on the building, infrastructure, and equipment requirements for medicinal maggot insectaries and laboratories (from now referred to as production laboratories). The establishment of any laboratory can be described as a process that begins with the decision to establish a laboratory, followed by preplanning, planning, design, construction, and post-construction activities. Prospective producers are advised to consult the literature on

https://doi.org/10.11647/OBP.0300.12

laboratory planning, construction, and management—particularly the following books:

- **Laboratory Design, Construction, and Renovation: Participants, Process, and Production.** Committee on Design, Construction, and Renovation of Laboratory Facilities; Board on Chemical Sciences and Technology; Commission on Physical Sciences, Mathematics, and Applications; National Research Council. National Academy Press, Washington D.C. (2000). [1]

- **The Sustainable Laboratory Handbook: Design, Equipment, Operation.** Dittrich, E. & ProQuest, Ebooks. Wiley-VCH, Weinheim, Germany (2015). [2]

- **Guidelines for Laboratory Design: Health, Safety, and Environmental Considerations.** DiBerardinis, L. J. & ProQuest, Ebooks. Wiley, Hoboken, New Jersey (2013). [3]

The first is an excellent guide on the planning of laboratories from predesign to postconstruction, and the technical aspects that need to be considered. As a free online resource, it should be essential reading for any prospective producer needing to build or refurbish laboratory facilities—ideally, before planning has commenced! The other two books are much more technical and detailed in nature and are intended to provide professionals involved in the planning, design, construction, and operation of laboratories with essential information to facilitate collaboration.

A detailed discussion of all aspects of laboratory planning, construction and operation are beyond the scope of this book. Instead, this chapter will focus on key considerations as they apply specifically to medicinal maggot production laboratories. First it is important to understand the different types of laboratories that are typically concerned with the production of medicinal maggots and related research, and how these differ depending on their primary objectives and history. This discussion also includes an introduction to the production of medicinal maggots in compromised healthcare settings with mobile and community-based do-it-yourself medicinal maggot laboratories [4]. The remainder of the chapter explains the building and space requirements for research- and commercial-production laboratories, and the equipment needed.

Production Laboratory Typology

Thanks to the robust and adaptable nature of calliphorid fly species suitable for maggot therapy, laboratory and equipment infrastructure can be tailored to suit conditions, needs and resources. What a production facility will look like depends on several factors including a) financial resources, b) pre-existing building infrastructure, c) proximity to the point of care, d) transport infrastructure and distribution logistics, e) the wound burden amenable to maggot therapy, f) access to trained medical or scientific workforce, and more social factors such as g) institutional support for maggot therapy, h) healthcare-worker endorsement of maggot therapy, i) patient acceptance, j) regulatory approval of maggot therapy, and k) insurance cover for maggot therapy either via national health insurance or private health cover.

In general, laboratories that produce medicinal maggots either conduct maggot therapy-related research, forensic research, or they are dedicated medicinal maggot production laboratories. Research laboratories may produce medicinal maggots on a small scale to supply lab experiments or small clinical trials. The market size for medicinal maggots is largely determined by the wound burden, the general acceptance of maggot therapy, regulatory approval, and reimbursement of treatment costs via health insurance schemes. It follows that the scale of operations depends on the actual and/or potential demand for maggot therapy, i.e. from small-scale, not-for-profit production by research laboratories to fully independent and for-profit enterprises. The latter may specialise exclusively in the production of medicinal maggots or have a diversified product range that includes medicinal maggots. Table 12.1 presents a typology of medicinal maggot production organisations and their characteristics.

It appears that commercial producers emerge more often than not from university medical research laboratories that investigate clinical and biochemical aspects of maggot therapy. Large institutions such as universities afford a safety net allowing budding producers to slowly test and build the market through awareness-raising and educational activities, and to initiate the regulatory approval process. Since the regulators require clinical evidence of safety and efficacy, such trials are also best conducted from within a biomedical research organisation with clinical trial support and infrastructure. However, once the regulatory agencies have approved maggot therapy, it is unlikely that the host research organisations have the agility, entrepreneurial mindset, and expertise required for start-up and commercialisation. At this point, the producer ought to create a largely independent spin-off company that still maintains strong research ties with the parent organisation.

Up to recently, there has been little effort to provide high-quality maggot therapy to hard-to-reach patient populations such as in remote locations, at times of disaster or in armed conflict. However, the author's group has developed a mobile shipping container that is fitted with an insectary and laboratory capable of producing medicinal maggots in remote locations and where logistics infrastructure is failing to guarantee 24- to 48-hour delivery of medicinal maggots. We also developed and tested production and treatment manuals that allow isolated communities to establish and run do-it-yourself (DIY) laboratories with limited resources so they can produce safe medicinal maggots for efficacious maggot therapy (Stadler et al. QVSA). All project material including container lab construction plans, DIY lab instructions, and the treatment manual are available online (www.medmaglabs.com). These resources provide all necessary information for isolated communities to produce safe medicinal maggots.

Mobile and Do-it-yourself Medicinal Maggot Laboratories for Compromised Healthcare Settings

The discussion of production facility establishment has largely focussed on fixed infrastructure such as existing labs, purpose built, or building infrastructure that can be converted into medicinal maggot production facilities. When production is tied to a specific place then this means that the availability of maggot therapy to patients will be dependent on their proximity to the production facility. In advanced economies with highly effective and reliable logistics networks, rapid 24-hour distribution of medicinal maggots over long distances and under cool chain conditions is feasible and standard practice [5]. However, this is not the case where economic disadvantage, poverty, war and conflict, or disasters disrupt logistics infrastructure and supply chains. The answer to this problem may well be mobile and low-resource do-it-yourself medicinal maggot laboratories as mentioned earlier.

Table 12.1 Typology of organisations that produce medicinal maggots.

Factor	Scale			
	Small-scale mostly not-for-profit			Large-scale or diversified and for-profit
	Research laboratory	Mobile laboratories	DIY laboratories	Commercial laboratory
Financial resources	Limited, not core business	Supported by aid agencies or government	Very limited	Investment capital and industry development grants
Pre-existing infrastructure	Biological, forensic, or biomedical laboratory	No building infrastructure	No building infrastructure	Laboratories, convertible buildings, new buildings
Proximity to point of care	Close, in-house or local hospitals	Close, but far from major population centres	Close, but far from major population centres	Irrespective of proximity
Distribution logistics	No need for sophisticated logistics	Container deployment logistics	No distribution logistics	Sophisticated distribution logistics
Wound burden	Low	Up to approx. 250 wounds per day	Low but flexible	High wound burden/ market size
Trained workforce	Present	Present	Untrained laypersons	Present
Institutional support	Within the scope of research	Strong institutional support	Grass-roots community support	Independent
Healthcare-worker endorsement	Limited to collaborating hospitals	Endorsement restricted to agency and care setting	Endorsed by local lay- and trained healthcare workers	Widely endorsed
Patient awareness and acceptance	Low in greater community but high in treating hospitals	High	High	Generally high
Regulatory approval	Not approved	Not necessarily approved	Not necessarily approved	Approved

The provision of medical services in the field close to the point of care is not a new idea. Portable healthcare facilities provide life-saving emergency care during war and disasters such as earthquakes, tsunamis, infectious disease outbreaks. They may include independently functioning medical units like airborne, floating, or terrestrial truck-mounted infrastructure. Temporary medical infrastructure is transported in parts and assembled and disassembled as required [6]. Tents have been traditionally used for temporary field hospital shelters to house emergency and surgical care, hospital wards, and support services, but their ease of deployment comes with significant disadvantages. For example, they have no rigid flooring and require level ground, they are prone to the elements because they are not insulated, they may leak during rain. In addition, they are difficult to keep clean [7].

In recent times, military field hospitals have been developed and deployed that are composed of a combination of soft and hard portable infrastructure. The new British Army front-line field hospitals use inflatable dome tents in conjunction with pre-configured, fully equipped, containerised units for services such as sterilisation departments [8]. Converted shipping containers have also proven cost-effective and practical solutions for the provision of medical and scientific laboratory services in low-income country healthcare settings [9, 10]. For example, 40-foot modified shipping containers are used by the President's Malaria Initiative to provide low-cost laboratory infrastructure for mosquito control programmes in Mozambique, Mali, Angola and Liberia [9]. These innovations in mobile healthcare and laboratory services provision suggest strongly that there is a place for mobile medicinal maggot production close to the point of care.

For extremely isolated communities that are cut off from clinical supplies and advanced clinical care by armed conflict, disaster, or simply remoteness, the only way to provide effective limb- and life-saving wound care may be via do-it-yourself medicinal maggot production and maggot therapy—similar to the way maggot therapy had been practiced for millennia in ancient and tribal cultures [11]. The overriding concern, of course, must be patient safety. In today's age, it would not be acceptable to let wild flies lay eggs on wounds for the maggots to treat the wound of their own accord without quality control—although, this is essentially what had been done in the past and what still happens today when wounds get accidentally colonised by fly maggots. Many cases of such fly colonisation (myiasis) are benign and even beneficial [12, 13], although maggot colonisation can be distressing for the patient, family, and carers because flies and maggots are usually associated with death, decay and filth. Controlled therapy rather than wild infestation is also desirable because of the potential risk of harmful microbes carried in by wild flies above and beyond the microbial burden that is already in the wound [14]. Moreover, a few species of fly such as screw worms can colonise wounds and cause damage to live tissue [15]. Chapter 7 [16] explains in detail the natural history of medicinal flies and related species and Chapters 4 to 6 [17–19] are concerned with the treatment of wounds with maggot therapy.

It follows that if isolated communities are to be encouraged and enabled to produce their own maggots and practice maggot therapy, then any instructions and guidelines need to be based on best practice. Community-based producers will need to be trained in the construction of basic production facilities and equipment, in the identification and culture of safe fly species, in the disinfection of eggs, and the safe treatment of wounds. Such training needs to overcome the material and social constraints of the low-resource setting. Instructions need to be provided in highly visual format to overcome language barriers. Any written material should ideally be provided in multi-lingual format. Minimum requirement would be instructional material in the official national language of the country and easy-to-understand English. The suggested solutions need to be supported by the resources that are locally available, which may vary from place to place. This means the instructions will need to be sufficiently flexible. This will give the end user the freedom to adopt and adapt local resources to achieve production and medicinal maggot quality objectives. The ingenuity and resourcefulness of communities in compromised healthcare settings must not be underestimated. For further information on our own efforts to give isolated communities the wherewithal to treat chronic wounds with safe maggot therapy, please go to www.medmaglabs.com.

Building and Space Requirements

Key activities conducted in the operation of a medicinal maggot production laboratory include the rearing and maintenance of fly colonies, the disinfection of fly eggs and rearing of larvae, the packaging of maggots into primary packaging containers, packaging of consignments for customers, quality control activities, storage of inventory, as well as office-based activities. Each of these has its own space, equipment and consumables requirements (Table 12.2 available at https://hdl.handle.net/20.500.12434/2f7d12xl). This chapter pre-empts by necessity some of the discussion that follows in subsequent chapters explaining fly colony establishment (Chapter 13) [20], medicinal maggot production (Chapter 14) [21], and packaging technology (Chapter 16) [22]. However, the focus is on space and equipment requirements for the establishment and operation of a medicinal maggot production laboratory.

Production spaces are less defined in shared research laboratories that are not exclusively set up for the purpose of medicinal maggot production. Research laboratories must often meet the needs of many users, and maggot therapy-related research and production activities sharing this space need to adapt accordingly. However, when dedicated production facilities are to be established, there is the opportunity to account and plan for the distinct work area requirements, and the workflows between them. It follows that a production facility should have:

Table 12.2 Production facility resources (e.g. equipment, space requirements and consumables) required to undertake production processes and sub-processes. https://hdl.handle.net/20.500.12434/2f7d12xl.

Insectary. An insectary for the rearing and maintenance of medicinal fly colonies. Its specifications arise from the environmental preferences of calliphorid flies, and the need to keep the space clean and pest-free. A constant temperature of 25°C and 12 hours of light per day will ensure that the flies continue to produce eggs over their useful life span and that their offspring do not enter a diapause or resting phase during pupariation [23]. Humidity should range between approximately 40 and 60% RH. If the air conditioning system is not able to maintain this range, additional humidification or de-humidification systems may need to be installed. If possible, circulated air should be filtered to remove fly-generated dust from the insectary atmosphere. If this is not possible, a stand-alone air purifier can be installed, or lack of air filtration can be compensated for with more frequent cleaning protocols and/or increased personal protection with gloves, dust masks, hair nets, and lab gowns for prolonged insectary activities. Ventilation ports for fresh air intake and air exhaust should be screened with fine insect screens and doors should be fitted with door sweeps to prevent vermin entering the room. All surfaces should be washable and all cracks, gaps, joints, etc. sealed to avoid refugia for vermin and build-up of dirt. The insectary should also have potable water taps and greywater plumbing for a lab sink to be fitted. The insectary is entered via a small room that serves as a change room for protective clothing. The same protective clothing must not be worn in the general and clean lab to maintain hygiene and avoid contamination of disinfected medicinal maggots.

Clean lab. Here, a clean lab is defined as the part of the production laboratory that is dedicated to disinfection of eggs, quality control, and packaging of medicinal maggots into primary packaging. It is 'clean' in the sense that no activities such as washing up of dirty equipment, fly diet preparation and regular lab maintenance tasks are performed in this space. The clean lab should not be confused with a clean room, which in medical and pharmaceutical production laboratories provides a sterile work environment. Although possible, clean rooms are not necessary in medicinal maggot production. The sterile environment for work activities is usually provided by laminar flow cabinets (clean benches) that fulfil the same role but cost only a fraction to establish and operate (see equipment requirements).

Overall, the specifications for the clean lab are similar to those for the insectary but lighting is not automatically controlled and there is less stringent requirement to keep temperature and humidity in the optimal range. However, if disinfected eggs and medicinal maggots are to be incubated in the clean lab without an incubator, the temperature must also be kept at around 25°C, unless accelerated growth and development of medicinal maggots at higher temperatures is required. Like the insectary, the clean lab is also entered via a small room used for workers to change into protective clothing.

General lab. A general lab space for food and media preparation, cleaning of laboratory utensils after use, autoclaving of equipment used for clean-bench work, and quality control work other than microbial assays of eggs and maggots. The basic space requirements are identical to those of the clean lab. Again, basic services such as air conditioning, adequate lighting, plumbing and potable water supply should be installed.

Packaging and dispatch room. Product packaging and dispatch room for order processing. Medicinal maggots that have been packed into vials (primary packaging) in various unit sizes and treatment modalities (free-range or bagged) are collated according to customer orders and packed into insulated cool-chain shippers (packaging) and processed for dispatch. Requirements for this space are not as stringent as for the lab spaces but worker comfort should be considered regarding lighting levels, ventilation and air conditioning.

Store room. To hold supplies until they are required. It is best to have separate store rooms for laboratory supplies and office/general operations supplies. This is mainly to locate them in close proximity to the respective work area and facilitate easy access by the main user groups. It may also be necessary for facilities with high production volumes and many courier shipments to store a significant volume of insulated shippers and cool elements. If the packaging and dispatch room is not large enough then an additional store for this inventory may be required. Although hazardous chemical use is minimal in medicinal maggot production laboratories, larger volumes of corrosive or flammable chemicals need to be stored in dedicated safety cabinets according to local regulations.

Restrooms. These may be unisex or separate male/female amenities.

Change and locker rooms. These may also be provided for staff to change into lab uniforms and protective clothing and to store valuables that staff cannot or will not want to take into the labs.

Meeting rooms. Meeting rooms provide staff the opportunity to gather and socialise during breaks and prepare and consume food. A separate board or business meeting room should also be considered. If space is at a premium, the staff room can also serve as a formal meeting room.

Offices. For management and administration of operations including marketing, sales, customer support and customer relations, finance/accounts, quality control, and regulatory compliance. An open-plan office accommodating most office staff may not be advisable due to the different functions performed by staff. For example, it is likely that the sales and marketing team members spend a lot of time on the phone which can be disruptive to colleagues sharing the same space. Therefore, it is necessary to consider ahead of facility establishment which arrangement is most productive.

Actual floor area is not being considered in this discussion because it depends, among other things, on the available overall space, the size of operation/production volume, the number of workers using each workspace at the same time, local health and safety regulations, and building codes. It is, however, a good idea to be generous with floor area allocation when planning a production facility so that future growth in staff and production volume can be accommodated without disruption to operations.

An important consideration that does demand some discussion is the relative position of each workspace in relation to the overall facility layout. The physical infrastructure must facilitate the efficient flow of workers, information, products, and materials. This also includes resources entering and leaving the organisation. Figure 12.1 illustrates this relationship for a medicinal maggot production facility and shows the major flows between the spaces. There should be a clear spatial separation between the production areas and the office and support areas. Access to the labs should be via a single point and the clean lab as well as the insectary should be accessible via the general lab area rather than directly from the office area. There are consequently two main hubs, the office area and the general lab area, for administrative and production facilities, respectively. The medicinal maggot production workflow should be one-directional: 1) eggs are passed from insectary to the general lab for separation and prewashing; 2) from there, they are passed to the clean lab where disinfection, incubation and primary packaging takes place; 3) finally, the packaged maggots are moved on to the dispatch room for order fulfilment and shipping. Other activities such as quality control processes involve workflows that are less directional. It is also desirable that the dispatch room is close to the facility reception and office areas. This ensures good communication with sales who will want to oversee order fulfilment. Shipping-ready consignments also need to be picked up by couriers who may access the premises via the main entrance and reception unless a dedicated service entry exists.

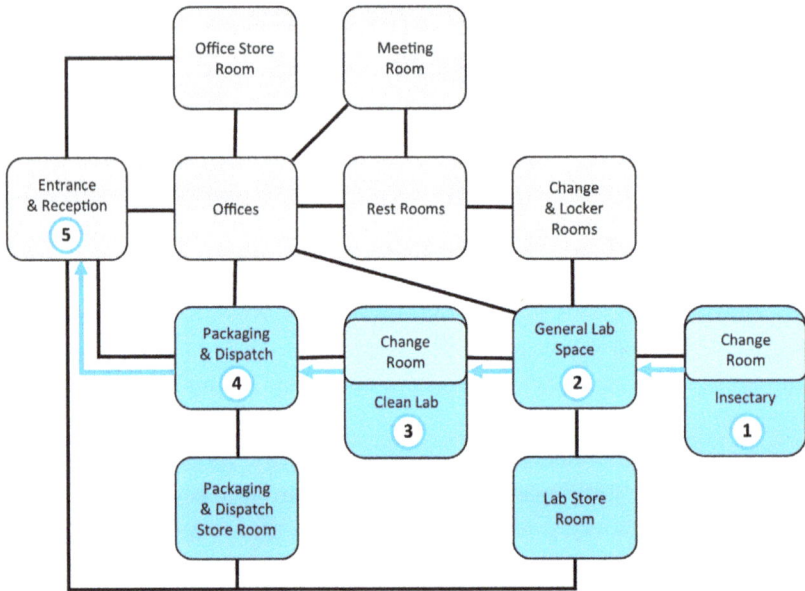

Figure 12.1 Proximity and workflow diagram for production facility. Relative position of bubbles in diagram suggests the spatial layout and proximity of workspaces in the facility. Black lines describe the movement of staff and materials around the facility according to production and administrative workflows. The blue arrows describe the unidirectional production path of medicinal maggots from (1) egg harvest in the insectary to (2) the general lab area for pre-cleaning and perhaps de-agglutination, to (3) the clean lab for disinfection, quality control, and primary packing, to (4) the packing and dispatch area, and (5) the reception for pickup by couriers.

Equipment Requirements

The equipment needs for medicinal maggot production are best discussed in relation to the specific work processes and functions they relate to. This chapter will provide an overview of the equipment needs without being prescriptive regarding specific brands, makes or suppliers. As has been explained earlier, medicinal maggot production affords a great deal of flexibility regarding the scale of operations and the production approaches. Much can be achieved with very little by way of facilities and equipment which makes maggot therapy such an attractive proposition for the low-resource healthcare setting.

The following discussion of equipment needs will guide the prospective producer through the production areas and specific process:

1. insectary activities (e.g. adult fly colony maintenance and maggot rearing)

2. general lab activities (e.g. diet preparation and quality control)

3. clean lab activities (e.g. disinfection, medicinal maggot rearing, and packaging)

4. packaging and dispatch activities (packaging of consignments).

The general equipment and furnishing needs for staff support areas (e.g. restrooms, locker rooms, meeting rooms), reception and offices is omitted here because these are not unique to medicinal maggot production facilities. By necessity, the following discussion of equipment and material needs for production facilities foreshadows content discussed in subsequent chapters, particularly those on medicinal maggot production (Chapter 14) [21] and transport packaging (Chapter 16) [22].

Insectary. The insectary is a dedicated space for the maintenance of medicinal flies and the rearing of new fly stock. Disinfected eggs and medicinal maggots should not be incubated in this space. Adult flies can be housed in a variety of cage systems [21]. The main consideration for choosing the right cage model, home-made or commercial, is adequate ventilation, light penetration, volume, and ease of handling and cleaning. These cages are best stored on easy-to-clean shelving that is water resistant and withstands a wide range of cleaning reagents such as bleach and alcohol-based disinfectants.

The maggots are conventionally reared in an inexpensive double-container system. A smaller plastic container holding the diet and maggots is placed inside a larger container holding a pupariation substrate such as sand, sawdust or vermiculite. The larger container is securely covered with fine-mesh muslin or synthetic fabric to provide ventilation but prevent wandering maggots from escaping. Once maggots have pupated, they need to be separated from the substrate by sieving. A variety of expensive metal sieves and inexpensive plastic colanders are readily available so long as they achieve separation of the puparia. This can be a dusty business and workers should wear dust masks or perform the sieving where particulates are quickly removed, either in the open air or under a laboratory exhaust system. Fly larvae shy away from light and therefore maggots are best reared in darkness. In addition, depending on the diet used, maggot rearing can be a smelly business. To make insectary work bearable, maggot containers can be stored in converted cupboards, fridge bodies or similar furniture that is fitted with ventilation that draws room air in and vents it to the outside. Alternatively, such units can be fitted with air filtration systems to limit odour in the room. If air is vented to the outside, it is important to ensure that the exhaust piping is screened with fine mesh to prevent wild flies and fly parasites from accessing the rearing cupboard.

Maintenance of fly colonies will require the removal of cages from the shelves and placement on a work bench. Like the shelving, the work bench or table should be sufficiently large to provide ample room for cages and other equipment. When flies have reached their useful life span and begin to die off, it is time to replace them with young flies. At this point the cage is placed in a freezer for a few hours to euthanise the flies and kill any pests such as mites. For more info on the humane treatment of flies please consult Chapter 19 [24]. The insectary should be fitted with a sink unit and drying racks to allow for easy cleaning of cages and food containers. Where feasible, shelving and other insectary furniture should be fitted with castors so it can be easily rolled about and moved for regular cleaning of the room surfaces.

Diets for maggots or bait to encourage egg laying may be prepared in the insectary or the general lab space. For most producers a household food blender will suffice to allow homogeneous mixing and maceration of various dietary ingredients for either plant- or meat-based diets. Adult flies are fed with a variety of protein-based and carbohydrate-rich food depending on the preference of the producer. These diets and egg-harvesting baits are usually offered with inexpensive and easy-to-clean or disposable plastic containers small enough to fit through the sleeve access in the fly cage. In order not to drown flies accidentally, liquid foods and water are offered with lidded plastic containers that are fitted with a cellulose sponge or rolled cellulose wicks (ideally organic and unstained to avoid poisoning of flies from residues).

Clean lab. The clean lab is where harvested and pre-cleaned fly eggs are disinfected and incubated, where hatched maggots are packaged into primary packaging containers, and where the microbial safety of medicinal maggots is examined via microbial assays. The clean lab should be as uncluttered as possible and may feature some cupboard and benchtop space as required for convenient operations. In practice, however, most activities undertaken in the clean lab take place within the laminar flow cabinet.

The production of medicinal goods such as medicinal maggots requires clean room conditions to maintain sterility during production processes, handling and packaging. There is no need to maintain the entire lab under clean room conditions. The comparatively small production volumes and the small size of the product handled in medicinal maggot production makes it feasible to use laminar flow cabinets, also known as clean benches, for the work that requires a sterile work environment. The number of laminar flow cabinets installed in a medicinal maggot clean lab depends on the volume of production and the time available to undertake required work. For most producers, one such work bench will suffice. When planning the clean lab, enough space should be allocated to be prepared for higher production volumes and to allow for additional clean benches.

There are a number of microbial testing protocols that may be employed by producers to make sure medicinal maggots are adequately disinfected [21]. These tests require a laboratory incubator that can be set and maintained at a constant temperature conducive to the growth of clinically relevant microbes (32°C to 37°C). Such an incubator is therefore an essential piece of equipment for any sophisticated production facility. It is also convenient to be able to store pre-prepared consumables such as egg incubation media and blood agar plates in a refrigerator within the clean lab to maximise efficient workflow and to maintain hygiene in the clean lab area. A sink and water supply to the clean lab is not essential because clean lab activities do not necessarily require access to running water. Eggs should be already separated and prewashed when they arrive in the clean lab and all water used during the disinfection and packaging processes must be autoclaved prior to use, which is taking place in the general lab space. The small amounts of waste water and disinfection solution are collected and disposed of afterward when the disinfection equipment and utensils are taken to the general lab space for cleaning and autoclaving.

The actual work processes of egg disinfection, quality control, and packaging of medicinal maggots generally require various reagent bottles, measuring cylinders and pipettes, various spatulas or applicators, and a vacuum filtration system (electric or handpump-driven) for the filtration of eggs and perhaps maggots. The exact equipment needs will have to be established through trial as they depend on the volume of work, the disinfection procedure chosen by the lab, and personal preference.

General lab. The general lab area is the central hub of the production laboratory. It provides the support for activities that take place in the insectary and the clean lab. Consequently, the lab should be equipped with cupboards and shelves to hold utensils and consumables and provide ample benchtop workspace for diet preparation and quality control activities.

The general lab has a dedicated wet area with tap, sink and drying racks to clean equipment and utensils. Diets for the incubation of disinfected eggs and for the rearing of fly stock are prepared in the general lab area. A fridge and a freezer should be available to store perishable, meat-based diet ingredients and pre-prepared diets. A kitchen food blender may be used for diet preparation. All sterilisation of equipment, diets and water is conducted with an autoclave, or a medical-grade steam steriliser which is a cost-effective alternative to expensive autoclaves [10].

Quality control work such as monitoring the fly colony performance requires an analytical scale with a sensitivity of at least 0.0001g [25] to be able to determine the weight of individual flies, pupae and older larvae. A stereo dissecting microscope with a magnification range of 10 to 40 times is essential for visual observation of flies and their life stages. Measurement of morphological characters such as wing features may be conducted with digital image analysis software [26] but the length of puparia or maggots can be measured relatively simply with a fine ruler (0.1mm scale) [27], or a geometrical micrometre [28].

Packing and dispatch. The equipment required to support the dispatch of orders will vary depending on the volume of consignments processed per day and the business logistics systems employed. At the very least, the room will have a good amount of bench space to comfortably handle products and packaging, and process orders. For producers shipping their maggots further afield using couriers, equipment is needed to package and handle cool chain consignments (e.g. tape dispensers). Vials holding medicinal maggots are placed into insulated shippers along with phase-change cool elements which have been pre-cooled in a fridge.

Summary

The take-home-message from this chapter is that there is no one typical production laboratory. Production laboratory infrastructure needs will depend on pre-existing building and laboratory infrastructure, on the current research and/or production activities, and on the production objectives—whether only for research or therapy, or a combination of both. There are clearly opportunities to optimise infrastructure and equipment and thereby also work processes when setting up a lab specifically for commercial production. However, it is important to understand that reliable production of safe and high-quality medicinal maggots does not necessarily require sophisticated and expensive laboratories and equipment. Maggot therapy has been performed for millennia in tribal cultures and innovations such as mobile laboratories and community-based laboratories utilising locally-available resources have the potential to produce safe medical-grade maggots where there is little to no access to reliable wound care.

References

1. Anonymous. *Laboratory Design, Construction, and Renovation: Participants, Process, and Production.* 2000. https://doi.org/10.17226/9799.

2. Dittrich, E., *The Sustainable Laboratory Handbook: Design, Equipment, Operation.* 2015, Weinheim: Wiley-VCH.

3. DiBerardinis, L.J., *Guidelines for Laboratory Design: Health, Safety, and Environmental Considerations.* 2013, Hoboken: Wiley.

4.   MedMagLabs. *MedMagLabs*. http://medmaglabs.com.

5.   Monarch Labs. *Order Form*. https://www.monarchlabs.com/Monarch-Labs-Order-Form.pdf.

6.   Bitterman, N. and Y. Zimmer, *Portable Health Care Facilities in Disaster and Rescue Zones: Characteristics and Future Suggestions*. Prehospital and Disaster Medicine, 2018: pp. 1–7, https://doi.org/10.1017/S1049023X18000560.

7.   Bricknell, M.C., *Organisation and Design of Regular Field Hospitals*. Journal of the Royal Army Medical Corps, 2001. 147(2): pp. 161–167, https://doi.org/10.1136/jramc-147-02-09.

8.   Apthorp, C. *Inside the British Army's New Front-line Field Hospital*. 2016, 30 March. https://www.army-technology.com/features/featureinside-the-british-armys-new-front-line-field-hospital-4809564/.

9.   Bridges, D.J., et al., *Perspective Piece Modular Laboratories-Cost-Effective and Sustainable Infrastructure for Resource-Limited Settings*. American Journal of Tropical Medicine and Hygiene, 2014. 91(6): pp. 1074–1078, https://doi.org/10.4269/ajtmh.14-0054.

10. Boubour, J., et al., *A Shipping Container-Based Sterile Processing Unit for Low Resources Settings*. PLoS ONE, 2016. 11(3): e0149624, https://doi.org/10.1371/journal.pone.0149624.

11. Kruglikova, A.A. and S.I. Chernysh, *Surgical Maggots and the History of Their Medical Use*. Entomological Review, 2013. 93(6): pp. 667–674, https://doi.org/10.1134/S0013873813060018.

12. Chan, Q.E., M.A. Hussain, and V. Milovic, *Eating out of the Hand, Maggots — Friend or Foe?* Journal of Plastic, Reconstructive and Aesthetic Surgery, 2012. 65(8): pp. 1116–1118, https://doi.org/10.1016/j.bjps.2012.01.014.

13. Terterov, S., et al., *Posttraumatic Human Cerebral Myiasis*. World Neurosurgery, 2010. 73(5): pp. 557–559, https://doi.org/10.1016/j.wneu.2010.01.004.

14. Snyder, S., P. Singh, and J. Goldman, *Emerging Pathogens: A Case of Wohlfahrtiimonas chitiniclastica and Ignatzschineria indica bacteremia*. IDCases, 2020. 19: e00723, https://doi.org/10.1016/j.idcr.2020.e00723.

15. Zhou, X., et al., *Human Chrysomya bezziana Myiasis: A Systematic Review*. PLOS Neglected Tropical Diseases, 2019. 13(10): e0007391, https://doi.org/10.1371/journal.pntd.0007391.

16. Harvey, M., *The Natural History of Medicinal Flies*, in *A Complete Guide to Maggot Therapy: Clinical Practice, Therapeutic Principles, Production, Distribution, and Ethics*, F. Stadler (ed.). 2022, Cambridge: Open Book Publishers, pp. 121–142, https://doi.org/10.11647/OBP.0300.07.

17. Sherman, R., *Indications, Contraindications, Interactions, and Side-effects of Maggot Therapy*, in *A Complete Guide to Maggot Therapy: Clinical Practice, Therapeutic Principles, Production, Distribution, and Ethics*, F. Stadler

(ed.). 2022, Cambridge: Open Book Publishers, pp. 63–78, https://doi.org/10.11647/OBP.0300.04.

18. Sherman, R., *Medicinal Maggot Application and Maggot Therapy Dressing Technology*, in *A Complete Guide to Maggot Therapy: Clinical Practice, Therapeutic Principles, Production, Distribution, and Ethics*, F. Stadler (ed.). 2022, Cambridge: Open Book Publishers, pp. 79–96, https://doi.org/10.11647/OBP.0300.05.

19. Sherman, R. and F. Stadler, *Wound Aetiologies, Patient Characteristics, and Healthcare Settings Amenable to Maggot Therapy*, in *A Complete Guide to Maggot Therapy: Clinical Practice, Therapeutic Principles, Production, Distribution, and Ethics*, F. Stadler (ed.). 2022, Cambridge: Open Book Publishers, pp. 39–62, https://doi.org/10.11647/OBP.0300.03.

20. Stadler, F., et al., *Fly Colony Establishment*, in *A Complete Guide to Maggot Therapy: Clinical Practice, Therapeutic Principles, Production, Distribution, and Ethics*, F. Stadler (ed.). 2022, Cambridge: Open Book Publishers, pp. 257–288 (p. 269), https://doi.org/10.11647/OBP.0300.13.

21. Stadler, F. and P. Takáč, *Medicinal Maggot Production*, in *A Complete Guide to Maggot Therapy: Clinical Practice, Therapeutic Principles, Production, Distribution, and Ethics*, F. Stadler (ed.). 2022, Cambridge: Open Book Publishers, pp. 289–330, https://doi.org/10.11647/OBP.0300.14.

22. Stadler, F., *Packaging Technology*, in *A Complete Guide to Maggot Therapy: Clinical Practice, Therapeutic Principles, Production, Distribution, and Ethics*, F. Stadler (ed.). 2022, Cambridge: Open Book Publishers, pp. 349–362, https://doi.org/10.11647/OBP.0300.16.

23. Barnes, K.M. and D.E. Gennard, *Rearing Bacteria and Maggots Concurrently: A Protocol Using Lucilia sericata (Diptera: Calliphoridae) as a Model Species.* Applied Entomology and Zoology, 2013. 48(3): pp. 247–253, https://doi.org/10.1007/s13355-013-0181-7.

24. Stadler, F., *The Ethics of Maggot Therapy*, in *A Complete Guide to Maggot Therapy: Clinical Practice, Therapeutic Principles, Production, Distribution, and Ethics*, F. Stadler (ed.). 2022, Cambridge: Open Book Publishers, pp. 405–430, https://doi.org/10.11647/OBP.0300.19.

25. Bala, M. and D. Singh, *Development of Two Forensically Important Blowfly Species (Chrysomya megacephala and Chrysomya rufifacies) (Diptera: Calliphoridae) at Four Temperatures in India.* Entomological Research, 2015. 45(4): pp. 176–183, https://doi.org/10.1111/1748-5967.12110.

26. Limsopatham, K., et al., *A Molecular, Morphological, and Physiological Comparison of English and German Populations of Calliphora vicina (Diptera: Calliphoridae).* PLoS ONE, 2018. 13(12), https://doi.org/10.1371/journal.pone.0207188.

27. Tarone, A.M. and D.R. Foran, *Generalized Additive Models and Lucilia sericata Growth: Assessing Confidence Intervals and Error Rates in Forensic*

Entomology. Journal of Forensic Sciences, 2008. 53(4): pp. 942–948, https://doi.org/10.1111/j.1556-4029.2008.00744.x.

28. Villet, M.H., *An Inexpensive Geometrical Micrometer for Measuring Small, Live Insects Quickly without Harming Them*. Entomologia Experimentalis et Applicata, 2007. 122(3): pp. 279–280, https://doi.org/10.1111/j.1570-7458.2006.00520.x.

13. Fly Colony Establishment, Quality Control and Improvement

Frank Stadler, Nikolas P. Johnston, Nathan J. Butterworth, and James F. Wallman

This chapter provides guidance on the collection and selection of species suitable for maggot therapy. All life stages are suitable for collection, except pupae that are generally hidden from view. Correct identification of the species that are collected and the correct selection of breeding stock is critical. Domestication of the newly established fly colony proceeds via adaptation to the insectary environment and the producers' operating procedures. Monitoring of fly colony life history and morphological traits enables producers to manage the adaptation of flies to the insectary environment and to improve performance through selective breeding, genetic replenishment, and genetic engineering.

Introduction

The first step in the establishment of a laboratory colony is the collection of flies and their subsequent maintenance in the laboratory or insectary [e.g. 1, 2, 3]. While in some instances blowfly strains have been reared continuously for decades [4], there is concern that relatively small population sizes, limited genetic diversity, rapid selection and adaptation to the laboratory [5] may require genetic replenishment and rejuvenation of lab colonies with newly caught flies on a regular basis to ensure productivity and health of the colonies [6].

https://doi.org/10.11647/OBP.0300.13

Moreover, maggot therapy treatment conditions vary between geographic areas and socio-economic conditions. For example, maggot therapy in Sub-Saharan Africa might benefit from the domestication of African fly species or strains such as *Lucilia sericata* or perhaps even the tropical African latrine fly *Chrysomya putoria*, that are already adapted to African environmental conditions. It is known that fly development is temperature-dependent and speeds up as temperature increases, up to a threshold temperature beyond which development is negatively impacted and may even lead to death [7]. While the laboratory and insectary conditions can be regulated, the wound temperature during treatment may be difficult to control. Average chronic wound temperature has been reported to be between 32 and 33ºC under mild climatic conditions [8–10]. Ambient atmospheric conditions in Sub-Saharan Africa may lead to a significant increase in the temperature medicinal maggots experience on the wound. Therefore, rather than importing flies from Europe, it will be beneficial to develop locally collected fly strains that are better adapted to higher developmental temperatures. However, further research to determine the influence of temperature on maggot therapeutic performance in tropical regions is required.

Finally, local quarantine laws and regulations may not permit the introduction of foreign insect material, which means that local flies will need to be collected. If the therapeutic efficacy of the species has not already been shown, its suitability for maggot therapy will need to be established. However, at times of great need when disaster or war is raging, or where there is no access to medical treatment, these restrictions may not apply, particularly regarding the use of local fly species [11, 12].

Chapter 11 is chiefly concerned with the bioprospecting and testing of new fly species for maggot therapy [13], while this chapter provides guidance on the collection and selection of species deemed suitable for maggot therapy. Not all of the species suggested here have been subject to robust testing as proposed in Chapter 11 but have a recorded history of successful medicinal use and at least one of the discussed species can be found in every major zoogeographic region. Because domestication is critical to the reliable supply of high-quality medicinal maggots, some attention must be given to the monitoring of fly colony life history and morphological traits. This will enable producers to manage the adaptation of flies to the insectary environment and to improve performance through selective breeding, genetic replenishment, and potentially genetic engineering.

Of course, it is not strictly necessary for maggot therapists to use maggots that were reared in the laboratory. Under extremely austere conditions and with no access to medical aid and purpose-produced medicinal maggots, it is possible to collect eggs from the wild or permit free-living females to deposit eggs on a wound [11, 12]. Such controlled myiasis is not without its risks but anecdotal and published case histories of maggot colonisation (myiasis) of necrotic wounds from surgery, violence, neglect, or misfortune demonstrate its potential benefit [14–16].

Medicinal Fly Species

There are many fly species worldwide that could potentially be employed to treat wounds. These belong mostly to the family Calliphoridae of which over 1,500 species have been described to date [17]. There are some prerequisites for species to be suitable for maggot therapy:

- In the first instance, any species used for maggot therapy must not consume or damage healthy tissue, but only debride dead or devitalised tissue.

- Ideally, the species used should not only debride dead tissue but also control infection and stimulate wound healing.

- The species should be easy to maintain in captivity and colonies should retain their vigour over many generations.

- The species should lay eggs and not give birth to live maggots. This is necessary to efficiently harvest and disinfect eggs and rear medicinal maggots prior to treatment.

Although a good number of fly species have been used to treat wounds (Table 13.1) the fly species most widely cited and regularly used for maggot therapy are the greenbottle blowfly *L. sericata* and to a lesser extent the sheep blowfly *Lucilia cuprina* [18–20]. However, other species are also under active experimental and clinical investigation for use in maggot therapy, including: i) the secondary screwworm *Cochliomyia macellaria* which is found from southern Canada to the South American tropics [21, 22], ii) the tropical African latrine fly *Ch. putoria* that is now also found across the Americas [23], and iii) the South American *Sarconesiopsis magellanica* [24]. There are likely to be many more fly species globally that could be employed to treat wounds and all except the harshest of environments should be home to candidate fly species for maggot therapy.

Table 13.1 Species that have been used in maggot therapy to date and associated references.

Species	Reference
Calliphora vicina	[25]
Lucilia caesar	[26]
Lucilia illustris	[27]
L. sericata	[24, 28–30]
L. cuprina	[20, 31–33]
Phormia regina	[26, 29, 34]
Protophormia terraenovae	[35]
Chrysomya megacephala	[36]
Ch. putoria	[23]
Co. macellaria	[21, 22, 37]
S. magellanica	[24]
Wohlfahrtia nuba	[38]
Musca domestica	[39]

Collecting Wild Flies

Several options are available to the collector of live flies for the establishment of laboratory colonies. Female flies can be encouraged to lay eggs on decomposing meat or other suitable bait [40], maggots may be hand-collected from wild carcasses and cadavers [7, 41, 42], and adult flies can be trapped [6, 43–45]. Common choices of bait include minced ovine (sheep), porcine (pork), or bovine (cattle) meat, but a wide range of other mammal and bird meats will attract medicinal fly species. It is best to use meat which has not been treated with preservatives. If fresh store-bought meat is used, give the meat up to 3 days to become putrid (depending on the ambient temperature), at which stage it will begin to attract significant numbers of blowflies. If using meat other than mince, to aid the process of decomposition and the release of volatile organic compounds, it can be beneficial to cut the meat into smaller pieces. The attractiveness of the decomposing meat can be further enhanced when it is mixed with sodium sulphide (Na_2S) [46]. Furthermore, the attractive potential of meat bait is also enhanced once blowfly adults and larvae begin to arrive, as they release attractive semiochemicals when feeding [47]. Occasionally stirring the bait can further aid in the release of volatile organic compounds.

Importantly, the occurrence and distribution of necrophagous calliphorids varies greatly depending on the season and habitat [48, 49]. While some species are cold-tolerant and will remain active in winter in low abundances (e.g. *C. vicina*) [48], the majority of necrophagous calliphorids are only active in the warmer months. As such, fly collection should be undertaken in the warmer months in most geographic regions.

Trapping of Adult Flies

The characteristic behaviour of flies can be used to efficiently trap adults without killing them [50]. Flies in search of food and cadavers on which to deposit eggs have no difficulty searching out small dark holes and crevices as would be found on a cadaver. However, when taking flight, blowflies invariably head straight up and towards light. Cone or funnel traps make use of this behaviour. There are various versions of this trap type, but all work the same. A bait is provided to attract the flies. Suspended above the bait station is a cone/funnel (wide at the bottom and narrowing to a small opening at the top) which ends in a holding compartment made of fabric, a plastic bag or such containment. Flies that visit the bait station fly off vertically into the cone and wander upward through the small opening into the holding compartment. The flies have difficulty finding the small opening again and remain trapped [50]. Although cone/funnel traps are easily constructed, there are now various types of these traps available online via entomological equipment suppliers and popular retail platforms such as eBay and

Alibaba (e.g. Figure 13.1). Traps that have been specifically designed for entomological investigations will allow easy access and collection of trapped flies while the inexpensive traps sold for pest control may be permanently closed and make access to the fly compartment difficult. This requires modification of the fly trap prior to use, or particular retrieval strategies as described in Figure 13.2.

A variant of this trap mechanism utilises the same inability of flies to escape through an inverted, funnel-shaped opening. Inexpensive plastic storage containers may be baited with meat or other attractants and furnished with inward-pointing cones [44]. Commercial traps exploit this approach to capture sheep blowflies that can cause significant stock loss and animal suffering [51]. Figure 13.3 explains how an inexpensive trap based on the same principle can be constructed from a simple plastic bottle.

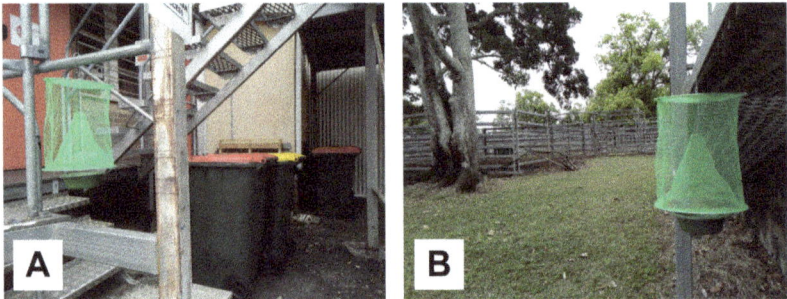

Figure 13.1 Inexpensive fly trap available from online retailers. The trap is best set up where flies naturally congregate. In an urban setting, this may be domestic or commercial garbage bins or near food businesses (A). In the rural environment, traps may be set up near livestock (B), but flies will detect attractive bait from afar and find the trap even if it is set up away from livestock or food waste. Photos by F. Stadler, CC BY-NC.

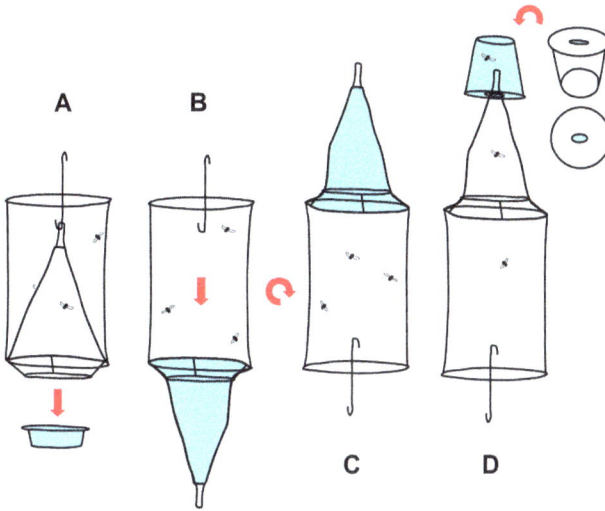

Figure 13.2 Retrieval of flies. Flies may be removed from the trap in Figure 13.1 by exploiting their natural inclination to move upward. Remove the bait tray from the trap (A). Unhook the net funnel and pull it out through the wire basket that held the bait tray (B). Turn the trap upside down (C). Use a transparent plastic container and cut an oval hole into the lid or bottom of it. It has to be wide enough to receive the narrow end of the trap's net funnel but thinner than the diameter of the funnel opening (D). When inserted, the metal-enforced funnel opening will sit on the inside edge of the hole without slipping out. Let the trap hang from the plastic container and make sure the funnel is untwisted to avoid obstruction. Flies will climb upward and through the funnel into the collection container (D).

Illustration by F. Stadler, CC BY-NC.

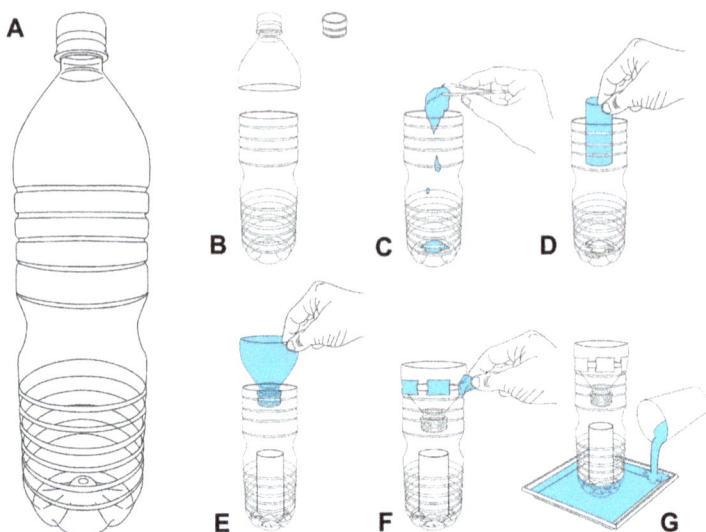

Figure 13.3 Instruction for a DIY plastic container cone trap. A standard soft drink plastic bottle (A). The tapered neck is cut off and the lid is removed (B). The bottle is baited with putrid meat to attract flies (C). A piece of cardboard such as a toilet paper roll is placed on top of the bait to provide a perch for flies as they may not be able to easily grip the plastic bottle walls after contact with the moist bait (D). The tapered neck is inverted and fitted back onto the bottle (without the lid) (E) and secured with a few strips of sticky tape (F). The trap is then placed in a dish of water to keep ants and other crawling insects out (G). The trap should be set up in a spot that is accessible to flies but protected from rain and direct sun. Illustration by P. Busana, MedMagLabs and Creating Hope in Conflict: A Humanitarian Grand Challenge, CC BY-ND.

Collecting Eggs

Female flies are attracted to cadavers to feed on protein-rich food and lay their eggs. It is therefore possible to collect eggs by placing meat bait in select locations during the day. Flies are not nocturnal and will not seek out the bait during the night. However, flies prefer to lay their eggs in dark recesses and orifices of cadavers such as the mouth or nostrils. Therefore, offering the bait in a dark container mimicking a cadaver and covering it while still allowing flies easy access via entry holes will make the bait more attractive. The bait must also be protected from larger animals and ants that will raid this free food. Birds and rats may be excluded with a wire mesh cage of sorts. Ants and other crawling invertebrates can be prevented from accessing the bait by placing the meat container into a larger tray/container partially filled with water. This creates a moat surrounding the meat that cannot be crossed by ants. Rain protection and a dark cover to mimic a cadaver can be achieved by placing a dark sheet of plastic material or similar cover onto the exclusion cage. The bait station may be set up in the morning and by late afternoon the eggs must be collected from the bait or else they are prone to dry out if it is hot, or hatch overnight. Unfortunately, it is not easy to discern what fly species has laid the eggs. One way to narrow down the species is by collecting egg masses from the bait used in a trap as described earlier and in Figure 13.1. It will be highly likely that the eggs will have been deposited by flies that were subsequently trapped. Irrespective of the method, it is best to place individual egg masses laid by a single female into separate rearing containers with larval diet. Once they have been raised to adult stage, they can be properly identified and placed into communal cages along with flies of the same species.

Hand Collecting of Adults, Eggs and Maggots

When hand collecting fly specimens, a bait such as an animal carcass, a quantity of putrid meat, or even faeces can be placed in a convenient spot to attract flies over a period of a few days. The collector returns regularly to the bait to collect adult flies with an entomological sweep net. The cadavers may also be examined periodically for egg masses and maggots. Various utensils such as spoons, forceps and applicator sticks may be used to pick eggs and maggots off the bait. Pathology specimen containers, various test tubes, or even empty food jars may be used to store and transport collected eggs and maggots to the insectary for identification and culture. Containers will not need to be ventilated if this transfer happens quickly. It is, however, best to use containers that are fitted with lids that permit air exchange. For this purpose, larger holes can be drilled into the lid and a sheet of fine-weave fabric can be sandwiched between lid and container-mouth prior to closing. This is especially necessary if very active, minute maggots are to be collected.

Taxonomic Identification and Confirmation of Species

Great care must be taken in accurate identification and selection of the desired fly species to ensure that the flies added to the existing laboratory stock are of the same species and that no harmful species is inadvertently selected. Morphological characteristics are used for the identification of adult flies [52–58], larvae [59–62], and pupae [63]. Even non-specialists can use reliable morphological character differences between *L. sericata* and *L. cuprina* [64]. In recent times a variety of molecular genetic techniques have been employed for taxonomic studies and identification of species, including *L. sericata*, and have been found to be as reliable as examination of morphological characters [55, 65–68]. Because many maggot therapy entrepreneurs will not have access to molecular laboratory facilities and may find it difficult to access the taxonomic literature, it follows an identification guide that highlights the most relevant medicinal fly species for each zoogeographic region (Figure 13.4).

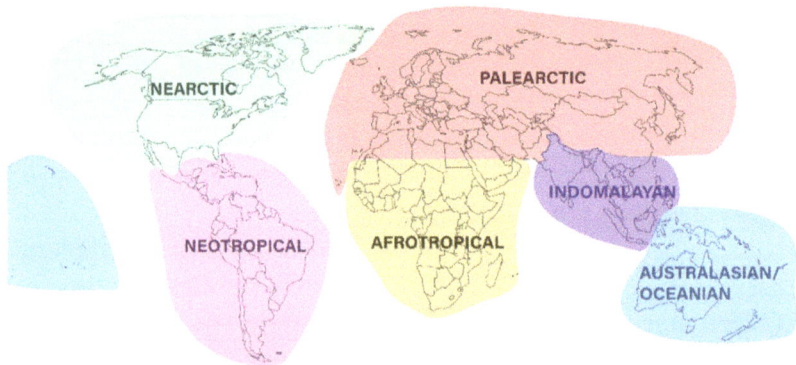

Figure 13.4 The six major zoogeographic regions of the world.

Although a range of species have been used in maggot debridement therapy (Table 13.1), we have chosen to provide identification guides to the following five species because they are well described biologically and broadly distributed throughout the world.

- *C. vicina*
- *L. cuprina*
- *Ch. megacephala*
- *L. sericata*
- *Co. macellaria*

At least one of these species can be found in every major zoogeographic region (Table 13.2). Importantly, the diagnoses provided here are only intended to be used as a general guide for identifying flies that are associated with and breed in carrion. There will be uncommon and non-carrion-breeding blowfly species that cannot be discriminated by the simplified diagnoses we provide here. It is therefore crucial that specimen identity be confirmed by reference to one of the many published resources such as those cited here (Table 13.2), or by sending your specimen to an expert entomologist at your closest research institution. For a list of recommended institutions refer to Table 13.2. For later reference throughout this section, the term 'bristles' refers to larger hairs (setae) located in a sunken pit in the exoskeleton. The term 'hairs' refers to smaller hairs (setulae) not located in such a pit.

Table 13.2 The six major zoogeographic regions of the world, and which of the five fly species (*C. vicina, L. sericata, L. cuprina, Co. macellaria, Ch. megacephala*) are found there. Also provided are suggested facilities that can provide specimen identification services. The last column lists the references to the relevant taxonomic keys for species identification.

Zoogeographic Region	Species	ID Facility	Key
Afrotropical	*L. sericata* *L. cuprina* *Ch. megacephala*	KwaZulu-Natal Museum, South Africa	[69]
Indomalayan	*Ch. megacephala* *L. cuprina*	Department of Parasitology, Faculty of Medicine, Chiang Mai University, Thailand	[70–72]
Palearctic	*C. vicina* *L. sericata*	Natural History Museum, UK	[58, 73]
Nearctic	*L. sericata* *L. cuprina* *Co. macellaria*	Smithsonian National Museum of Natural History, USA	[74, 75]
Australasian-Oceanian	*L. sericata* *L. cuprina* *Ch. megacephala* *C. vicina*	Australian National Insect Collection, Australia	[76, 77]

Zoogeographic Region	Species	ID Facility	Key
Neotropical	Co. macellaria L. cuprina Ch. megacephala	Laboratory of Integrative Entomology, Department of Animal Biology, University of Campinas, Brazil	[74, 78]

Calliphorid Fly Morphology Relevant to the Identification of Species

In order to facilitate the identification of flies using the information and figures provided in this section, it will be helpful to first locate the relevant morphological characters on a fly (Table 13.3 and Figure 13.5). The blue highlighting is omitted in subsequent species plates in order not to obstruct the features.

Table 13.3 Key to morphological characters used for species identification.

Head		
Fo.P	fronto-orbital plate	Figure 13.5a, b
G	genae	Figure 13.5a, e
Pa.V	paravertical	Figure 13.5c
Pf	parafacials	Figure 13.5e
Vi.S	vibrissal setulae	Figure 13.5e
Pl	palpi	Figure 13.5e

Thorax		
H.C.	humeral calli	Figure 13.5a, b
Lo.C	lower calypter	Figure 13.5a

Wing		
St.V	stem vein	Figure 13.5d
B	basicosta	Figure 13.5a, b

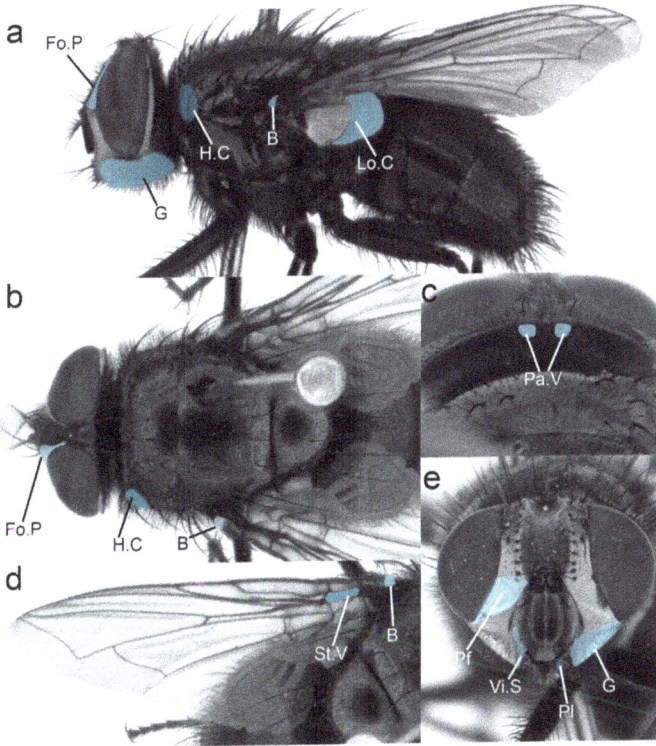

Figure 13.5 Morphological characters required for the identification of the five medicinal fly species. Head: Fo.P fronto-orbital plate, G genae, Pa.V paravertical, Pf parafacials, Vi.S vibrissal setulae, Pl palpi. Thorax: H.C. humeral calli, Lo.C lower calypter. Wing: St.V stem vein, B basicosta. CC BY-NC.

Genus *Calliphora*

Genus Diagnosis. Flies of the genus *Calliphora* (Figure 13.6) are generally black or brown in colour with a blue-metallic abdomen (rarely green), and a powdery coating on their thorax and abdomen. The genus *Calliphora* can be distinguished from *Lucilia*, *Chysomya* and *Cochliomya* by the combination of the following characters: lower parafacial area without strong bristles (Figure 13.6d), stem vein without bristles on dorsal surface (Figure 13.6e), dorsal surface of lower calypter hairy (Figure 13.6b). Note that some of these characters may be present in the other mentioned genera, but the combination of all three is unique to the genus *Calliphora*.

Calliphora vicina. C. *vicina* can be distinguished from other carrion-breeding members of the genus *Calliphora* through the combination of following characteristics: abdomen metallic blue with a silver powdery coating that changes with viewing angle (Figure 13.6c), eyes without any hairs (Figure 13.6a, c, d), parafacials and genae orange, with black hairs on genae (Figure 13.6a, d), basicosta yellow/orange-brown (can appear darker but not black) (Figure 13.6c, e).

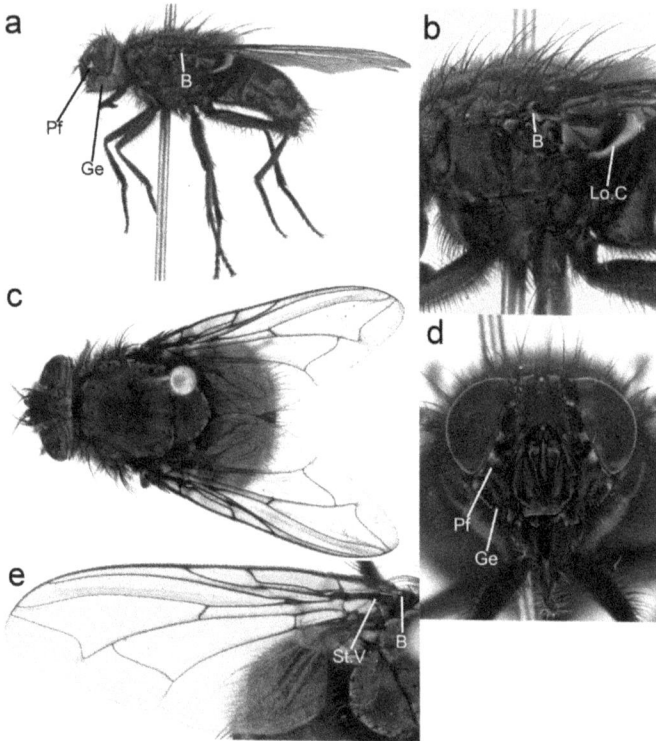

Figure 13.6 *Calliphora vicina.* Pf: parafacials, Ge: genae, B: basicosta, Lo.C: lower calypter. CC BY-NC.

Genus *Lucilia*

Genus Diagnosis. Flies of the genus *Lucilia* can be distinguished from *Calliphora* by the bright metallic green, blue or copper thorax and abdomen without any significant powdery coating (Figure 13.7c, 13.8c). In addition, this genus can be distinguished from *Chrysomya* and *Cochliomya* by the combination of wing stem vein without hairs on dorsal surface (Figure 13.7e, 13.8e) and lower calypter without hairs on dorsal surface (Figure 13.7b, 13.8b).

Lucilia cuprina. This fly has an abdomen and thorax ranging in colour from metallic green to copper (Figure 13.7a, b) with a white head (fronto-orbital and parafacial regions) (Figure 13.7f). Wings are clear (Figure 13.7e), basicosta yellow not fuscous or black (Figure 13.7a–c). This species closely resembles *L. sericata* but can be distinguished from this species through the combination of occipital area with one (rarely 0 or 2) paravertical hairs (Figure 13.7d) and humeral callus (anterior lateral region of the thorax) with three strong bristles and very few hairs (0–4) (Figure 13.7c).

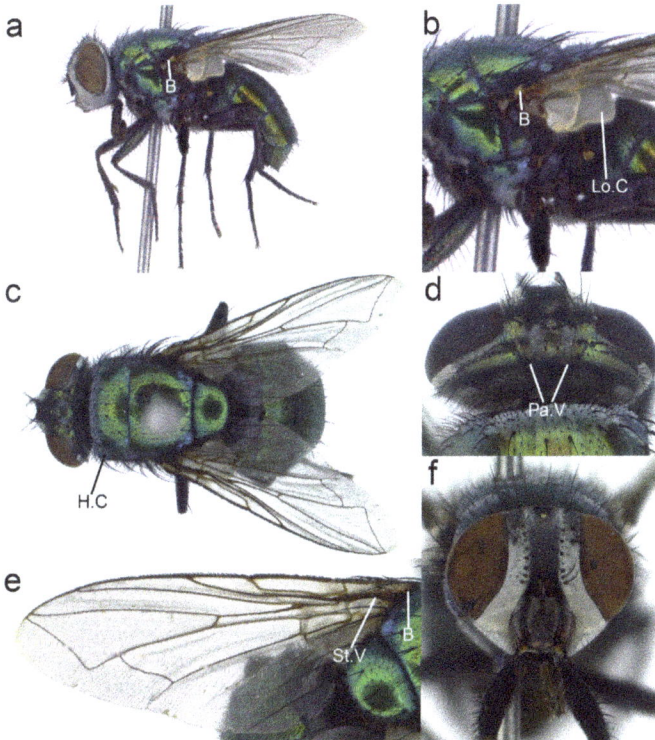

Figure 13.7 *Lucilia cuprina.* B: basicosta, Lo.C: lower calypter, H.C: humeral calli, Pa.V: paravertical, St.V: stem vein. CC BY-NC.

Lucilia sericata. This fly has an abdomen and thorax ranging from metallic green to copper in colour with a white head (fronto-orbital and parafacial regions) (Figure 13.8a, c, e). Wings are clear (Figure

13.8c), basicosta yellow not fuscous or black (Figure 13.8a-c). This species closely resembles *L. cuprina* but can be distinguished from it by the combination of central occipital area with many hairs (2–8) (Figure 13.8d) and humeral callus (anterior lateral region of the thorax) with three strong bristles and many fine hairs (>5) (Figure 13.8c).

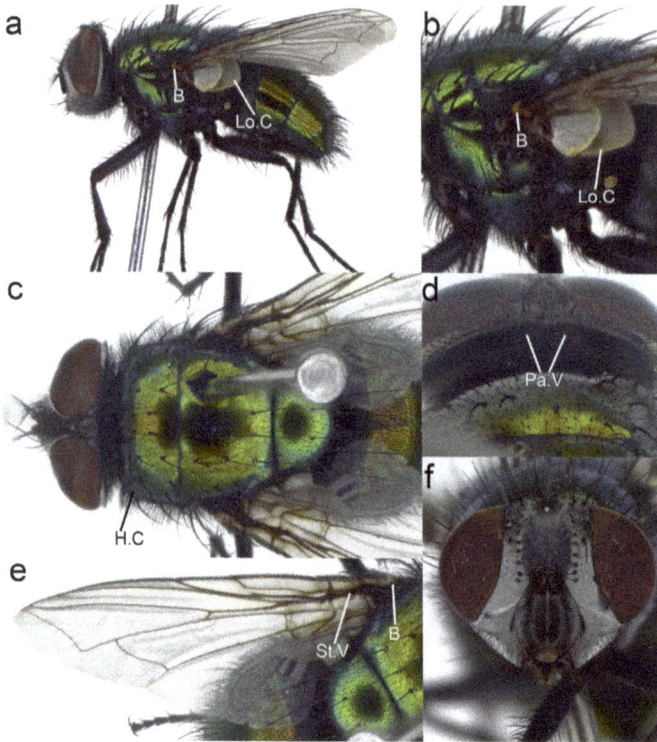

Figure 13.8 *Lucilia sericata*. B: basicosta, Lo.C: lower calypter, H.C: humeral calli, Pa.V: paravertical, St.V: stem vein. CC BY-NC.

Genus *Cochliomyia*

Genus Diagnosis. The genus *Cochliomyia* can be distinguished from *Calliphora*, *Chrysomya* and *Lucilia* by the combination of three black longitudinal stripes on the thorax (Figure 13.9c), short thread-like palpi (Figure 13.9a, f), and at least some yellow hairs on the genae (Figure 13.9a, f). It is most closely related to *Chrysomya* and both genera can be distinguished from *Calliphora* and *Lucilia* through the presence of a row of hairs on the dorsal surface of the stem vein (Figure 13.9e).

Cochliomya macellaria. This species can be distinguished from all other species of *Cochliomya* by the combination of genae with only yellow hairs (Figure 13.9a, f), fronto-orbital area with both a row of black bristles (Figure 13.9f) and fine pale hairs, particularly in the lower half (Figure 13.9a, d, f) (if fine black hairs are present, proceed with caution—the specimen could be *Co. hominivorax* and should NOT be used for maggot debridement therapy). The entire abdomen is metallic green or blue (with each segment being identical in colour) (Figure 13.9c).

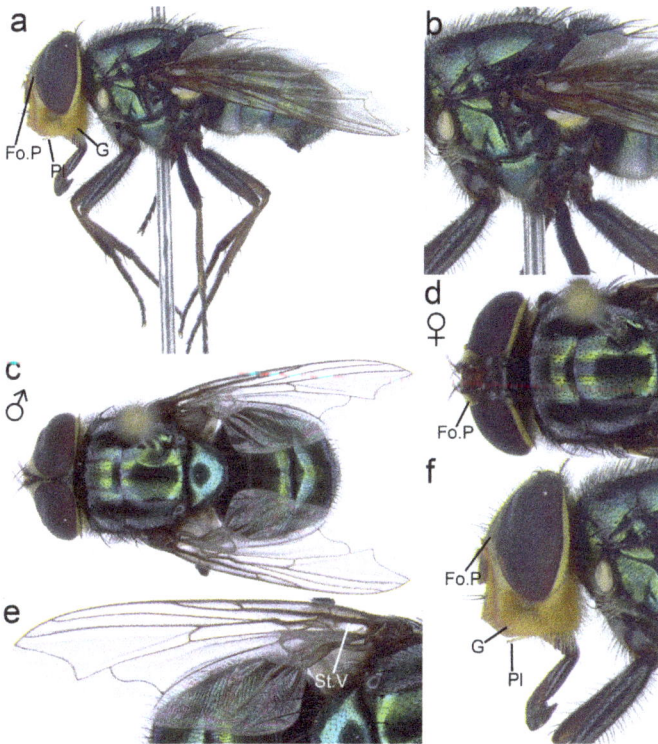

Figure 13.9 *Cochliomyia macellaria.* Fo.P: fronto-orbital plate, Pl: palpi, G: genae, St.V: stem vein. CC BY-NC.

Genus *Chrysomya*

Genus Diagnosis. The genus *Chrysomya* is most closely related to *Cochliomya* and both genera can be distinguished from *Calliphora* and *Lucilia* by the presence of a row of hairs on the dorsal surface of the stem vein (Figure 13.10e). *Chrysomya* can be distinguished from *Cochliomya* by the absence of any longitudinal black stripes on the thorax (Figure 13.10c).

Chrysomya megacephala. This species can be distinguished from other *Chrysomya* by the combination of entirely clear wings (Figure 13.10e), a blackish-brown anterior spiracle (Figure 13.10b), lower calypter brownish (not white or black) (Figure 13.10b), and many black vibrissal setulae on the face and parafacialia (Figure 13.10f). Males of this species possess touching eyes (holoptic) with sharply distinguished upper and lower facets (Figure 13.10c). In the female, the eyes are separated (dichoptic) (Figure 13.10d), and the fronto-orbital plate is dark rather than red (Figure 13.10d).

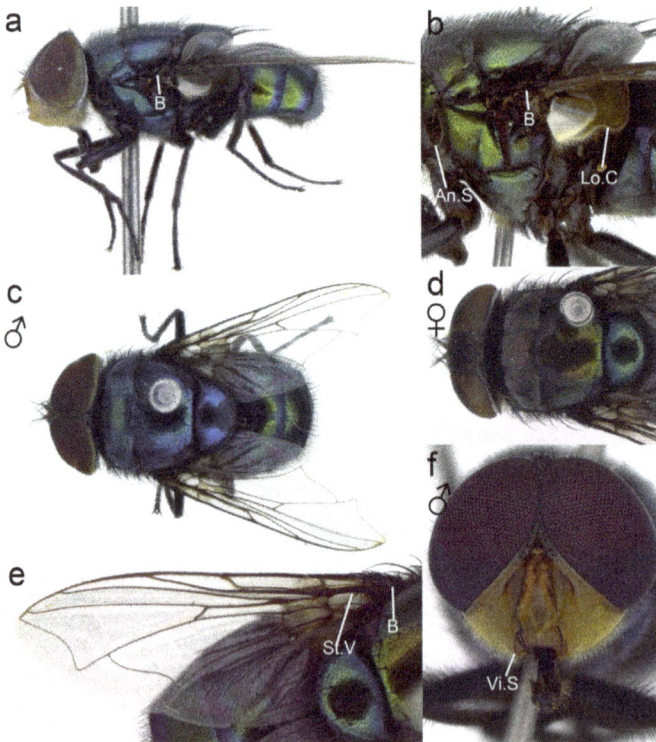

Figure 13.10 *Chrysomya megacephala.* B: basicosta, An.S: anterior spiracle, Lo.C: lower calypter, St.V: stem vein, Vi.S: vibrissal setulae. CC BY-NC.

Colony Replenishment

While some laboratory colonies of fly species that are of interest to forensic, agricultural, or medical entomologists have been kept successfully for many years without adding wild flies to the colonies [4], it may be necessary to periodically restock in order to replenish colony genetics and vigour. For consistent performance of production colonies, it will be best to always collect replenishment stock from the same location as that of the founder colony [79–81]. This will avoid introduction of vastly different genetics and resulting life history traits. The aim is to maintain uniform fly performance characteristics in the laboratory.

When collecting from the wild, there is always a danger that flies have been exposed to toxins, and carry disease or parasites, making preliminary quarantine necessary. Careless introduction of these newly caught flies into the laboratory environment can harm established colonies. Many flies including *L. sericata* are also prone to pupal parasites [82] and various fungi and nematodes that kill insects. These diseases must not be introduced into the laboratory and insectary [83, 84]. In practical terms this means that newly collected flies should be kept apart from the established laboratory colonies for at least one life-cycle until their health has been confirmed.

Domestication of Fly Stock

Domestication is the process of cultivating or rearing plant and animal species for human use, pleasure or companionship. During domestication, the animal or plant population adjusts to the new environmental conditions under human cultivation. This is also the case when wild flies are brought into the laboratory. They will need to adjust to the laboratory environment, constant temperature and light regimens, diets, cages, and higher population densities. Initially, individuals of newly collected fly stock will vary in their life history characteristics such as development times, number of eggs produced and timing of maturation. Over a number of generations and as laboratory processes impose selection pressure on the fly population, this variation will diminish, performance will become more and more uniform, and fitness may even increase [85], provided the negative effects of inbreeding can be managed.

The objectives regarding colony performance may vary depending on the purpose of the colony. For example, if flies are to be reared in the laboratory for the purpose of controlled-release field experiments or pest control, it will be important to maintain their natural fitness and resilience in the field [86]. In contrast, the objectives for medicinal fly production are:

1. Optimisation of the therapeutic performance of medicinal fly species or strains.

2. Reliability of colony performance via homogenous life history traits, meaning that the individuals in the colony have very similar development times and growth rates, for example.

3. Maximisation of the number of eggs produced by females.

Unfortunately, there has not been much published research on optimal domestication and management of medicinal fly populations in the laboratory and insectary [87]. Much of this information and practical knowledge, as far as it exists, is of proprietary nature and held by medicinal maggot producers. Chapter 14 provides comprehensive guidance on how medicinal flies are best maintained in the insectary and how medicinal maggots are prepared for treatment [88].

Quality Control

Newly collected flies and established colonies should be carefully monitored, and their life history parameters measured on a regular basis. Species-specific characteristics such as morphology, life-history, physiology, and genetic characteristics can all be used as performance indicators. Which sampling regimen and performance indicators are chosen will depend on the producer's resources. For example, it is fairly easy to measure how many eggs females produce, how many of these hatch, how fast maggots grow and how many survive to adulthood. Table 13.4 lists some easily monitored quality control activities that may be included in the standard operating procedures. However, wing morphology or genetic investigations are more complex and demand sophisticated instrumentation, software, and skilled laboratory technicians that may not be available to all producers [89–91].

The easiest way for a producer to monitor therapeutic efficacy of medicinal maggots over time is to communicate frequently with maggot therapy practitioners to receive feedback on clinical performance. This must also include an adverse-events reporting system so that any potential quality issues that have led to adverse treatment outcomes can be addressed quickly. The therapeutic performance with respect to debridement can also be tested in the laboratory with a meat-based test that simulates debridement in a wound. A protocol for such a debridement activity assay is given by Thyssen and Masiero [13] in Chapter 11 based on studies published in the literature.

Table 13.4 Quality control activities.

Life history characteristic	Measurement
Adult fly performance	
Sex ratio	Ratio of males to females. Determine the sex of 100 randomly sampled adult flies.
Adult weight	Measure the weight of adults directly after emergence and before first meal. There should be a strong correlation between this weight and that of pupae.
First oviposition	Time (hours) it takes from emergence for females to lay their first egg mass (assuming that males are present for mating as soon as females are receptive)
Number of oviposition events	Number of times a female lays eggs (oviposition).
Egg mass size	Number of eggs per oviposition (per egg batch).
Fecundity	Total number of eggs laid in a lifetime.
Adult longevity	Life span (days) of an adult fly from emergence.
Egg development	
Development time	Time (hours) from oviposition to emergence of larvae at a specific temperature.
Survival rate (in %)	Number of emerged larvae divided by the total number of eggs incubated and multiplied by 100.
Larval development	
Development time	Time (hours) from hatching to post-feeding period (when they leave the larval food substrate).

Life history characteristic	Measurement
Body length at post-feeding	Length of maggots (mm) at the beginning of the post-feeding period. Immerse maggots in boiling water to rapidly kill them and then preserve in 70–80% ethanol prior to measurement [92].
Weight at post-feeding	Weight of maggots (mg) at beginning of post-feeding period.
Time to pupariation	Time (hours) it takes for post-feeding maggots to pupariate.
Pupariation rate (in %)	Number of pupariated maggots divided by the total number of maggots studied, multiplied by 100.
Pupal development	
Pupal weight	Weight (mg) of pupae just after pupariation (when puparia have hardened and darkened to a glossy brown colour).
Development time	Time (hours) it takes for the fly to emerge after pupariation.
Emergence rate (in %)	Number of healthy flies divided by the number of pupae studied, multiplied by 100.

Strain Improvement

In addition to selecting suitable species with maggots that are benign and highly effective in debriding necrotic tissue, clinical performance could also be improved, and new therapeutic benefits introduced to maggot therapy, if fly strains were to be genetically enhanced. Traditionally, such enhancement is done through animal breeding based on selecting individuals with favourable characteristics. There have been recent attempts to genetically engineer *L. sericata* so that the flies express human growth hormone in larval excretions and secretions. Such genetically modified strains could deliver a variety of growth factors and anti-microbial substances during maggot therapy and thereby enhance wound healing [93]. However, due to the negative perception of genetic modification, regulatory approval for genetically modified flies may be difficult to obtain even if *in vitro* and clinical trials demonstrate efficacy. Therefore, until regulatory barriers have been overcome, the best strategy will be to improve medicinal maggot performance and efficacy through conventional animal breeding approaches.

Summary

There are potentially many fly species that could be utilised for maggot therapy and several species have been successfully applied to treat wounds. Nevertheless, it is recommended that producers and researchers starting medicinal fly colonies only collect species of known efficacy. For the most part this will involve the production of *L. sericata* and *L. cuprina* thanks to their near-global distribution. Producers and therapists interested in developing maggot therapy with other fly species will find Chapter 11 on the identification and testing of new maggot therapy species essential reading [13].

All life stages are suitable for collection, except pupae that are generally hidden from view because maggots bury into the ground for pupariation. Correct identification of the species that are collected and the correct selection of breeding stock is critical. Identification guides provided in this chapter and identification keys published in the literature should be consulted. In addition, identification services offered by natural history museums or molecular barcoding methods should be used where accessible to confirm species identity.

Domestication of the newly established fly colony will proceed via adaptation to the laboratory/insectary environment and the producer's operating procedures. Producers must implement routine quality-monitoring protocols during colony establishment and, beyond that, track life history characteristics like the ones suggested in Table 13.4. There is largely unexplored scope for selective breeding of desirable characteristics of medicinal fly species and molecular tools may also offer opportunities for genetic enhancement of medicinal flies. However, the latter will require considerable research, regulatory approval and patient acceptance before transgenic maggots reach the bedside.

References

1. Firoozfar, F., et al., *Mass Rearing of Lucilia sericata Meigen (Diptera: Calliphoridae)*. Asian Pacific Journal of Tropical Biomedicine, 2011. 1(1): pp. 54–56, https://doi.org/10.1016/S2221-1691(11)60068-3.

2. Firoozfar, F., et al., *Laboratory Colonization of Lucilia sericata Meigen (Diptera: Caliphoridae) strain from Hashtgerd, Iran*. Journal of Vector Borne Diseases, 2012. 49(1): pp. 23–26.

3. Sanei-Dehkordi, A., et al., *Anti Leishmania Activity of Lucilia sericata and Calliphora vicina Maggots in Laboratory Models.* Experimental Parasitology, 2016. 170: pp. 59–65, https://doi.org/10.1016/j.exppara.2016.08.007.

4. Leopold, R.A., R.R. Rojas, and P.W. Atkinson, *Post Pupariation Cold Storage of Three Species of Flies: Increasing Chilling Tolerance by Acclimation and Recurrent Recovery Periods.* Cryobiology, 1998. 36(3): pp. 213–224, https://dx.doi.org/10.1006/cryo.1998.2081.

5. Pinilla, Y.T., M.A. Patarroyo, and F.J. Bello, *Sarconesiopsis magellanica (Diptera: Calliphoridae) Life-cycle, Reproductive and Population Parameters Using Different Diets under Laboratory Conditions.* Forensic Science International, 2013. 233(1–3): pp. 380–386, https://doi.org/10.1016/j.forsciint.2013.10.014.

6. Anderson, G.S., *Minimum and Maximum Development Rates of Some Forensically Important Calliphoridae (Diptera).* Journal of Forensic Sciences, 2000. 45(4): pp. 824–832.

7. Grassberger, M. and C. Reiter, *Effect of Temperature on Lucilia sericata (Diptera: Calliphoridae) Development with Special Reference to the Isomegalen- and Isomorphen-diagram.* Forensic Science International, 2001. 120(1–2): pp. 32–36, https://doi.org/10.1016/S0379-0738(01)00413-3.

8. Blake, F.A.S., et al., *The Biosurgical Wound Debridement: Experimental Investigation of Efficiency and Practicability.* Wound Repair and Regeneration, 2007. 15(5): pp. 756–761, https://doi.org/10.1111/j.1524-475x.2007.00298.x.

9. McGuiness, W., E. Vella, and D. Harrison, *Influence of Dressing Changes on Wound Temperature.* Journal of Wound Care, 2004. 13(9): pp. 383–385, 10.12968/jowc.2004.13.9.26702.

10. Dini, V., et al., *Correlation between Wound Temperature Obtained with an Infrared Camera and Clinical Wound Bed Score in Venous Leg Ulcers.* Wounds, 2015. 27(10): pp. 274–278.

11. US Army, *ST 31–91B US Army Special Forces Medical Handbook.* 1982: United States Army Institute for Military Assistance.

12. Sherman, R.A. and M.R. Hetzler, *Maggot Therapy for Wound Care in Austere Environments.* Journal of Special Operations Medicine, 2017. 17(2): pp. 154–162.

13. Thyssen, P.J. and F.S. Masiero, *Bioprospecting and Testing of New Fly Species for Maggot Therapy*, in *A Complete Guide to Maggot Therapy: Clinical Practice, Therapeutic Principles, Production, Distribution, and Ethics*, F. Stadler (ed.). 2022, Cambridge: Open Book Publishers, pp. 195–234, https://doi.org/10.11647/OBP.0300.11.

14. Chan, Q.E., M.A. Hussain, and V. Milovic, *Eating out of the Hand, Maggots — Friend or Foe?* Journal of Plastic, Reconstructive and Aesthetic Surgery, 2012. 65(8): pp. 1116–1118, https://doi.org/10.1016/j.bjps.2012.01.014.

15. Giri, S.A., et al., *Cerebral Myiasis Associated with Artificial Cranioplasty Flap: A Case Report.* World Neurosurg, 2016. 87: p. 661.e13–6, https://doi.org/10.1016/j.wneu.2015.09.046.

16. Terterov, S., et al., *Posttraumatic Human Cerebral Myiasis.* World Neurosurgery, 2010. 73(5): pp. 557–559, https://doi.org/10.1016/j.wneu.2010.01.004.

17. Bickel, D.J., T. Pape, and R. Meier, *Appendix. Diptera per Family for All Regions*, in *Diptera Diversity: Status Challenges and Tools*, D.J. Bickel, T. Pape, and R. Meier, Editors. 2009, Brill: Boston; Leiden. pp. 439–444.

18. Paul, A.G., et al., *Maggot Debridement Therapy with Lucilia cuprina: A Comparison with Conventional Debridement in Diabetic Foot Ulcers.* International Wound Journal, 2009. 6(1): pp. 39–46, https://doi.org/10.1111/j.1742-481X.2008.00564.x.

19. Yeong, Y.S., et al., *Scanning Electron Microscopic Evaluation of the Successful Sterilization of Lucilia cuprina (Wiedemann) Utilized in Maggot Debridement Therapy (mdt).* Tropical Biomedicine, 2011. 28(2): pp. 325–332. https://www.msptm.org/files/325_-_332_Yeong_Y_S.pdf.

20. Tantawi, T.I., K.A. Williams, and M.H. Villet, *An Accidental but Safe and Effective Use of Lucilia cuprina (Diptera: Calliphoridae) in Maggot Debridement Therapy in Alexandria, Egypt.* Journal of Medical Entomology, 2010. 47(3): pp. 491–494, https://doi.org/10.1093/jmedent/47.3.491.

21. Nassu, M.P. and P.J. Thyssen, *Evaluation of Larval Density Cochliomyia macellaria F. (Diptera: Calliphoridae) for Therapeutic Use in the Recovery of Tegumentar Injuries.* Parasitology Research, 2015. 114(9): pp. 3255–3260, https://doi.org/10.1007/s00436-015-4542-8.

22. Alvarez Garcia, D.M., A. Pérez-Hérazo, and E. Amat, *Life History of Cochliomyia macellaria (Fabricius, 1775) (Diptera, Calliphoridae), a Blowfly of Medical and Forensic Importance.* Neotropical Entomology, 2017. 46(6): pp. 606–612, https://doi.org/10.1007/s13744-017-0496-0.

23. Dallavecchia, D.L., R.G. da Silva Filho, and V.M. Aguiar, *Sterilization of Chrysomya putoria (Insecta: Diptera: Calliphoridae) Eggs for Use in Biotherapy.* Journal of Insect Science, 2014. 14, https://doi.org/10.1093/jisesa/ieu022.

24. Diaz-Roa, A., et al., *Evaluating Sarconesiopsis magellanica Blowfly-derived Larval Therapy and Comparing it to Lucilia sericata-derived Therapy in an Animal Model.* Acta Tropica, 2016. 154: pp. 34–41, https://doi.org/10.1016/j.actatropica.2015.10.024.

25. Teich, S. and R.A.M. Myers, *Maggot Therapy for Severe Skin Infections.* Southern Medical Journal, 1986. 79(9): pp. 1153–1155.

26. Baer, W.S., *The Treatment of Chronic Osteomyelitis with the Maggot (Larva of the Blow Fly).* The Journal of Bone and Joint Surgery. American Volume, 1931. 13: pp. 438–475.

27. Sherman, R.A. and E.A. Pechter, *Maggot Therapy: A Review of the Therapeutic Applications of Fly Larvae in Human Medicine, Especially for Treating Osteomyelitis.* Medical and Veterinary Entomology, 1988. 2(3): pp. 225–230, https://doi.org/10.1111/j.1365-2915.1988.tb00188.x.

28. Andersen, A.S., et al., *A Novel Approach to the Antimicrobial Activity of Maggot Debridement Therapy.* The Journal of Antimicrobial Chemotherapy, 2010. 65(8): pp. 1646–1654, https://doi.org/10.1093/jac/dkq165.

29. Sherman, R.A., M.J.R. Hall, and S. Thomas, *Medicinal Maggots: An Ancient Remedy for Some Contemporary Afflictions.* Annual Review of Entomology, 2000. 45(1): pp. 55–81, https://doi.org/10.1146/annurev.ento.45.1.55.

30. Sun, X., et al., *A Systematic Review of Maggot Debridement Therapy for Chronically Infected Wounds and Ulcers.* International Journal of Infectious Diseases, 2014. 25: pp. 32–37, https://doi.org/10.1016/j.ijid.2014.03.1397.

31. Nair, H.K.R., et al., *Maggot Debridement Therapy in Malaysia.* The International Journal of Lower Extremity Wounds, 2020: p. 1534734620932397, https://doi.org/10.1177/1534734620932397.

32. Paul, A.G., et al., *Maggot Debridement Therapy with Lucilia cuprina: A Comparison with Conventional Debridement in Diabetic Foot Ulcers.* International Wound Journal, 2009. 6(1): pp. 39–46, https://doi.org/10.1111/j.1742-481X.2008.00564.x.

33. Yeong, Y.S., et al., *Scanning Electron Microscopic Evaluation of the Successful Sterilization of Lucilia cuprina (Wiedemann) Utilized in Maggot Debridement Therapy (mdt).* Tropical Biomedicine, 2011. 28(2): pp. 325–332.

34. Horn, K.L., A.H. Cobb, and G.A. Gates, *Maggot Therapy for Subacute Mastoiditis.* Archives of otolaryngology (1960), 1976. 102(6): pp. 377–379, https://doi.org/10.1001/archotol.1976.00780110089013.

35. Durán, D., et al., *Histological and Immunohistochemical Study of Wounds in Sheep Skin in Maggot Therapy by Using Protophormia terraenovae (Diptera: Calliphoridae) Larvae.* Journal of Medical Entomology, 2019. 57(2): pp. 369–376, https://doi.org/10.1093/jme/tjz185.

36. Pinheiro, M.A.R.Q., et al., *Use of Maggot Therapy for Treating a Diabetic Foot Ulcer Colonized by Multidrug Resistant Bacteria in Brazil.* The Indian Journal of Medical Research, 2015. 141(3): pp. 340–342, https://doi.org/10.4103/0971-5916.156628.

37. Masiero, F.S., et al., *First Report on the Use of Larvae of Cochliomyia macellaria (Diptera: Calliphoridae) for Wound Treatment in Veterinary Practice.* Journal of Medical Entomology, 2019. 57(3): pp. 965–968, https://doi.org/10.1093/jme/tjz238.

38. Grantham-hill, C., *Preliminary Note on the Treatment of Infected Wounds with the Larva of Wohlfartia nuba.* Transactions of the Royal Society of Tropical Medicine and Hygiene, 1933. 27(1): pp. 93–98, https://doi.org/10.1016/S0035-9203(33)90138-8.

39. Li, Q., et al., *Maggots of Musca domestica in Treatment of Acute Intractable Wound*. Surgery, 2009. 145(1): pp. 122–123, https://doi.org/10.1016/j.surg.2008.08.016.

40. Gallagher, M.B., S. Sandhu, and R. Kimsey, *Variation in Developmental Time for Geographically Distinct Populations of the Common Green Bottle Fly, Lucilia sericata (Meigen)*. Journal of Forensic Sciences, 2010. 55(2): pp. 438–442, https://doi.org/10.1111/j.1556-4029.2009.01285.x.

41. El-Moaty, Z.A. and A.E.M. Kheirallah, *Developmental Variation of the Blow Fly Lucilia sericata (Meigen, 1826) (diptera: Calliphoridae) by Different Substrate Tissue Types*. Journal of Asia-Pacific Entomology, 2013. 16(3): pp. 297–300, https://doi.org/10.1016/j.aspen.2013.03.008.

42. Warren, J.A. and G.S. Anderson, *Effect of Fluctuating Temperatures on the Development of a Forensically Important Blow Fly, Protophormia terraenovae (Diptera: Calliphoridae)*. Environmental Entomology, 2013. 42(1): pp. 167–172, https://doi.org/10.1603/EN12123.

43. Klong-Klaew, T., et al., *Impact of Abiotic Factor Changes in Blowfly, Achoetandrus rufifacies (Diptera: Calliphoridae), in Northern Thailand*. Parasitology Research, 2014. 113(4): pp. 1353–1360, https://doi.org/10.1007/s00436-014-3774-3.

44. Lindsay, T.C., et al., *Development of Odour-Baited Flytraps for Sampling the African Latrine Fly, Chrysomya putoria, a Putative Vector of Enteric Diseases*. PLoS ONE, 2012. 7(11), https://doi.org/10.1371/journal.pone.0050505.

45. Warren, J.A. and G.S. Anderson, *The Development of Protophormia terraenovae (Robineau-Desvoidy) at Constant Temperatures and Its Minimum Temperature Threshold*. Forensic Science International, 2013. 233(1–3): pp. 374–379, https://doi.org/10.1016/j.forsciint.2013.10.012.

46. Harvey, M., et al., *Dipteran Attraction to a Variety of Baits: Implications for Trapping Studies as a Tool for Establishing Seasonal Presence of Significant Species*. Journal of Medical Entomology, 2019. 56(5): pp. 1283–1289, https://dx.doi.org/10.1093/jme/tjz050.

47. Brodie, B.S., et al., *Is Aggregated Oviposition by the Blow Flies Lucilia sericata and Phormia regina (Diptera: Calliphoridae) Really Pheromone-mediated?* Insect Science, 2015. 22(5): pp. 651–660, https://doi.org/10.1111/1744-7917.12160.

48. Hwang, C. and B.D. Turner, *Spatial and Temporal Variability of Necrophagous Diptera from Urban to Rural Areas*. Medical and Veterinary Entomology, 2005. 19(4): pp. 379–391, https://doi.org/10.1111/j.1365-2915.2005.00583.x.

49. Zabala, J., B. Díaz, and M.I. Saloña-Bordas, *Seasonal Blowfly Distribution and Abundance in Fragmented Landscapes. Is It Useful in Forensic Inference about Where a Corpse Has Been Decaying?* PloS one, 2014. 9(6): e99668, https://doi.org/10.1371/journal.pone.0099668.

50. Hall, M.J.R., *Trapping the Flies that Cause Myiasis: Their Responses to Host-stimuli*. Annals of Tropical Medicine and Parasitology, 1995. 89(4): pp. 333–357.

51. BioGlobal. *LuciLure Sheep Blowfly Attractant.* www.bioglobal.com.au/images/stories/lucilow.pdf.

52. Akbarzadeh, K., et al., *Species Identification of Middle Eastern Blowflies (Diptera: Calliphoridae) of forensic importance.* Parasitology Research, 2015. 114(4): pp. 1463–1472, https://doi.org/10.1007/s00436-015-4329-y.

53. Langer, S.V., C.J. Kyle, and D.V. Beresford, *Using Frons Width to Differentiate Blow Fly Species (Diptera: Calliphoridae) Phormia regina (Meigen) and Protophormia terraenovae (Robineau-Desvoidy).* Journal of Forensic Sciences, 2017. 62(2): pp. 473–475, https://doi.org/10.1111/1556-4029.13281.

54. Szpila, K. and J.F. Wallman, *Morphology and Identification of First Instar Larvae of Australian Blowflies of the Genus Chrysomya of Forensic Importance.* Acta Tropica, 2016. 162: pp. 146–154, https://doi.org/10.1016/j.actatropica.2016.06.006.

55. Tourle, R., D. Downie, and M.H. Villet, *Flies in the Ointment: A Morphological and Molecular Comparison of Lucilia cuprina and Lucilia sericata (Diptera: Calliphoridae) in South Africa.* Medical and Veterinary Entomology, 2009. 23(1): pp. 6–14, http://dx.doi.org/10.1111/j.1365-2915.2008.00765.x.

56. Vairo, K.P.e., C.A.d. Mello-Patiu, and C.J.B.d. Carvalho, *Pictorial Identification Key for Species of Sarcophagidae (Diptera) of Potential Forensic Importance in Southern Brazil.* Revista Brasileira de Entomologia, 2011. 55(3): pp. 333–347, https://doi.org/10.1590/S0085-56262011005000033.

57. Waterhouse, D.F. and S.J. Paramonov, *The Status of the Two Species of Lucilia (Diptera: Calliphoridae) Attacking Sheep in Australia.* Australian Journal of Biological Sciences, 1950. 3(3): pp. 310–336, http://dx.doi.org/10.1071/BI9500310.

58. Sivell, O., *Blow Flies (Diptera: Calliphoridae, Polleniidae, Rhiniidae), Handbooks for the Identification of British Insects 10 (16).* 2021, St Albans: Royal Entomological Society.

59. Erzinclioglu, Y.Z., *The Early Larval Instars of Lucilia sericata and Lucilia cuprina (Diptera, Calliphoridae) — Myiasis Blowflies of Africa and Australia.* Journal of Natural History, 1989. 23(5): pp. 1133–1136, https://doi.org/10.1080/00222938900771021.

60. Niederegger, S., K. Szpila, and G. Mall, *Muscle Attachment Site (MAS) Patterns for Species Determination in European Species of Lucilia (Diptera: Calliphoridae).* Parasitology Research, 2015. 114(3): pp. 851–859, https://doi.org/10.1007/s00436-014-4248-3.

61. Niederegger, S., et al., *Connecting the Dots: From an Easy Method to Computerized Species Determination.* Insects, 2017. 8(2): pp. 1–16, https://doi.org/10.3390/insects8020052.

62. Niederegger, S., K. Szpila, and G. Mall, *Muscle Attachment Site (MAS) Patterns for Species Determination in Five Species of Sarcophaga (Diptera:*

Sarcophagidae). Parasitology Research, 2016. 115(1): pp. 241–247, https://doi.org/10.1007/s00436-015-4740-4.

63.   Samerjai, C., et al., *Morphology of Puparia of Flesh Flies in Thailand.* Tropical Biomedicine, 2014. 31(2): pp. 351–361 https://www.msptm.org/files/351_-_361_Sukontason_KL.pdf.

64.   Holloway, B.A., *Morphological Characteristics to Identify Adult Lucilia sericata (Meigen, 1826) and L. cuprina (Wiedemann, 1830) (Diptera, Calliphoridae).* New Zealand Journal of Zoology, 1991. 18(4): pp. 415–420, https://dx.doi.org/10.1080/03014223.1991.10422847.

65.   Olekšáková, T., et al., *DNA Extraction and Barcode Identification of Development Stages of Forensically Important Flies in the Czech Republic.* Mitochondrial DNA Part A: DNA Mapping, Sequencing, and Analysis, 2017. 29(3): pp. 427–430, https://doi.org/10.1080/24701394.2017.1298102.

66.   Salem, A.M., F.K. Adham, and C.J. Picard, *Survey of the Genetic Diversity of Forensically Important Chrysomya (diptera: Calliphoridae) from Egypt.* Journal of Medical Entomology, 2015. 52(3): pp. 320–328, https://doi.org/10.1093/jme/tjv013.

67.   Williams, K.A., et al., *Identifying Flies Used for Maggot Debridement Therapy.* South African Medical Journal, 2008. 98(3): pp. 196–197.

68.   Shayya, S., et al., *Forensically Relevant Blow Flies in Lebanon Survey and Identification Using Molecular Markers (Diptera: Calliphoridae).* Journal of medical entomology, 2018. 55(5): pp. 1113–1123, https://doi.org/10.1093/jme/tjy068.

69.   Lutz, L., et al., *Species Identification of Adult African Blowflies (Diptera: Calliphoridae) of Forensic Importance.* International Journal of Legal Medicine, 2018. 132(3): pp. 831–842, https://doi.org/10.1007/s00414-017-1654-y.

70.   Kurahashi, H. and N. Bunchu, *The Blow Flies Recorded from Thailand, with the Description of a New Species of Isomyia WALKER (Diptera, Calliphoridae).* Japanese Journal of Systematic Entomology, 2011. 17: pp. 237–278.

71.   Kurahashi, H. and L. Chowanadisai, *Blow Flies (Insecta: Diptera: Calliphoridae) from Indochina.* Species Diversity, 2001. 6(3): pp. 185–242.

72.   Yang, S.-T., H. Kurahashi, and S.-F. Shiao, *Keys to the Blow Flies of Taiwan, with a Checklist of Recorded Species and the Description of a New Species of Paradichosia Senior-White (Diptera, Calliphoridae).* ZooKeys, 2014(434): pp. 57–109, https://doi.org/10.3897/zookeys.434.7540

73.   Rognes, K., *Blowflies (Diptera, Calliphoridae) of Fennoscandia and Denmark.* Vol. 24. 1991: Brill.

74.   Whitworth, T., *Keys to the Genera and Species of Blow Flies (Diptera: Calliphoridae) of America North of Mexico.* Proceedings of the Entomological Society of Washington, 2006. 108: pp. 689–725.

75. Whitworth, T., *Keys to the Genera and Species of Blow Flies (Diptera: Calliphoridae) of the West Indies and Description of a New Species of Lucilia Robineau-Desvoidy*. Zootaxa, 2010. 2663: pp. 1–35, https://doi.org/10.11646/zootaxa.2663.1.1.

76. Dear, J.P., *Calliphoridae (Insecta: Diptera)*. Fauna of New Zealand, 1986. 8.

77. Wallman, J.F., *A Key to the Adults of Species of Blowflies in Southern Australia Known or Suspected to Breed in Carrion*. [corrigendum in Medical and Veterinary Entomology 16(2): 223] Medical and Veterinary Entomology, 2001. 15(4): pp. 433–437, https://doi.org/10.1046/j.0269-283x.2001.00331.x.

78. Carvalho, C.J.B.d. and C.A.d. Mello-Patiu, *Key to the Adults of the Most Common Forensic Species of Diptera in South America*. Revista Brasileira de Entomologia, 2008. 52: pp. 390–406.

79. Hwang, C.C. and B.D. Turner, *Small-scaled Geographical Variation in Life-history Traits of the Blowfly Calliphora vicina between Rural and Urban Populations*. Entomologia Experimentalis et Applicata, 2009. 132(3): pp. 218–224, https://doi.org/10.1111/j.1570-7458.2009.00891.x.

80. Martínez-Sánchez, A., et al., *Geographic Origin Affects Larval Competitive Ability in European Populations of the Blow Fly, Lucilia sericata*. Entomologia Experimentalis et Applicata, 2007. 122(2): pp. 93–98, https://doi.org/10.1111/j.1570-7458.2006.00497.x.

81. Picard, C.J. and J.D. Wells, *The Population Genetic Structure of North American Lucilia sericata (Diptera: Calliphoridae), and the Utility of Genetic Assignment Methods for Reconstruction of Postmortem Corpse Relocation*. Forensic Science International, 2010. 195(1–3): pp. 63–67, https://doi.org/10.1016/j.forsciint.2009.11.012.

82. Voss, S.C., H. Spafford, and I.R. Dadour, *Temperature-dependant Development of Nasonia vitripennis on Five Forensically Important Carrion Fly Species*. Entomologia Experimentalis et Applicata, 2010. 135(1): pp. 37–47, https://doi.org/10.1111/j.1570-7458.2010.00966.x.

83. Tóth, E.M., et al., *Evaluation of Efficacy of Entomopathogenic Nematodes against Larvae of Lucilia sericata (Meigen, 1826) (Diptera: Calliphoridae)*. Acta Veterinaria Hungarica, 2005. 53(1): pp. 65–71, https://doi.org/10.1556/AVet.53.2005.1.7.

84. Wright, C., A. Brooks, and R. Wall, *Toxicity of the Entomopathogenic Fungus, Metarhizium anisopliae (Deuteromycotina: Hyphomycetes) to Adult Females of the Blowfly Lucilia sericata (Diptera: Calliphoridae)*. Pest Management Science, 2004. 60(7): pp. 639–644, https://doi.org/10.1002/ps.808.

85. Hoffmann, A.A. and P.A. Ross, *Rates and Patterns of Laboratory Adaptation in (Mostly) Insects*. Journal of Economic Entomology, 2018. 111(2): pp. 501–509, https://doi.org/10.1093/jee/toy024.

86. Berkebile, D.R., et al., *Laboratory Environment Effects on the Reproduction and Mortality of Adult Screwworm (Diptera: Calliphoridae)*. Neotropical

Entomology, 2006. 35(6): pp. 781–786, https://doi.org/10.1590/S1519-566X2006000600010.

87. Stadler, F., *The Maggot Therapy Supply Chain: A Review of the Literature and Practice*. Med Vet Entomol, 2020. 34(1): pp. 1–9, https://doi.org/10.1111/mve.12397.

88. Stadler, F. and P. Takáč, *Medicinal Maggot Production*, in *A Complete Guide to Maggot Therapy: Clinical Practice, Therapeutic Principles, Production, Distribution, and Ethics*, F. Stadler (ed.). 2022, Cambridge: Open Book Publishers, pp. 289–330, https://doi.org/10.11647/OBP.0300.14.

89. Laparie, M., et al., *Wing Morphology of the Active Flyer Calliphora vicina (Diptera: Calliphoridae) during its Invasion of a Sub-Antarctic Archipelago Where Insect Flightlessness Is the Rule*. Biological Journal of the Linnean Society, 2016. 119(1): pp. 179–193, https://doi.org/10.1111/bij.12815.

90. Hayes, E.J., R. Wall, and K.E. Smith, *Measurement of Age and Population Age Structure in the Blowfly, Lucilia sericata (Meigen) (Diptera: Calliphoridae)*. Journal of Insect Physiology, 1998. 44(10): pp. 895–901, https://doi.org/10.1016/S0022-1910(98)00067-5.

91. Diakova, A.V., et al., *Assessing Genetic and Morphological Variation in Populations of Eastern European Lucilia sericata (Diptera: Calliphoridae)*. European Journal of Entomology, 2018. 115: pp. 192–197, https://doi.org/10.14411/eje.2018.017.

92. Adams, Z.J.O. and M.J.R. Hall, *Methods Used for the Killing and Preservation of Blowfly Larvae, and Their Effect on Post-mortem Larval Length*. Forensic Science International, 2003. 138: pp. 50–61.

93. Linger, R.J., et al., *Towards Next Generation Maggot Debridement Therapy: Transgenic Lucilia sericata Larvae that Produce and Secrete a Human Growth Factor*. BMC Biotechnology, 2016. 16:30, pp. 1–12, https://doi.org/10.1186/s12896-016-0263-z.

14. Medicinal Maggot Production

Frank Stadler and Peter Takáč

This chapter discusses the requirements for adult fly rearing, high-volume egg production, larval rearing and pupariation, and it explains the production of disinfected medicinal maggots for maggot therapy, the quality control procedures that are required to ensure safe and efficacious maggot therapy, and supply chain management considerations arising from the perishability of medicinal maggots. The chapter draws on a broad range of sources including the literature on maggot therapy, forensic entomology, and general entomology. For compromised healthcare settings with limited resources, point-of-care production solutions are discussed that do not rely on sophisticated laboratory and logistics infrastructure.

Introduction

Having covered the laboratory and insectary infrastructure and equipment needs in Chapter 12 [1], as well as the process of medicinal fly colony establishment in Chapter 13 [2], the next step is to provide the information necessary to produce high-quality, efficacious, and safe medicinal maggots. This chapter discusses the requirements for adult fly rearing, high-volume egg production, larval rearing and pupariation. The chapter also explains the production of disinfected medicinal maggots for maggot therapy, the quality control procedures that are required to ensure safe and efficacious maggot therapy, and the

 https://doi.org/10.11647/OBP.0300.14

supply chain management considerations arising from the perishability of medicinal maggots. The information presented has been drawn from a broad range of sources such as the literature on maggot therapy, forensic entomology, and general entomology. Much of the information relates to the most commonly used medicinal fly species *Lucilia sericata* and *Lucilia cuprina* but literature on other calliphorid fly species with comparable life histories was also consulted. The information presented in this chapter will equip the novice producer with all that is needed to produce high-quality, safe, and efficacious medicinal maggots. Although the guidance provided here should ensure appropriate husbandry that optimises fly health and minimises any fly suffering, Chapter 19 of this book will discuss in more detail the animal ethics of medicinal maggot production [3].

How to Care for Adult Flies

Cages

Cage set-ups for adult flies vary from wire and gauze to cages constructed from various plastic containers covered with mesh fabric or nylon stocking, and rearing cages offered by specialist entomology suppliers (Figure 14.1). The size of cages used and, therefore, the space available for flight also varies depending on what the keeper of flies has in mind. Researchers have reared flies in cages as small as 15 cm diameter by 9 cm deep, up to large setups of 120 x 60 x 60 cm [4, 5].

Flies in the wild occur at low densities with plenty of room to avoid each other, which is impractical in captive rearing. Therefore, the relationship between fly density in cages and performance needs to be considered. Laboratory experiments seem to suggest that there is little evidence for adult competition in *L. sericata* [6]. It appears that high larval density (rather than high adult density) has a detrimental impact on adult longevity and reproductive output [6]. This is because the level of larval nutrition and larval size at the point of pupation determines adult body size and the number of eggs a female can produce. Large adult fly cages mean increased flight activity and therefore increased energy expenditure by flies when the objective is to direct as much of the metabolic energy as possible into egg production. In addition, the laboratory infrastructure and space availability, as well as convenience of maintenance and handling, will place limits on the practical size of cages. An important consideration in the design and size of adult fly cages is the ease with which they can be cleaned and disinfected because, over the course of a colony's short lifetime, the cage gets badly soiled with fly faeces [7]. Considering then the health and welfare needs of flies and the practical aspects of insectary management, we recommend a stocking density of one fly per approximately 100 to 150 cm^3 of cage space [8]. For example, a commercially available, off-the-shelf 47.5 x 47.5 x 47.5 cm insect cage can be stocked with approximately 1000 flies (Figure 14.1).

Cage designs for adult flies must support maintenance which means that daily changes of food and water, and the harvesting of eggs can be done quickly and easily. For this purpose, cages must have a net sleeve that is easy to open, accommodates an adult hand holding a food dish, and is easy to close once the work has been done. As opposed to hinged cage doors, the tried and tested net sleeves maintain a snug fit around hand and arm and thus largely preventing the escape of flies during maintenance. In addition, a light source at the opposite side to the cage access will draw flies away from the opening and therefore also reduce escapes.

A cost-effective option for fly cages is a plastic storage container of convenient size in which the plastic lid is replaced with a nylon panty hose (Figure 14.1). The panty hose is slipped over the container and its elastic nature provides a secure hold around the rim of the plastic container. In order to create a sleeve for maintenance work, one leg of the panty hose is cut off to leave a stump of about 20 cm and the other leg is shortened and tied off with a knot. The container can be placed either on one of its sides offering front access or placed upright as intended which will facilitate top access for maintenance. After use, the container can be easily dismantled, and the nylon stocking can be washed and sterilised in bleach for re-use. From experience, this plastic container cage works well, provided the ambient relative humidity is low and condensation or build-up of fly-generated moisture on the container walls can be avoided. If the container walls become moist the flies lose grip of the plastic surface and crash-land continuously when flying about. This leads to stress, injury, and premature colony decline.

In contrast, cages that have mesh-covered sides are well-ventilated which prevents moisture build-up. They also provide flies with sufficiently secure footing and prevent frequent crash landing. When cages are used that do not have a solid impervious floor surface then it might be necessary to place cages onto a tray of sorts to keep shelving clean, capture dust generated by fly activity and permit the handling and relocation of cages without having to remove food, water and oviposition containers.

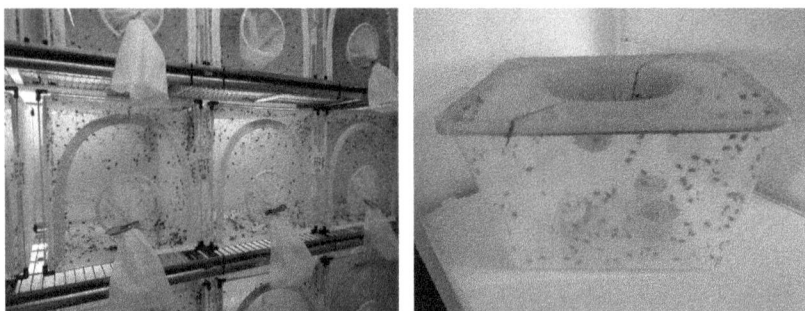

Figure 14.1 Examples of cages for the maintenance of adult fly colonies. A) A suitable cage model from an entomological equipment supplier (BugDorm Insect Cage, MegaView Science Co. Ltd.). B) A low-cost cage made of a household plastic storage box fitted with a nylon panty hose lid. Cut one panty hose leg for sleeved access to the cage. Photos by F. Stadler, MedMagLabs and Creating Hope in Conflict: A Humanitarian Grand Challenge, CC BY-ND.

Environmental Conditions

Like all organisms, medicinal fly species have their preferred environmental conditions as dictated by their evolutionary and ecological history. However, the various species used for maggot therapy (predominantly, but not exclusively, *L. sericata* and *L. cuprina*) exhibit remarkable robustness and adaptability in the laboratory environment and can be maintained at a wide range of environmental conditions, at least short-term over a few generations. However, the objective for a medicinal maggot producer is to establish and maintain highly productive fly colonies that are well-adapted to the laboratory environment and retain vigour over many generations. It is therefore important to meet the environmental and physiological needs of the flies as much as is practical.

As mentioned earlier, adult flies are best kept in cages that are well-ventilated and successful colony maintenance has been reported for relative humidity ranges from 30 to 70%. It is therefore advisable to maintain a steady humidity of 50 to 60% for adult flies, with constant provision of drinking water [7, 9, 10]. Temperature modulates activity levels in blowflies. Higher temperatures result in greater activity but shorter lifespan, and lower temperatures in less activity and decreased fertility, but a longer lifespan. In the laboratory a suitable compromise must be found that maximises the production of eggs over a relatively long period before flies age and die. The demand for reliable and predictable egg production makes it necessary to avoid any interruptions to reproductive activity. If flies are subjected to short day lengths and low temperatures, they may enter reproductive diapause and stop laying eggs. This can be avoided by providing summer climatic and photoperiodic conditions, meaning sufficiently high temperature and long day lengths [11]. A common regime is to maintain *L. sericata* adult colonies between 25°C and 27°C and at 12 to 16 hours light per day [4, 12–17]. The nature of the light provided also influences the wellbeing of flies. While regular incandescent and fluorescent light sources suffice, light sources are recommended that resemble as closely as is practical the natural daylight, particularly regarding the quantum of UV radiation.

Diet

Without access to energy-rich foods either in the form of lipids or carbohydrates, *L. sericata* flies expend all their energy reserves within a matter of days and die [18]. It is essential that adult flies have access at all times to carbohydrates such as table sugar or honey. In addition, females require protein meals in order to be able to mature ovaries and produce viable eggs [19–21]. Protein for ovary maturation and egg production is provided directly after adult emergence. Under natural conditions blowflies obtain protein from a variety of sources including from live animals, carcasses, or faeces. In the laboratory, flies are best fed with sugar, water, and a protein source. There is a great range of possible human foods that could be used (Table 14.1). Convenient foods include table sugar and a blend of dried protein sources such as milk powder, whey protein, and brewer's yeast. If meat such as liver is offered, it may be presented in pieces, or blended and mixed 1:1 with wheat bran and some water. However, continuous presentation of a moist, high-protein diet will lead to females depositing eggs on these feeding stations prior to planned egg harvesting. If this is a common occurrence, then it might be best to only offer dry protein sources between egg harvests. This is perfectly feasible because flies can regurgitate digestive secretions and dissolve dry food matter for ingestion. Feeding flies with a limited range of foods may result in vitamin deficiency which may be compensated by offering the flies a weak solution of multi-vitamin supplements as used for human consumption with a feeding station as described in Figure 14.2.

There have also been efforts to develop plant-based, heat-sterilisable diets for adult *L. sericata* [17]. Ingredients include dried yeast, wheat germ, agar powder and water, with or without whole milk powder (Table 14.2). Although absence of a high-protein meat diet delays ovary development and oviposition, all other performance indices in relation to longevity and reproductive success are much the same. Therefore, it is important to settle on one diet, whether meat-based or not, and consistently use it in order to establish a routine with predictable life-cycle and laboratory-process timing.

It is important that flies always have access to plenty of water. However, in order to prevent drowning in water and other liquid foods, these should be offered via small plastic containers (70–200 mL) furnished with absorbent wicks or inverted on tissue paper pads as shown in Figure 14.2. Note that moist and liquid fly foods will become quickly soiled and contaminated with microbial growth. These food stations should be replaced every two to three days and either disposed of or thoroughly washed and disinfected.

Egg Production

As discussed, *L. sericata*, *L. cuprina*, and other species used for maggot therapy rely on protein meals for egg development. In the case of *L. cuprina*, females need to consume at least 3.6 mg of liver exudate for completion of one ovarian cycle, and it is likely that similar amounts of protein are also required by closely related *L. sericata* flies [22]. In the event that *L. sericata* females cannot find enough protein as they enter reproductive maturity, they have the ability to partially invest in egg

Table 14.1 Food types for adult flies according to physiological need.

Protein diets	Carbohydrate diets	Hydration
• Ovine or bovine liver in pieces, or blended and mixed 1:1 with wheat bran and some water • Full cream milk powder • Whey powder • Brewer's yeast powder • Any other protein-rich food source such as tinned cat or dog food	• Honey dissolved in water • Sugar and sugar-containing foods (table sugar, sugar cubes, raw sugar, sweetened caffeine-free beverages, molasses, etc.)	• Water (as much as flies like to consume)

Table 14.2 Synthetic adult fly diets [17]

Meat-free adult diet with whole milk powder	Plant-based adult diet without milk powder
50g whole milk powder	75g dried yeast/brewer's yeast
50g dried yeast/brewer's yeast	75g wheat germ
50g wheat germ	5g agar powder
5g agar powder	1000 mL water
1000 mL water	

Note: All ingredients are mixed and boiled for ten minutes. To facilitate rapid cooling and convenient handling, the diet is best divided up into portions stored in single or multi-use plastic containers. To prevent spoilage, diets are stored in the refrigerator.

development by either depositing some yolk in all eggs followed by a pause in egg development, or by favouring the maturation of only a small number of eggs [20]. While this is an important ecological adaptation to resource insecurity and unpredictability, from an insect-rearing and egg-production standpoint, protein limitation must be avoided to maximise egg production over a female's lifetime. Moreover, reproductive output

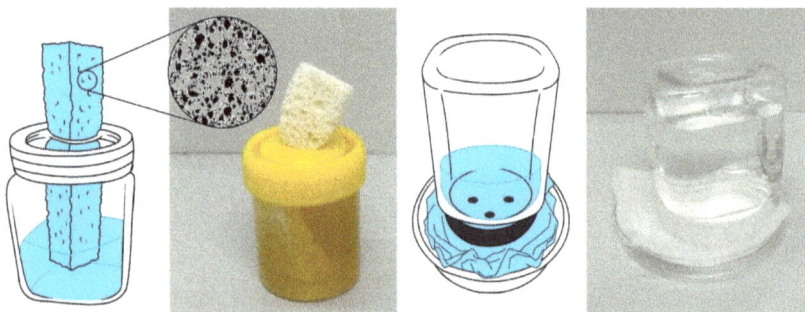

Figure 14.2 Liquid food dispensers (including water) for adult flies. A) Water and other liquids can be offered conveniently with a container fitted with a sponge wick. B) Alternatively, an inverted container with holes in the lid can be placed on a shallow dish lined with tissue paper. Solid foods like sugar or meat are best placed on shallow dishes such as reused food container lids or petri dishes. Illustrations by P. Busana and photos by F. Stadler, MedMagLabs and Creating Hope in Conflict: A Humanitarian Grand Challenge, CC BY-ND.

in blowfly females not only depends on the nutrition of the adult fly, it will also vary in response to nutrition during larval life, for example in the presence of larval competition over a limited food source [23].

Female *L. cuprina* usually mate only once, storing the sperm required for all their eggs [24]. Males, on the other hand, seek to mate soon after emergence and throughout their lifetime [25]. Consequently, the operational sex ratio in *L. cuprina* is heavily male-biased, meaning that there are far more males for any one receptive female. In captivity this leads to increased sexual harassment of females, a common issue in lab-reared colonies of blowflies [26]. It would be beneficial to skew the sex ratio toward females to maximise reproductive output and longevity of females [27], but this is not practical.

There is a great variation in reproductive output between species, and between strains within species. Research on the reproductive output of *L. sericata* and *L. cuprina* found lifetime reproductive outputs between 500 and over 2000 eggs per female [28]. Eggs are deposited in batches forming egg masses. The number of batches varied between six and 13 egg masses per female. Each egg mass contains around 200 or so eggs [29]. In the laboratory at 25°C constant temperature *L. sericata* could theoretically produce their first egg batch at around four to five days after emergence, and then at two- to three-day intervals, provided nutrition and all other environmental conditions are optimal [30]. However, delays to first oviposition and other life history events are to be expected because each fly strain and laboratory setup is different. Regardless, the female fly physiology has practical implications for the maintenance of medicinal flies and production of medicinal maggots: firstly, a protein-rich diet has to be offered to adult flies as soon as they emerge; secondly, colonies produce reasonable numbers of eggs around two weeks after emergence (personal experience with *L. sericata*); and thirdly, harvesting of eggs from the same flies may be repeated every three days, or twice per week.

Blowflies, and in particular *L. sericata* and *L. cuprina*, have a diurnal activity pattern which means that in the laboratory egg harvesting should be undertaken during daylight hours [31]. Egg laying has been observed between 17.5°C and 40°C [32] but this range is of little relevance to laboratory rearing of medicinal flies because it is necessary to maintain optimal and predictable rearing conditions. For this reason, the temperature in the insectary should be kept at a constant temperature between 25°C and 27°C.

The most common method for the harvesting of eggs is to place non-sterile decomposing liver in the adult fly cage [7], but this can vary between species with *Chrysomya* species preferring minced and wool-covered meat (personal communication). Blowflies like to deposit their eggs on animal carcasses in dark, protected places. In order to simulate the carcass environment and to stimulate egg laying in the laboratory, this behaviour can be encouraged by placing an opaque container with sufficiently large holes on top of the protein bait. The females promptly climb in and lay eggs. Once the first egg masses have been deposited on or near the bait, other females are encouraged to follow suit [7, 33]. Harvesting is best done first thing in the morning to ensure there is sufficient time in the day to disinfect the eggs and place them on sterile media if they are destined for maggot therapy.

Egg development has been studied for a variety of calliphorid fly species as part of general developmental studies. Investigations with *L. cuprina* and *L. sericata* have shown that optimal embryo development after oviposition and subsequent successful eclosion (hatching) of eggs needs to occur in a moist environment with a relative humidity in excess of 80%, and that relative humidity below 50% results in no eggs hatching

[34, 35]. If eggs should accidentally dehydrate in the laboratory, their hatching rate will greatly improve if they are soaked in water for a minute or kept for an hour or so in a container lined with wet tissue paper, creating a high-humidity environment. In *L. sericata*, as in other calliphorid flies, higher temperatures lead to faster egg development post oviposition and earlier hatching. For *L. sericata* at 25°C to 27°C hatching takes place after approximately 18 hours from oviposition [7]. In nature on a living sheep, the wound temperature does not drop below 31°C, and at such temperatures over 30°C, egg development is greatly accelerated, taking only 12 hours or less. To conclude, for rearing of medicinal flies in the laboratory it is critical that egg harvest is a speedy process so that eggs are not allowed to dehydrate. After harvest, eggs should be kept close to 100% relative humidity or at the very least on a moist substrate. In addition, the temperature at which eggs are incubated may be varied to speed up or slow down egg development to suit laboratory work processes. Low temperatures around 5 or 6°C can be utilised to store eggs for two to three days, with up to 50% mortality to be expected at 5°C [34, 36].

How to Care for Maggots

Rearing Cage Setup

The captive rearing setup for blowfly larvae has to facilitate their rapid growth and feeding over a period of three to five days, and subsequent pupariation. For the latter, post-feeding maggots in the wild wander off the carcass and burrow into soil or leaf litter [37]. To facilitate this process in the insectary, the most convenient method is to house maggots in a double container system where a smaller, open-topped container is placed into a larger container which is covered tightly with a fine-weave fabric mesh. The smaller container holds the diet and feeding larvae whilst the larger container is partially filled with a pupariation medium that can be wheaten chaff, sawdust, sand, or vermiculite (Figure 14.3). Sawdust and vermiculite are inhalation irritants and should be avoided if other substrates are available. Sand is a convenient substrate because it facilitates the separation and collection of pupae with a sieve. It has the added advantage that it can be periodically washed, dried, and heat-sterilised, although it might be more convenient to discard the sand after several maggot-rearing cycles. The use of cat litter made from extruded recycled paper (e.g. Breeders Choice, FibreCycle™, https://fibrecycle.com/breederschoice) has also proven to be a convenient, clean, and largely dust-free alternative (Figure 14.4). It is highly absorbent, which maintains a dry pupariation environment. Like sand, it also facilitates easy separation of the pupae from the substrate because the extruded, sausage-like litter particles are much larger than the pupae.

Larvae will feed on the diet inside the diet container until they are fully-grown or the food is exhausted. Upon entering the post-feeding stage, the maggots leave the food and wander up the side of the diet container and drop onto the pupariation substrate into which they bury themselves ahead of pupariation.

Blowfly maggots have a scrambling, exploitative feeding strategy that sees them compete intensely for food resources [38]. Therefore, food limitation is an undesirable consequence of overstocking and underfeeding and must be avoided. Should larvae be starved of food, they will enter the post-feeding stage and pupate prematurely, which leads to smaller adult flies with reduced fitness that produce fewer offspring [6, 23]. In medicinal fly rearing, laboratory standard operating procedures need to establish procedures for larval rearing regarding the amount of larval diet and stocking density. Irrespective of such protocols, insectary workers must regularly monitor larval development to spot food shortages early enough before they lead to post-feeding behaviour.

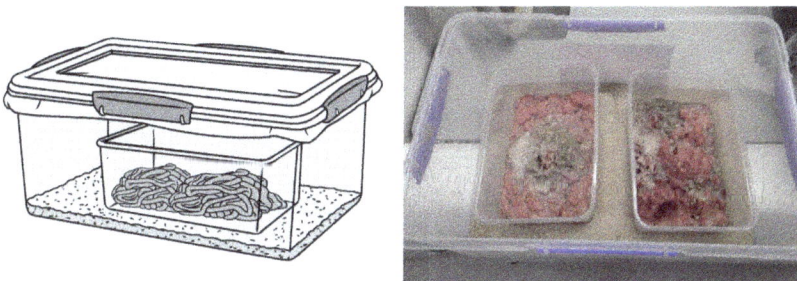

Figure 14.3 Setup for the rearing of maggots. A) and B) Meat-filled smaller containers are placed into a larger container that has been partially filled with sand or another medium for maggots to pupariate in when leaving the diet. A) The outer container is securely closed with a tight-fitting but well-ventilated lid.

A large hole cut into the lid with a fine-weave fabric sandwiched between lid and outer container is an easy way to provide such ventilation. Illustration by P. Busana and photo by F. Stadler, MedMagLabs and Creating Hope in Conflict: A Humanitarian Grand Challenge, CC BY-ND.

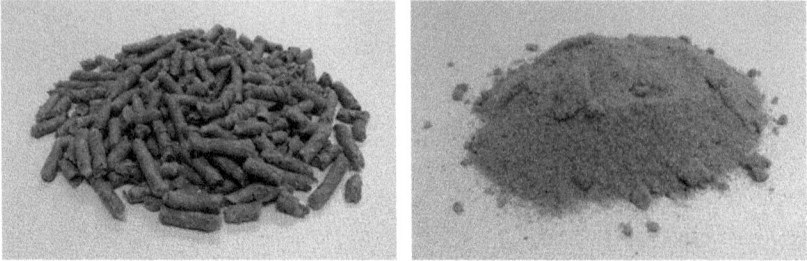

Figure 14.4 Suitable pupariation substrates. A) Extruded cat litter pellets made from recycled paper. B) Fine sand. Both substrates make separation of pupae with a sieve or strainer easy. Mesh or hole size of the sieve/strainer may be chosen to either capture pupae when sand is used, or the cat litter pellets which are larger than pupae. The same basic principle applies to other substrates as well. Photos by F. Stadler, MedMagLabs and Creating Hope in Conflict: A Humanitarian Grand Challenge, CC BY-ND.

Types of Maggot Diet

Many researchers advocate the use of liver as a suitable larval food. However, the evidence from feeding experiments shows that ovine, bovine or porcine liver are nutritionally inferior compared with various other tissues such as heart, lung, brain and meat which result in better larval growth performance [12] [10]. There are many reasons why it might not be feasible to use heart, lung or brain for maggot rearing. In this case commercially available liver or minced meat from a range of species including cattle, pig, and poultry will suffice. Once again, it is important to be consistent with the nature and quality of the larval food in order to be able to predict consumption and development rates. Interestingly in forensic entomology, a feeding study with *Calliphora vicina* found no developmental differences between pork and human tissue [39]. This raises the question of whether medicinal flies might be best reared on pork to breed fly strains that are better adapted for human maggot therapy.

Artificial diets for the rearing of blowflies have been developed over the years, not least because there was the need to reduce the odour associated with larvae rearing on putrid raw meat [7, 40]. Moreover, the plethora of diets used in forensic and medical entomology make it difficult to compare results between studies [41]. More recently, research investigating the antimicrobial activity of larval excretions and secretions has led to the development of various agar-based artificial diets [11]. However, the use of sterilisable semisynthetic diets for the aseptic rearing of medicinal maggots can be traced back to William S. Baer, who pioneered maggot therapy in the 1930s and '40s [42]. Semi-synthetic sterilised diets for fly larvae contain animal protein, various other nutritional ingredients and an agar base [40, 41]. The diet can be stored at room temperature and it generates a less bad odour when rearing maggots.

Rearing of large numbers of flies for maggot therapy and other purposes, including pollination services, may turn out to be rather expensive, or impractical if ingredients are unavailable in resource-constrained settings. An alternative diet was developed for *Lucilia caesar* in West Africa, using locally available ingredients such as garri (processed cassava root, *Manihot esculenta*), soybeans, palm wine and liver [43]. In India a cheap diet for the rearing of *Chrysomya megacephala* was developed using soya flour, milk powder, and egg [44].

Completely meat-free diets have also been developed for *L. sericata* containing whole milk powder, dried yeast, wheat germ, agar powder, propionic acid, and distilled water (Table 14.3). Apart from a slightly longer larval development time, there appears to be no difference in mortality or pupal weight and pupal development compared with that of a liver diet [4]. Producers are encouraged to experiment with locally available and affordable resources to develop convenient diets that meet the nutritional needs of the medicinal fly species chosen. Synthetic or semi-synthetic diet performance for each fly species and strain should be tested against a known, reliable meat diet such as minced pork meat [12].

The therapeutic use of living organisms poses cultural, religious, and clinical challenges. To make the treatment acceptable to the widest possible patient cohort, it is critical that cultural and faith-appropriate medicinal maggots are available. For example, Malaysian biotech firms consider their halal-appropriate technologies as a market differentiator [45]. Allergic reactions to flies themselves, as well as to the dietary ingredients on which the flies have been reared, may occur [46]. In an ideal world, producers would offer allergen-free medicinal maggots on demand. It is also advisable that producers maintain excellent customer relationship management systems and stay in close contact with medical practitioners, to obtain feedback on medicinal maggot quality, performance and adverse reactions. Should clusters or patterns of complications such as allergic reactions be identified, then alternative rearing methods may be used, and quality control and quality assurance improvements made. The various diets already developed and the tolerance of medicinal flies to a range of rearing conditions make such customisation possible if it is required.

Table 14.3 Synthetic maggot diet [4].

Meat-free maggot diet with whole milk powder
50g whole milk powder
50g dried yeast/brewer's yeast
50g wheat germ
14g agar powder
5mL propionic acid
1000 mL water

Note: All ingredients are mixed and boiled for ten minutes. Propionic acid is added once the diet has cooled but not set. To facilitate rapid cooling and convenient handling, the diet is best divided up into portions stored in single- or multi-use plastic containers. To prevent spoilage, diets are stored in the refrigerator.

Pupariation

As with all life stages, pupariation is dependent on adequate ambient temperature. *L. sericata* require temperatures above 20°C for consistently high pupariation rates [35]. Once most larvae have left the food and have pupated in the pupariation substrate, the pupae are collected by sieving. The pupae are then stored within the temperature-controlled insectary environment until adult eclosion. If necessary, pupae can be refrigerated at 4°C for some time in order to delay development [47].

Dehydration is a concern during pupal development, particularly where the ambient relative humidity is difficult to control. Studies have shown that *L. sericata* pupae contain about 70% water and tolerate up to 28% dehydration [48]. Emergence of flies is also determined by the temperature during development, and it increases to approximately 80% for a temperature range between 20°C and 30°C. Extremely high temperatures above 35°C are lethal for pupae who would naturally reside in temperature-buffered soil for the period of pupal development [35].

Pupae are a convenient life stage for shipment between laboratories. *L. sericata* pupae require 0.2 mL of air per day per 1 mg of pupae, which needs to be provided either via ventilation or provision of sufficient air volume in sealed containers [49].

Disinfection of Medicinal Maggots

Adult flies and maggots inhabit many unsanitary environments and utilise microbe-rich food sources. Therefore, blowflies can harbour a range of harmful microbes, such as *Staphylococcus aureus*, *Escherichia coli*, *Corynebacteria dipththeria*, *Aspergillus* and *Fusarium*, which they potentially introduce to wounds during myiasis [50]. Consequently, there is a need to ensure that fly larvae used for medicinal wound treatment are sterile. However, it must be noted that anecdotes and academic case reports of myiasis [51, 52] point toward highly effective microbial control under most austere and unhygienic circumstances. Nevertheless, it is necessary to minimise the microbial burden of medicinal maggots to avoid the introduction of harmful microbes that can exacerbate already-existing infections or even lead to bloodstream infection [53].

There is a growing realisation among the maggot therapy research community that completely sterile maggots are unachievable and perhaps undesirable from a therapeutic efficacy point of view [54–56]. There is good evidence to suggest that bacteria are internally transferred from adult fly to egg, from egg to larva, from one larval stage to another [55]. This means that currently practiced 'sterilisation' methods for medicinal maggots achieve at best surface sterilisation [57]. In other words, recommended rapid sterility testing over 24 to 48 hours for disinfected eggs and emerging maggots has its limits because some microbes may be difficult to culture and/or hide in internal maggot tissues and organs, and thus remain undetected. The exact relationship and ecology of the microbes inside and on the body of medicinal fly species and their environment is still little understood and requires further investigation. However, what current evidence and centuries-long practice of maggot therapy in tribal and modern wound care can tell us is that medicinal maggot species effectively reduce the microbial burden in their wound environment and control microbes that impair wound healing [58]. This should also include the microbes introduced to the wound by medicinal maggots unless they are co-adapted symbionts [55], which are likely to enhance the therapeutic activity of maggots. Beneficial cases of myiasis provide further support for this hypothesis [42, 51, 52].

In summary, current practice of disinfecting the eggs and subsequent aseptic incubation of emerging maggots [59] has proven to be safe for both maggots and patients. The maggots remain therapeutically efficacious and do not cause or exacerbate wound infections.

Disinfection Methods

The most convenient and most common way to produce largely germ-free maggots involves the disinfection of the fly eggs and subsequent rearing of larvae on sterile media. Conversely, some workers advocate the disinfection of only the larvae [60], or a two-stage process involving sterilisation of both the eggs and young larvae [61]. A range of successful sterilisation procedures have been reported in the literature.

Because eggs in an egg mass are glued together as they are deposited by the female, the eggs must be first mechanically separated from each other in order to permit total surface disinfection. The importance of this step cannot be overemphasised if complete surface disinfection is to be achieved. The deglutination process can be enhanced with chemical reagents such as sodium hydroxide, potassium hydroxide, or sodium carbonate [62]. Sterilisation protocols vary regarding the chemicals used but also regarding the efficacy of the disinfection process and the egg survival rate [59]. The protocol described in Box 14.1 is a synthesis of protocols reported in the literature. They describe the same general process which includes separation and prewash of eggs, followed by the actual disinfection step. After each treatment, eggs must be washed or rinsed to remove treatment chemicals, liberated debris, and microbes. Although this generic method is based on reliable disinfection protocols published in the literature, it is recommended that producers try a few and finetune their own protocol. A summary of common disinfection methods and their efficacy is given by Brundage and colleagues [59]. Finally, it is important to use generous amounts of solution for the deglutination, disinfection, and rinsing steps because the chemicals in solution lose potency proportional to the number of eggs and amount of contamination present, and because the greater the dilution of contaminants and chemicals, the more effective the cleansing process.

In line with Good Manufacturing Practices, the entire sterilisation process ought to be conducted in a Grade A zone clean room [63]. Instead of an entire room being maintained as a Grade A zone, the same microbial protection can be achieved for much cheaper with a laminar flow cabinet that prevents contamination of eggs and larvae from germs suspended in the laboratory air. Each production batch of sterilised eggs and emerging sterile larvae must be tested for sterility before it can be released for maggot therapy.

Incubation of Eggs

For the incubation of eggs and rearing of larvae to late-first or early-second instar, the sterilised eggs are placed on a sterile larval diet which may be chicken egg-yolk, a semi-synthetic diet, or a fully artificial larval diet [4, 7, 11, 13, 40, 65]. For instance, a basic semi-synthetic diet consisting of 20 g/L agar, 20% horse blood, and added yeast supports *L. sericata* larval growth comparable to that of a meat diet [11, 13]. Chocolate agar, sabouraud dextrose agar, and brucella blood agar also provide adequate nutrition to hatching maggots.

At 25–27°C eggs hatch within 18 hours and reach the second-instar life stage within 24–48 hours of egg incubation. Therefore, rearing at 25–27°C allows for harmonisation of production timing with quality control testing. If need be, first- and second-instar larval development can be paused with refrigeration at 6–8°C to await test results or in anticipation of maggot therapy [66]. Temperatures below 6°C may cause unsustainable mortality of fragile first- and early second-stage maggots.

Box **14.1** Synthesised protocol for the sterilisation of medicinal fly eggs.

Step 1: Separation of eggs and prewash [#]

1. Soak and agitate (stir/shake) eggs in <u>one</u> of these deglutination solutions for 5-10 minutes until the eggs are fully separated [62].
    - 1% sodium hydroxide
    - 2% potassium hydroxide
    - 4% sodium carbonate

    Alternatively, separate eggs mechanically in clean water by vigorous stirring or shaking, or with the help of utensils such as paintbrushes.

2. Let eggs settle to the bottom of the container.

3. Decant solution.

4. Rinse eggs two to three times with sterile saline or sterile water to reduce microbial contaminants and deglutination chemicals.

Step 2: Disinfection

5. Soak eggs in <u>one</u> of these disinfectants for 5 minutes and make sure to stir/agitate the eggs during the soaking process:
    - 0.5% sodium hypochlorite (NaClO) [64]
    - 3% Lysol® (Reckitt Benckiser) [7]

6. Let eggs settle to the bottom of the container.

7. Decant disinfectant.

8. Rinse the eggs two to three times with sterile saline or sterile water.

Transfer disinfected eggs for incubation

9. Use part of the saline/water from the last rinse to pour out eggs and collect them on sterile filter paper or fine mesh.

10. Transfer disinfected eggs to sterile larval diet.

[#] It is vital that eggs are fully separated to allow disinfection solution to contact entire egg surface area.

Quality Control

Testing of disinfection efficacy. Microbial quality control may occur at all stages of the disinfection and rearing process for maggots destined for maggot therapy to minimise the microbes carried by medicinal maggots and to avoid harmful microbial contamination. In line with aseptic laboratory practice, all disinfection processes are undertaken in the laboratory inside a laminar flow cabinet or clean room with sterile reusable or disposable laboratory equipment and consumables in order to minimize contamination of solutions, media, and samples via the laboratory air [63]. In addition, it is good practice to also monitor the laboratory environment, especially the clean room facilities, on a regular basis for microbial contamination [67].

Disinfection is tested at the very least directly after the disinfection of eggs and ideally again after the eclosion of maggots. Because medicinal maggots are highly perishable, and cannot be stored over extended periods, there is insufficient time to conduct sterility testing as advised by the Pharmacopoeia [68] and expected in medical goods manufacturing [69]. Therefore, microbial testing may be done using blood agar (trypticase soy agar) plates in an incubator at 35°C for 24–48 hours [7, 70]. Alternatively, the sterility testing methodology specified in the Pharmacopoeia and related guidelines may be employed but test samples are assessed after 24 and 48 hours to facilitate rapid dispatch of medicinal maggots. Personal experience suggests that if culturable microbes have been sampled, they proliferate rapidly and are readily detectable after 24 to 48 hours. The precise quality assurance and quality control procedures for medicinal maggot production demanded by the regulators may vary from jurisdiction to jurisdiction as will the regulators' general approach to maggot therapy [71].

Colony and medicinal maggot performance monitoring. Blowflies in general, and *L. sericata* and *L. cuprina* in particular, have proven to be well-suited for laboratory maintenance as they tolerate a wide variety of diets and rearing conditions. However, declines in laboratory fly strains kept at constant conditions have been reported, and have manifested in reduced fecundity, cessation of egg production and abnormal pupation [72]. This is not acceptable in a production context where reliable and consistent colony performance is required. Therefore, there is a need to monitor life history parameters on a regular basis. Species-specific characteristics such as morphological and life-history, physiological, and genetic characteristics can all be used to monitor colony performance [73, 74]. The sampling regimen and parameters to obtain these performance measurements must be carefully considered but may include data on adult fly performance, egg development, larval development, and pupal development.

The capacity of medicinal maggots to debride necrotic tissue may also differ from fly strain to fly strain or over time. The debridement activity of medicinal maggots can be assessed clinically by monitoring their therapeutic action in the wound or in the laboratory with a simple meat-based assay [75–77]. Recently, a radial diffusion enzymatic assay (RDEA) has been developed in order to obtain more reliable performance data in medicinal maggot production and to support good manufacturing and laboratory practice [78].

Supply Management and Perishability of Medicinal Maggots

It would be desirable to store eggs, pupae, or adult flies over extended periods of time. This would support supply and demand management of medicinal maggots, particularly regarding regular demand fluctuations and rapid demand spikes in the aftermath of, for example, an earthquake which would bring about many injuries and related wound infections that can be treated with maggot therapy [79]. Unfortunately, longer-term cold storage or cryopreservation of eggs, maggots, or flies is not yet available. Indeed, medicinal maggots are a highly perishable commodity in terms of their vulnerability to adverse environmental conditions such as hot temperatures, very cold temperatures, or low humidity. In addition, medicinal maggots grow rapidly and have corresponding energetic requirements. Provided with enough food, the development rate of medicinal maggots is largely determined by the temperature. This has far-reaching implications for production scheduling, supply management, distribution, and clinical practice. In the context of supply-chain management, medicinal maggots can be considered perishable [80] because:

11. if environmental conditions are not conducive, or if nutrition is withheld from the maggots for too long, they will lose vitality and efficacy and may even die;

12. the longer medicinal maggots are held in cold storage and transit, the less time is available to the healthcare provider to arrange for treatment in the clinical setting which reduces convenience and thus value of medicinal maggots as a commodity;

13. to safeguard against the use of lower-quality medicinal maggots and associated reputational damage, and also to assist in treatment scheduling, producers set a safe expiry or best-before-date which also influences perishability and its implications for supply chain management.

In the absence of long-term egg storage technology and fluctuating demand, the response time for a single facility to increase production is in excess of 20 days, unless the facility maintains production capacity buffer in the form of surplus fly stock of all development stages. This incurs additional costs in feed and maintenance which under a lean production strategy would have to be avoided. It is then a matter for the producer to reconcile the benefits of responsiveness and agility with the additional costs incurred by the maintenance of surplus inventory in the form of fly stock. In other words, a more suitable supply chain model would be 'agile' rather than 'lean'.

Seamless delivery of medicinal maggots to healthcare providers requires careful management of the disinfection and quality control process. Hence these disinfection and quality control procedures potentially form a bottleneck in the production of sterile maggots. If sterility testing with agar plates is to be performed at the time of egg disinfection and again when maggots hatch, then sterile maggot production (from egg harvest to shipment of maggots) takes two to three days. Given that larval growth is rapid and full larval development can take less than 2 days under optimal conditions, there may be a need to refrigerate first- or second-instar larvae at 6–8°C in order to arrest their development until sterility is confirmed. Likewise, maggots are shipped overnight at between 6°C and 25°C to healthcare providers and may be stored within this temperature range for up to 24 hours at the point of care [66, 77, 81].

There may be instances where delivery times are expected to exceed 48 hours or there is reason to believe that treatment cannot proceed within 48 hours from dispatch of maggots from the lab, even if delivered in time. If this is the case and there is a strong argument in favour of maggot therapy treatment, then producers can send disinfected eggs rather than first- or second-instar maggots. For this purpose, disinfected eggs may be placed on a sterile, moist gauze pad for shipment. This buys some time, especially when shipped with extra supply of cool elements to prolong the cool period, but the eggs will hatch eventually. The emerging maggots require food immediately and there is a risk that they will perish if not applied to the wound shortly thereafter. To extend the safe shipment and storage duration even further, it will be necessary to provide the first-instar maggots with a sterile protein food source. This combination of egg shipment, longer cool conditions during transit, and the provision of food for emerging maggots has been shown to extend the shelf-life of medicinal maggots to five days (personal communication). One drawback of this shipment method is that both the chorion ('egg shell') from which maggots emerge and any uneaten food will be applied to the wound along with the medicinal maggots. Although there is no evidence of adverse treatment outcomes when disinfected eggs have been applied directly [82], healthcare providers may nevertheless be concerned. Moreover, producers must be careful to operate within the licence conditions for the production and supply of medicinal maggots as negotiated with their ministry of health or other regulator. It appears that the extension of medicinal maggot shelf-life in this manner, although practiced from time to time (personal communication), has not yet received any formal attention in the scientific literature. For a detailed discussion of the distribution logistics for medicinal maggots please consult Chapter 17 of this book [83].

Scheduling of Production Activities

Scheduling production activities to ensure reliable supply from week to week and throughout the year is no trivial undertaking. However, with available information from the literature and existing producers, it is possible to draw up a weekly production schedule [84]. The schedule in Table 14.4A considers a 7-day production week and assumes that courier and distribution services are available on the weekend. In this case medicinal maggots can be delivered daily for application on any day of the week. However, adherence to a Monday-to-Friday working week as in Table 14.4B will interrupt production and dispatch. Consequently, treatment will not be possible on Mondays. In practice, variations to these schedules are likely depending on local circumstances [84].

Quality Management

Laboratory operation. Of the many ISO standards relevant to medicines and medical devices, ISO 9001:2015 *Quality management systems*, and ISO 15189:2012 *Medical laboratories—Requirements for quality and competence* are of particular importance. ISO 9001 specifies requirements for consistent delivery of products and services according to statutory and regulatory requirements. Many pre-existing organisations operating laboratories such as clinics, pathology, and research laboratories, may well comply with ISO 9001 and ISO 17025:2005 *General requirements for the competence of testing and calibration laboratories* but may also need, depending on the maggot therapy approval process, to consider accreditation for ISO 15189. Moreover, if medicinal maggots are considered a medical device by the respective regulator, then ISO 9001 may need to be replaced with a more comprehensive quality assurance standard. For example, Malaysian medical device manufacturers had successfully adopted ISO 9001:2000 but were compelled to transition to ISO 13485:2003 *Medical devices—Quality management systems—Requirements for regulatory purposes* [85] in order to access the harmonised export markets of Europe and elsewhere [86]. Since producers mostly supply medicinal maggots to national or regional healthcare providers (e.g. within the EU), such regulatory pressure may not apply in all cases, but it illustrates the complexity of the regulatory landscape for producers. Moreover, regulatory compliance can be a large burden to a producer, both in terms of time commitment and cost, and full accreditation may not be affordable to many laboratories in low- and middle-income countries [84]

Table 14.4 Sterile maggot production schedules. The theoretical schedule for a 7-day production operation with harvesting of eggs, quality control, and shipment taking place every day of the week is shown in Table 14.4A. Importantly, this schedule allows for maggot therapy every day of the week. In contrast, the schedule in Figure 14.4B shows the impact of weekend-interruptions (Saturday and Sunday) to production and distribution. As a consequence, maggot therapy treatment may not be possible on Sundays if couriers don't operate on the weekend, and will not be possible on Mondays. These are only example schedules and actual schedules will vary from producer to producer depending on local circumstances, operating procedures, and demand fluctuations.

A) Sterile maggot production schedule for 7-day production operations and no prolonged cool storage of maggots over the weekend.

Harvest day	Mon	Tue	Wed	Thu	Fri	Sat	Sun	Mon	Tue	Wed
Mon	H		S	T	T					
Tue		H		S	T	T				
Wed			H		S	T	T			
Thu				H		S	T	T		
Fri					H		S	T	T	
Sat						H		S	T	T
Sun							H		S	T
Treatment	T	T	T	T	T	T	T			

B) Sterile maggot production schedule for 5-day production operations with cool storage of maggots over the weekend.

Harvest day	Mon	Tue	Wed	Thu	Fri	Sat	Sun	Mon	Tue	Wed
Mon	H		S	T	T					
Tue		H		S	T	T				
Wed			H		s	t	t			
Thu				H		Storage		S	T	T
Treatment	T	T	T	t				T	T	

Note: H = harvest of eggs and disinfection; S = quality control clearance and shipment; T = treatment; Storage = cool storage of maggots in-house; s = potential shipment and t = potential treatment, provided courier service is available for delivery on Saturday and care provider / patient is willing to pay surcharge. © F. Stadler, https://doi.org/10.25904/1912/3170.

Barriers aside, there are clear benefits to accreditation and adherence to standards. For example, ISO 9001 enforces consistency and efficiency of processes which increases quality and reduces errors. Customers and international regulators look to ISO 9001 as a quality assurance for supplied products, and accreditation can convey competitive advantage. Implementation of ISO 9001 will also assist in solving and avoiding problems in the manufacturing process and will lead to leaner, more efficient companies [87].

Occupational Health and Safety

The health and wellbeing of insectary and laboratory workers throughout the rearing, quality control and packaging process is of utmost importance. Occupational health and safety (OH&S) considerations specific to the rearing of medicinal flies include the potential of allergies and/or fly-borne diseases. If air purification systems cannot be fitted in the insectary due to practical or financial constraints, then dust allergens from adult fly colonies can be managed by frequent wet wiping of insectary surfaces and by suspending fly cages over trays of water to catch the fly-generated dust.

Adult wild calliphorid flies are potential animal- and human-disease vectors and may deliver pathogens via their body surface or excretions, including anthrax, *Clostridium botulinum*, and the causal agents for paratuberculosis and avian influenza [88–90]. Long-term culturing of flies in captivity should, over time, lead to less harmful bacterial burdens, particularly when synthetic and semi-synthetic diets are used in the rearing of larvae. Nevertheless, it is important to minimise the potential for transmission of fly-borne diseases with good insectary and laboratory hygiene, protective clothing and best-practice hand-hygiene. This goes hand-in-hand with dust control as insectary shelving, benchtops and floors should be wet-wiped with disinfectant surface cleaner (e.g. domestic bleach) several times per week. Production workers should use two sets of protective clothing, one dedicated to the insectary and the other to lab work. This is to avoid cross-contamination between the two production environments. Protective clothing includes hair caps, face masks, and gloves in order to reduce dust and germ exposure in the insectary and to minimise the potential for contamination of medicinal maggots during the sterilisation process.

Sustainable Production and Waste Management

From a medical and therapeutic point of view, maggot therapy is highly sustainable because it is a low-tech therapy that is effective under the most austere conditions and it significantly reduces the need for antibiotic treatment of wound infections. Thus, it does not contribute to the growing problem of antibiotic resistance in human pathogens. Indeed, maggot therapy effectively controls antibiotic-resistant bacteria [91].

As far as the sustainability of medicinal maggot production itself is concerned, it depends among other things on producer location, available resources and infrastructure, and general awareness. It cannot be assumed that producers globally have guaranteed access to clean water, reliable energy, ready supply of equipment and consumables, and a reliable municipal sewage and waste service, especially in the case of impoverished and remote locations. Out of necessity, this provides an opportunity to implement sustainable water and energy solutions. Paradoxically it may be harder for producers in high-resources settings to become more sustainable. For example, the reuse of materials, as opposed to the use of disposable items, is associated with more time-consuming cleaning and maintenance which results in higher labour costs, especially in high-income, high-resource economies. Therefore, a producer must carefully weigh up whether it is of benefit financially, operationally, and safety-wise to re-use materials. Indeed, the additional labour, electricity, water, and reagent inputs required for on-site cleaning and disinfection may be more costly and environmentally unsustainable than opting for disposable materials. For commercial producers, increased costs associated with sustainable production may either reduce the profit margin or will be passed on to the consumer through higher product prices. However, for producers aiming to supply cheap and affordable medicinal maggots to the poor and underserved, any production cost increase is difficult to pass on and may undermine their business model and viability.

Fortunately, medicinal maggot production is not very resource intensive compared with other industries. Setting up a production facility in a building with high environmental performance (insulation, air conditioning, lighting, plumbing, etc.) immediately increases operational sustainability. Where possible (or necessary), solar energy generation may be utilised to meet all or at least some of the production requirements, and to reduce reliance on the grid or generator power.

Waste management is an important component of sustainability. Neither liquid nor solid waste streams in production can be classified as containing clinical infectious waste since no clinical treatment is being performed and no patient-generated waste is being disposed. However, leftover putrid meat and other fly-diet waste is undoubtedly laden with pathogens and must therefore be disposed of in a safe manner according to local regulations. In practice, production waste does not differ significantly from municipal waste. Odour is of course a concern when collecting insectary waste prior to disposal, but it can be minimised by storing putrid meat waste in a dedicated freezer or cool room until the day of collection by waste services. The added benefit of this is that any eggs, maggots or flies among the waste are euthanised prior to disposal. For peace of mind, producers may want to adhere to the World Health Organisation's *Safe Management of Wastes from Health-care Activities* guidelines [92] and of course any local laboratory management guidelines where they exist.

In the insectary, most materials can be re-used after thorough cleaning including the maggot-rearing containers, the adult diet-dispensing dishes and containers, as well as the fly cages themselves. This is also true for the laboratory materials and equipment. However, as mentioned earlier, producers should carefully evaluate whether re-use of lab materials makes financial sense and is indeed more sustainable. When it comes to disposable personal protective gear such as gloves, gowns and face masks, there is room to be less wasteful. Here, waste is mostly due to the behaviour of lab and insectary workers. For example, thorough planning and streamlining of activities will reduce the need for frequent removal and disposal of gloves. The same face mask may be re-used several times throughout a day if convenient and safe to do so. Replacing single-use gloves with multi-use heavy duty gloves for some insectary work such as cleaning activities will also reduce waste.

The greywater waste generated during regular insectary and laboratory operations does not require special segregation or treatment. It can be disposed of in municipal sewage and stand-alone septic systems, provided chemicals such as from egg disinfection and lab cleaning activities are heavily diluted during disposal. Please note that irrespective of this advice, it is the responsibility of producers to comply with local rules and regulations.

Medicinal Maggot Production in Healthcare Settings with Poor Medical Services

The approaches and methods for medicinal maggot production described in this chapter assume that the materials and resources such as laboratory equipment, cages, and rearing diets can be readily purchased from suppliers either in shops or online, and that they are delivered in a timely fashion. It has also been assumed that the producers of medicinal maggots and their staff have qualifications in entomology and laboratory sciences. Unfortunately, this is not the case everywhere and the impacts of war, disasters, and deep economic depression create conditions in many parts of the world that result in the collapse of ordinary trade and commerce, broken supply chains, and the departure of scientists and other educated workers seeking opportunities elsewhere. Even emergency and development aid from governments and non-governmental organisations may fail to reach affected communities. If isolated communities want to take advantage of highly efficacious maggot therapy to treat patients, they must produce the medicinal maggots themselves. Highly perishable as they are, a reliable supply of medicinal maggots can only be guaranteed with local production.

To that end, MedMagLabs (www.medmaglabs.com) has developed instructions that allow communities in compromised healthcare settings to establish and operate do-it-yourself laboratories (DIY-Labs) and produce safe medicinal maggots. The guidance includes a Production Manual that explains the production process in some detail, and a User Manual that mirrors the content of the Production Manual (Figure 14.5). However, the difference is that the User Manual and its 20 fact sheets provide step-by-step descriptions of the production processes with clear illustrations in order to make the information more accessible.

The DIY-Lab is not a radical reimagining of medicinal maggot production. Instead, the MedMagLabs team have translated best-practice know-how as reported in the scientific literature into methods that can be implemented with very few locally available resources and without prior knowledge of fly husbandry. First, assumptions regarding the availability of resources that can be appropriated for medicinal maggot production were triangulated with five interviews of people who have lived or worked in conflict-affected communities. Then, a set of basic visual and textual instructions were prepared for lay producers. Without access to communities in conflict zones, MedMagLabs sought proxy communities to collaborate with. Four teams of citizen scientists (Year 9 and 10 high-school students) helped to establish whether lay persons can produce medicinal maggots and what guidance is required [93]. The students built adult fly cages, cared for fly colonies, reared maggots, disinfected eggs, and incubated young medicinal maggots with only basic resources such as repurposed water drums or jam jars. The outcomes of this collaboration had a material influence on what guidance was included in the Production and User Manuals, and how instructions were presented.

Both the Production and User Manual are creative commons (CC BY-ND) and can be accessed for free via www.medmaglabs.com along with a Treatment Manual for healthcare providers and lay carers (Figure 14.5).

Production Manual—Part B

MedMagLabs
Medicinal
Maggot
Laboratories

MML

How to harvest and separate eggs

Eggs are best harvested with some liver or other meat that is starting to go off. Flies will quickly lay eggs onto this smelly bait. Flies usually lay their eggs in clumps with eggs sticking to each other. This makes removing them from the meat easy. Use either forceps, a fork, or any similar tool to pick the egg clumps from the meat bait. Try to collect only clean eggs and remove bits of meat that are stuck to the eggs.

It is important to separate these eggs before they are disinfected so that the chemicals can reach all parts of the egg and kill all germs that are stuck to the eggs.

Break up the larger egg clumps into smaller ones in a shallow dish to which you add some water. A fork is a useful tool as it allows you to gently squash the egg clumps. It will also allow you to further remove pieces of meat bait that have remained on the eggs.

Alternatively, you can transfer the eggs directly from the bait to a container to which you add some clean water. It does not need to be boiled before use. Take a pair of forceps, some chopsticks, a fork, or a spoon, and vigorously stir the egg clumps in the water. You can also close the container and shake the content vigorously. This will separate most of the eggs, but some will stay stuck to each other. These remaining egg clumps float at the surface but separated eggs will sink to the bottom of the container. Pour the remaining egg clumps and the dirty water out into a waste container. Be careful not to pour out the separated eggs. A few drops of water may remain in the jar.

Add clean water to these separated eggs and gently stir them for a minute. Let the eggs settle to the bottom of the jar and pour the water out as before. Repeat this step at least once.

Go to User Manual B5 for illustrated guidance on how to harvest and separate fly eggs.

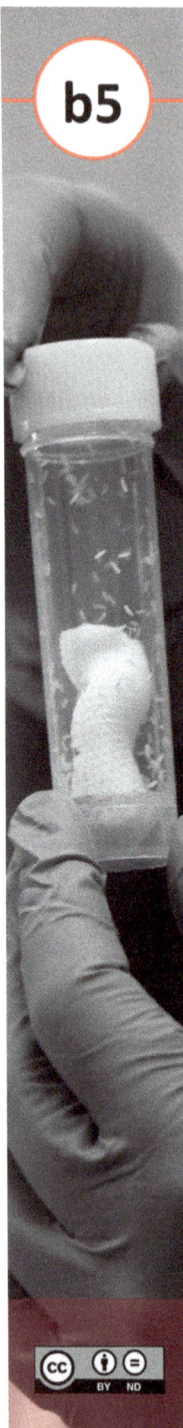

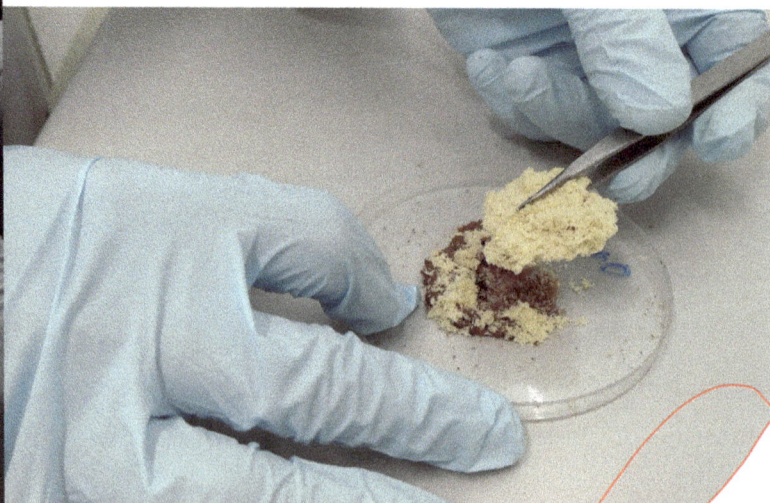

CREATING
HOPE
IN CONFLICT:
A HUMANITARIAN
GRAND CHALLENGE

How to harvest and separate eggs

B5

Flies lay their eggs in clumps and eggs stick to each other. For proper disinfection to be possible, eggs must be first separated.

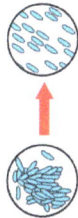

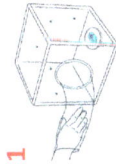

1 Place smelly old liver or other meat on a dish into the fly cage.

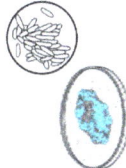

2-3 hrs

2 After two to three hours the flies will have laid many whitish eggs.

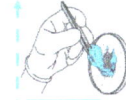

Steps 4-6 are optional

3 Remove the eggs from the meat. Make sure to collect only eggs and not meat.

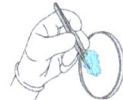

4 Place the eggs into a shallow clean dish.

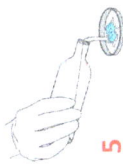

5 Pour clean water into the dish.

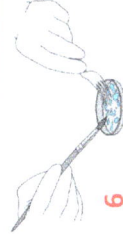

6 Carefully separate the eggs into smaller clumps or even individual eggs.

Steps 7-11 are compulsory

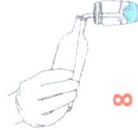

7 Place the separated or unseparated egg clumps into a container such as a food jar.

8 Add some more clean water.

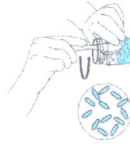

9 With a utensil such as a spoon or fork, stir the eggs vigorously.

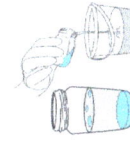

10 Any eggs still stuck together float on the surface. Pour them and the water out but keep the eggs on the bottom.

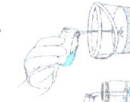

11 Wash the separated eggs with clean water and let them sink to the bottom. Then pour the water out as before.

2 x

B6

[U-B05-EN/2021-06] User Manual B5: How to harvest and separate fly eggs.
This document is provided as an information source only and without warranties of any kind, expressed or implied (except any which cannot be excluded by law). Go to www.medmaglabs.com for a full disclaimer.

CREATING HOPE IN CONFLICT
A HUMANITARIAN GRAND CHALLENGE

MedMagLabs
Medicinal
Maggot
Laboratories

MML

✖ When maggot therapy should be avoided or used with great caution

No informed consent
Informed consent from the patient or guardian is required before maggot therapy.

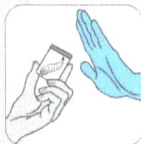

Allergy
If patients have allergies to flies or the food with which medicinal maggots are raised.

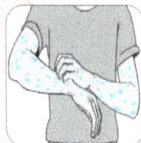

Rapidly progressing infections
If infection is spreading too fast and the wound must be monitored closely.

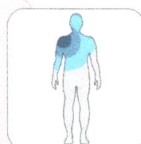

Dry necrotic tissue
Wounds with large amounts of dry hard eschar are not immediately suitable for maggot therapy. First, the eschar needs to be softened or at least partially removed.

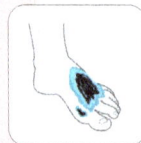

Body cavities and organs
Confinement (free-range) maggot dressings must not to be used near body cavities or exposed organs. Only maggots that are safely enclosed in net bags (bagged maggots) may be used near open body cavities and near eyes, ears, mouth, the urogenital and the rectal area.

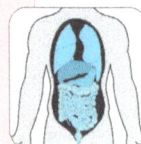

Risk of bleeding
For example, in patients who have impaired coagulation or where major blood vessels are exposed. If maggot therapy is performed, patients must be carefully monitored.

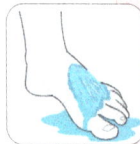

Internal use
Maggot therapy is not to be used in eyes, the gastrointestinal tract, and the respiratory tract.

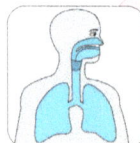

Fistulae
The full extent of the wound must be visible, maggot activity must be observable, and maggots must be easily accessible for removal.

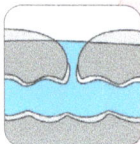

Pseudomonas infections
Maggot therapy may not be able to control Pseudomonas infection. Antibiotic therapy may be necessary in place of, or in addition to, maggot therapy.

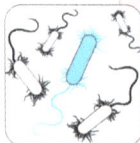

Pain
If patients experience pain and medication does not ease the pain, then maggot therapy must be discontinued.

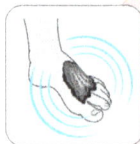

CREATING
HOPE
IN CONFLICT.
A HUMANITARIAN
GRAND CHALLENGE

Figure 14.5 Example pages from the MedMagLabs medicinal maggot Production Manual (b5), the corresponding highly-visual User Manual (B5), and the Treatment Manual (T4). These resources were developed to empower isolated, conflict-affected communities to produce medicinal maggots and perform maggot therapy with local resources and expertise.

Summary

This chapter provides a detailed description of both insectary and laboratory activities for the maintenance of fly colonies and the production of medicinal maggots. It describes how the care of adult flies and maggots depends on caging, environmental conditions, and diet. Of critical importance to the reliable and responsive production of high-quality, safe maggots for maggot therapy is the thorough knowledge of the reproductive and developmental performance of medicinal flies. Producers must have a reliable quality-management system in place and implement routine quality control not only to ensure the sterility of medicinal maggots destined for treatment but also for colony performance overall. Paramount to any workplace is the health and wellbeing of its workers. Insectaries provide special challenges, particularly regarding allergies and respiratory health, that need to be carefully managed. It is the objective of the producer as the focal organisation in the supply chain to ensure supply security and responsiveness to demand fluctuations which requires scheduling of production activities. Unfortunately, there is a tradeoff between responsiveness and lean supply management. In other words, the limited availability of cool or cold storage of eggs or other life stages makes lean and responsive supply management difficult to achieve. Moreover, it is incumbent on producers to limit their environmental footprint in terms of resource consumption and waste. This may be associated with savings and increased operational resilience but may also incur greater costs, which would need to be passed on to patients or absorbed by the producer.

Finally, the guidance provided here is based on available production information from the scientific literature and producers. Adherence is not mandatory, and it is indeed expected that producers will experiment and tailor methods to their own needs and local circumstances. Communities in compromised healthcare settings are no longer excluded. Free Production and User Manuals are available to empower lay persons to produce safe medicinal maggots with local resources. However, this does not mean that producers have complete freedom. There are rules and regulations that apply to and govern the production of medicines and medical goods in all but the most austere and isolated healthcare settings.

References

1. Stadler, F., *Laboratory and Insectary Infrastructure and Equipment*, in *A Complete Guide to Maggot Therapy: Clinical Practice, Therapeutic Principles, Production, Distribution, and Ethics*, F. Stadler (ed.). 2022, Cambridge: Open Book Publishers, pp. 237–256, https://doi.org/10.11647/OBP.0300.12.

2. Stadler, F., et al., *Fly Colony Establishment*, in *A Complete Guide to Maggot Therapy: Clinical Practice, Therapeutic Principles, Production, Distribution, and Ethics*, F. Stadler (ed.). 2022, Cambridge: Open Book Publishers, pp. 257–388 (p. 269), https://doi.org/10.11647/OBP.0300.13.

3. Stadler, F., *The Ethics of Maggot Therapy*, in *A Complete Guide to Maggot Therapy: Clinical Practice, Therapeutic Principles, Production, Distribution, and Ethics*, F. Stadler (ed.). 2022, Cambridge: Open Book Publishers, pp. 405–430, https://doi.org/10.11647/OBP.0300.19.

4. Tachibana, S.I. and H. Numata, *An Artificial Diet for Blow Fly Larvae, Lucilia sericata (Meigen) (Diptera: Calliphoridae)*. Applied Entomology and Zoology, 2001. 36(4): pp. 521–523.

5. Bugelli, V., et al., *Effects of Different Storage and Measuring Methods on Larval Length Values for the Blow Flies (Diptera: Calliphoridae) Lucilia sericata and Calliphora vicina*. Science and Justice, 2017. 57(3): pp. 159–164, https://doi.org/10.1016/j.scijus.2016.10.008.

6. Moe, S.J., N.C. Stenseth, and R.H. Smith, *Density Dependence in Blowfly Populations: Experimental Evaluation of Non-parametric Time-series Modelling*. Oikos, 2002. 98(3): pp. 523–533, https://doi.org/10.1034/j.1600-0706.2002.980317.x.

7. Sherman, R.A. and F.A. Wyle, *Low-cost, Low-maintenance Rearing of Maggots in Hospitals, Clinics, and Schools*. American Journal of Tropical Medicine and Hygiene, 1996. 54(1): pp. 38–41, https://doi.org/10.4269/ajtmh.1996.54.38.

8. Parry, N.J., E. Pieterse, and C.W. Weldon, *Longevity, Fertility and Fecundity of Adult Blow Flies (Diptera: Calliphoridae) Held at Varying Densities: Implications for Use in Bioconversion of Waste*. Journal of Economic Entomology, 2017. 110(6): pp. 2388–2396, https://doi.org/10.1093/jee/tox251.

9. Rosati, J.Y., et al., *Estimating the Number of Eggs in Blow Fly (Diptera: Calliphoridae) Egg Masses Using Photographic Analysis.* Journal of Medical Entomology, 2015. 52(4): pp. 658–662, https://doi.org/10.1093/jme/tjv053.

10. El-Moaty, Z.A. and A.E.M. Kheirallah, *Developmental Variation of the Blow Fly Lucilia sericata (Meigen, 1826) (Diptera: Calliphoridae) by Different Substrate Tissue Types.* Journal of Asia-Pacific Entomology, 2013. 16(3): pp. 297–300, https://doi.org/10.1016/j.aspen.2013.03.008.

11. Barnes, K.M. and D.E. Gennard, *Rearing Bacteria and Maggots Concurrently: A Protocol Using Lucilia sericata (Diptera: Calliphoridae) as a Model Species.* Applied Entomology and Zoology, 2013. 48(3): pp. 247–253, https://doi.org/10.1007/s13355-013-0181-7.

12. Clark, K., L. Evans, and R. Wall, *Growth Rates of the Blowfly, Lucilia sericata, on Different Body Tissues.* Forensic Science International, 2006. 156(2–3): pp. 145–149, https://doi.org/10.1016/j.forsciint.2004.12.025.

13. Daniels, S., K. Simkiss, and R.H. Smith, *A Simple Larval Diet for Population Studies on the Blowfly Lucilia sericata (Diptera: Calliphoridae).* Medical and Veterinary Entomology, 1991. 5(3): pp. 283–292, https://doi.org/10.1111/j.1365-2915.1991.tb00554.x.

14. Gallagher, M.B., S. Sandhu, and R. Kimsey, *Variation in Developmental Time for Geographically Distinct Populations of the Common Green Bottle Fly, Lucilia sericata (Meigen).* Journal of Forensic Sciences, 2010. 55(2): pp. 438–442, https://doi.org/10.1111/j.1556-4029.2009.01285.x.

15. Gasz, N.E. and M.L. Harvey, *A New Method for the Production of Sterile Colonies of Lucilia sericata.* Medical and Veterinary Entomology, 2017. 31(3): pp. 299–305, https://doi.org/10.1111/mve.12232.

16. Moe, S.J., N.C. Stenseth, and R.H. Smith, *Density-dependent Compensation in Blowfly Populations Give Indirectly Positive Effects of a Toxicant.* Ecology, 2002. 83(6): pp. 1597–1603, https://dx.doi.org/10.1890/0012-9658(2002)083[1597:DDCIBP]2.0.CO;2.

17. Zhang, B., et al., *A Simple, Heat-sterilizable Artificial Diet Excluding Animal-derived Ingredients for Adult Blowfly, Lucilia sericata.* Medical and Veterinary Entomology, 2009. 23(4): pp. 443–447, https://doi.org/10.1111/j.1365-2915.2009.00835.x.

18. Muntzer, A., et al., *Temperature-dependent Lipid Metabolism in the Blow Fly Lucilia sericata.* Medical and Veterinary Entomology, 2015. 29(3): pp. 305–313, https://doi.org/10.1111/mve.12111.

19. Linhares, A.X. and R.P. Avancini, *Ovarian Development in the Blowflies Chrysomya putoria and C. megacephala on Natural Diets.* Medical and Veterinary Entomology, 1989. 3(3): pp. 293–295, https://dx.doi.org/10.1111/j.1365-2915.1989.tb00231.x.

20. Wall, R., V.J. Wearmouth, and K.E. Smith, *Reproductive Allocation by the Blow Fly Lucilia sericata in Response to Protein Limitation.* Physiological Entomology, 2002. 27(4): pp. 267–274, https://doi.org/10.1046/j.1365-3032.2002.00296.x.

21. Wardhaugh, K.G., et al., *The Relationship between Dung Quality and Oocyte Resorption in Laboratory and Field Populations of Lucilia cuprina.* Entomologia Experimentalis et Applicata, 2008. 126(3): pp. 179–193, https://doi.org/10.1111/j.1570-7458.2007.00659.x.

22. Wall, R., N. French, and K.L. Morgan, *Effects of Temperature on the Development and Abundance of the Sheep Blowfly Lucilia sericata (Diptera: Calliphoridae).* Bulletin of Entomological Research, 1992. 82(1): pp. 125–131.

23. Williams, H. and A.M.M. Richardson, *Life History Responses to Larval Food Shortages in Four Species of Necrophagous Flies (Diptera: Calliphoridae).* Australian Journal of Ecology, 1983. 8(3): pp. 257–263, https://dx.doi.org/10.1111/j.1442-9993.1983.tb01323.x.

24. Smith, P.H., L. Barton Browne, and A.C.M. van Gerwen, *Sperm Storage and Utilisation and Egg Fertility in the Sheep Blowfly, Lucilia cuprina.* Journal of Insect Physiology, 1988. 34(2): pp. 125–129, https://doi.org/10.1016/0022-1910(88)90164-3.

25. Browne, L.B., A.C.M. Vangerwen, and P.H. Smith, *Relationship between Mated Status of Females and Their Stage of Ovarian Development in Field Populations of the Australian Sheep Blowfly, Lucilia cuprina (Wiedemann) (Diptera, Calliphoridae).* Bulletin of Entomological Research, 1987. 77(4): pp. 609–615, https://doi.org/10.1017/S0007485300012116.

26. Butterworth, N.J., P.G. Byrne, and J.F. Wallman, *The Blow Fly Waltz: Field and Laboratory Observations of Novel and Complex Dipteran Courtship Behavior.* Journal of Insect Behavior, 2019. 32(2): pp. 109–119, https://doi.org/10.1007/s10905-019-09720-1.

27. Queiroz, M.M.D.C., R.P. De Mello, and N.M. Da Serra Freire, *The Effect of Different Proportions of Males and Females over the Chrysomya albiceps (Wiedemann 1819) (Diptera, Calliphoridae) Biotic Potential and Longevity under Laboratory Conditions.* Memorias do Instituto Oswaldo Cruz, 1996. 91(2): pp. 243–247, https://dx.doi.org/10.1590/S0074-02761996000200023.

28. Mackerras, M.J., *Observations on the Life-histories, Nutritional Requirements and Fecundity of Blow-flies.* Bulletin of Entomological Research, 1933. 24: pp. 353–362, https://dx.doi.org/10.1017/S0007485300031680.

29. Wall, R., *The Reproductive Output of the Blowfly Lucilia sericata.* Journal of Insect Physiology, 1993. 39(9): pp. 743–750, https://doi.org/10.1016/0022-1910(93)90049-W.

30. Hayes, E.J., R. Wall, and K.E. Smith, *Mortality Rate, Reproductive Output, and Trap Response Bias in Populations of the Blowfly Lucilia sericata.* Ecological Entomology, 1999. 24(3): pp. 300–307, https://doi.org/10.1046/j.1365-2311.1999.00194.x.

31. Wooldridge, J., L. Scrase, and R. Wall, *Flight Activity of the Blowflies, Calliphora vomitoria and Lucilia sericata, in the Dark*. Forensic Science International, 2007. 172(2–3): pp. 94–97, https://doi.org/10.1016/j.forsciint.2006.12.011.

32. Ody, H., M.T. Bulling, and K.M. Barnes, *Effects of Environmental Temperature on Oviposition Behavior in Three Blow Fly Species of Forensic Importance*. Forensic Science International, 2017. 275: pp. 138–143, https://doi.org/10.1016/j.forsciint.2017.03.001.

33. Archer, M.S. and M.A. Elgar, *Female Breeding-site Preferences and Larval Feeding Strategies of Carrion-breeding Calliphoridae and Sarcophagidae (Diptera): A Quantitative Analysis*. Australian Journal of Zoology, 2003. 51(2): pp. 165–174, https://doi.org/10.1071/ZO02067.

34. Vogt, W.G. and T.L. Woodburn, *The Influence of Temperature and Moisture on the Survival and Duration of the Egg Stage of the Australian Sheep Blowfly, Lucilia cuprina (Wiedemann) (Diptera, Calliphoridae)*. Bulletin of Entomological Research, 1980. 70(4): pp. 665–671, https://dx.doi.org/10.1017/S0007485300007951.

35. Wall, R., K.M. Pitts, and K.E. Smith, *Pre-adult Mortality in the Blowfly Lucilia sericata*. Medical and Veterinary Entomology, 2001. 15(3): pp. 328–334, https://doi.org/10.1046/j.0269-283X.2001.00316.x.

36. Bo, Z., et al., *Short-term Cold Storage of Blowfly Lucilia sericata Embryos*. Insect Science, 2008. 15(3): pp. 225–228, https://doi.org/10.1111/j.1744-7917.2008.00204.x.

37. Gomes, L., W.A.C. Godoy, and C.J. Von Zuben, *A Review of Postfeeding Larval Dispersal in Blowflies: Implications for Forensic Entomology*. Naturwissenschaften, 2006. 93(5): pp. 207–215, https://doi.org/10.1007/s00114-006-0082-5.

38. von Zuben, C.J., F.J. von Zuben, and W.A.C. Godoy, *Larval Competition for Patchy Resources in Chrysomya megacephala (Dipt., Calliphoridae): Implications of the Spatial Distribution of Immatures*. Journal of Applied Entomology, 2001. 125(9–10): pp. 537–541, https://doi.org/10.1046/j.1439-0418.2001.00586.x.

39. Bernhardt, V., et al., *Of Pigs and Men-Comparing the Development of Calliphora vicina (Diptera: Calliphoridae) on Human and Porcine Tissue*. International Journal of Legal Medicine, 2017. 131(3): pp. 847–853, https://doi.org/10.1007/s00414-016-1487-0.

40. Sherman, R.A. and J.M. My-Tien Tran, *A Simple, Sterile Food Source for Rearing the Larvae of Lucilia sericata (Diptera: Calliphoridae)*. Medical and Veterinary Entomology, 1995. 9(4): pp. 393–398, https://doi.org/10.1111/j.1365-2915.1995.tb00011.x.

41. Rabêlo, K.C.N., et al., *Bionomics of Two Forensically Important Blowfly Species Chrysomya megacephala and Chrysomya putoria (Diptera: Calliphoridae) Reared on Four Types of Diet*. Forensic Science International, 2011. 210(1–3): pp. 257–262, https://doi.org/10.1016/j.forsciint.2011.03.022.

42. Baer, W.S., *The Treatment of Chronic Osteomyelitis with the Maggot (Larva of the Blow Fly)*. The Journal of Bone and Joint Surgery. American Volume, 1931. 13: pp. 438–475, https://doi.org/10.1007/s11999-010-1416-3.

43. Okorie, T.G. and J. Okeke, *Comparative Studies on the Blowfly Lucilia caesar (Diptera, Calliphoridae) Reared from 3 Rearing Media Prepared from Local Materials and the Standard Snyder Medium*. Insect Science and Its Application, 1990. 11(2): pp. 143–148, https://dx.doi.org/10.1017/S1742758400010493.

44. Reddy, P.V.R., V.V. Rajan, and A. Verghese, *A Non-meat-based Artificial Diet and Protocol for Mass searing of Chrysomya megacephala (Fab.) (Diptera: Calliphoridae), an Important Pollinator of Mango*. Current Science, 2015. 108(1): pp. 17–19.

45. Anonymous. *Malaysian Biotechnology Corporation: Interview With The CEO, Iskandar Mizal Mahmood. Scientific American worldVIEW. A Global Biotechnology Perspective*. 2011.

46. Carreno, S.P., et al., *Protophormia terraenovae. A New Allergenic Species in Amateur Fishermen of Caceres, Spain*. Allergologia et Immunopathologia, 2009. 37(2): pp. 68–72, http://dx.doi.org/10.1016/S0301-0546(09)71107-3.

47. Wolff, H. and C. Hansson, *Rearing Larvae of Lucilia sericata for Chronic Ulcer Treatment — An Improved Method*. Acta Dermato-Venereologica, 2005. 85(2): pp. 126–131, https://doi.org/10.1080/00015550510025533.

48. Rivers, D.B., et al., *Water Balance Characteristics of Pupae Developing in Different Size Maggot Masses from Six Species of Forensically Important Flies*. Journal of Insect Physiology, 2013. 59(5): pp. 552–559, https://doi.org/10.1016/j.jinsphys.2013.03.002.

49. Mądra-Bielewicz, A., K. Frątczak-Łagiewska, and S. Matuszewski, *Blowfly Puparia in a Hermetic Container: Survival under Decreasing Oxygen Conditions*. Forensic Science, Medicine, and Pathology, 2017. 13(3): pp. 328–335, https://doi.org/10.1007/s12024-017-9892-3.

50. Aigbodion, F.I., I.N. Egbon, and A.J. Obuseli, *Pathogens of Medical Importance Isolated from Phaenicia (Lucilia) sericata (Diptera:Calliphoridae) in Benin City, Nigeria*. Pakistan Journal of Biological Sciences, 2013. 16(23): pp. 1791–1795, https://doi.org/10.3923/pjbs.2013.1791.1795.

51. Chan, Q.E., M.A. Hussain, and V. Milovic, *Eating out of the Hand, Maggots — Friend or Foe?* Journal of Plastic, Reconstructive and Aesthetic Surgery, 2012. 65(8): pp. 1116–1118, https://doi.org/10.1016/j.bjps.2012.01.014.

52. Terterov, S., et al., *Posttraumatic Human Cerebral Myiasis*. World Neurosurgery, 2010. 73(5): pp. 557–559, https://doi.org/10.1016/j.wneu.2010.01.004.

53. Connelly, K., et al., *Wohlfahrtiimonas chitiniclastica Bloodstream Infection Due to a Maggot-infested Wound in a 54-year-old Male*. Journal of Global Infectious Diseases, 2019. 11(3): pp. 125–126, http://dx.doi.org/10.4103/jgid.jgid_58_18.

54. Kawabata, T., et al., *Induction of Antibacterial Activity in Larvae of the Blowfly Lucilia sericata by an Infected Environment.* Medical and Veterinary Entomology, 2010. 24(4): pp. 375–381, https://doi.org/10.1111/j.1365-2915.2010.00902.x.

55. Maleki-Ravasan, N., et al., *New Insights Into Culturable and Unculturable Bacteria Across the Life History of Medicinal Maggots Lucilia sericata (Meigen) (Diptera: Calliphoridae).* Frontiers in Microbiology, 2020. 11(505), https://doi.org/10.3389/fmicb.2020.00505.

56. Jiang, K.C., et al., *Excretions/Secretions from Bacteria-pretreated Maggot Are More Effective against Pseudomonas aeruginosa Biofilms.* PLoS ONE, 2012. 7(11): e49815, https://doi.org/10.1371/journal.pone.0049815.

57. Yeong, Y.S., et al., *Scanning Electron Microscopic Evaluation of the Successful Sterilization of Lucilia cuprina (Wiedemann) Utilized in Maggot Debridement Therapy (mdt).* Tropical Biomedicine, 2011. 28(2): pp. 325–332, https://www.msptm.org/files/325_-_332_Yeong_Y_S.pdf.

58. Kaplun, O., M. Pupiales, and G. Psevdos, *Adjuvant Maggot Debridement Therapy for Deep Wound Infection Due to Methicillin-resistant Staphylococcus aureus.* Journal of Global Infectious Diseases, 2019. 11(4): pp. 165–167, https://doi.org/10.4103/jgid.jgid_30_19.

59. Brundage, A.L., T.L. Crippen, and J.K. Tomberlin, *Methods for External Disinfection of Blow Fly (Diptera: Calliphoridae) Eggs prior to Use in Wound Debridement Therapy.* Wound Repair and Regeneration, 2016. 24: pp. 384–393, https://doi.org/10.1111/wrr.12408.

60. Paul, A.G., et al., *Maggot Debridement Therapy with Lucilia cuprina: A Comparison with Conventional Debridement in Diabetic Foot Ulcers.* International Wound Journal, 2009. 6(1): pp. 39–46, https://doi.org/10.1111/j.1742-481X.2008.00564.x.

61. Wang, S.Y., et al., *Clinical Research on the Bio-debridement Effect of Maggot Therapy for Treatment of Chronically Infected Lesions.* Orthopaedic Surgery, 2010. 2(3): pp. 201–206, https://doi.org/10.1111/j.1757-7861.2010.00087.x.

62. Berkebile, D.R. and S.R. Skoda, *Chemicals Useful for Separating Egg Masses of the Screwworm (Diptera : Calliphoridae).* Southwestern Entomologist, 2002. 27(3–4): pp. 297–299.

63. PIC/S, *Guide to Good Manufacturing Practice for Medicinal Products — Annexes.* 2017, Pharmaceutical Inspection Convention Pharmaceutical Inspection Co-operation Scheme. https://picscheme.org/en/publications?tri=gmp#zone.

64. Sherman, R.A., C.E. Shapiro, and R.M. Yang, *Maggot Therapy for Problematic Wounds: Uncommon and Off-label Applications.* Advances in Skin & Wound Care, 2007. 20(11): pp. 602–610, https://doi.org/10.1097/01.ASW.0000284943.70825.a8.

65. Limsopatham, K., et al., *Sterilization of Blow Fly Eggs, Chrysomya megacephala and Lucilia cuprina, (Diptera: Calliphoridae) for Maggot Debridement Therapy*

Application. Parasitology Research, 2017. 116(5): pp. 1581–1589, https://doi.org/10.1007/s00436-017-5435-9.

66. Nuesch, R., et al., *Clustering of Bloodstream Infections during Maggot Debridement Therapy Using Contaminated Larvae of Protophormia terraenovae.* Infection, 2002. 30(5): pp. 306–309, https://doi.org/10.1007/s15010-002-3067-0.

67. Merck. *Wound Treatment with Larvae — Stories.* https://www.merckgroup.com/en/stories/wound-treatment-with-larvae.html.

68. WHO. *The International Pharmacopoeia*, 3.2 Test for sterility. http://apps.who.int/phint/en/p/docf/.

69. TGA. *TGA Guidelines for Sterility Testing of Therapeutic Goods.* 2006. https://www.tga.gov.au/sites/default/files/manuf-sterility-testing-guidelines.pdf.

70. Thyssen, P.J., et al., *Sterilization of Immature Blowflies (Calliphoridae) for Use in Larval Therapy.* Journal of Medicine and Medical Sciences, 2013. 4(10): pp. 405–409 https://www.interesjournals.org/articles/sterilization-of-immature-blowflies-calliphoridae-for-use-in-larval-therapy.pdf.

71. Collier, R., *Medicinal Maggots Cross Border at a Crawl.* Canadian Medical Association Journal, 2010. 182(2): pp. E123-E124, https://doi.org/10.1503/cmaj.109-3134.

72. Vinogradova, E.B., *Some Principles of Selecting Natural Material for Rearing and the Endogenous Processes in Laboratory Strains of the Blowfly Calliphora vicina R.-D. (Diptera, Calliphoridae).* Entomological Review, 2011. 91(1): pp. 1–6, https://doi.org/10.1134/S0013873811010015.

73. Allen, M.L., D.R. Berkebile, and S.R. Skoda, *Postlarval Fitness of Transgenic Strains of Cochliomyia hominivorax (Diptera: Calliphoridae).* Journal of Economic Entomology, 2004. 97(3): pp. 1181–1185.

74. Allen, M.L. and P.J. Scholl, *Quality of Transgenic Laboratory Strains of Cochliomyia hominivorax (Diptera: Calliphoridae).* Journal of Economic Entomology, 2005. 98(6): pp. 2301–2306.

75. Blake, F.A.S., et al., *The Biosurgical Wound Debridement: Experimental Investigation of Efficiency and Practicability.* Wound Repair and Regeneration, 2007. 15(5): pp. 756–761, https://doi.org/10.1111/j.1524-475x.2007.00298.x.

76. Wilson, M.R., et al., *The Impacts of Larval Density and Protease Inhibition on Feeding in Medicinal Larvae of the Greenbottle Fly Lucilia sericata.* Medical and Veterinary Entomology, 2016. 30(1): pp. 1–7, https://doi.org/10.1111/mve.12138.

77. Čičková, H., et al., *Growth and Survival of Bagged Lucilia sericata Maggots in Wounds of Patients Undergoing Maggot Debridement Therapy.* Evidence-based Complementary and Alternative Medicine, 2013. https://doi.org/10.1155/2013/192149.

78. Pickles, S.F. and D.I. Pritchard, *Quality Control of a Medicinal Larval (Lucilia sericata) Debridement Device Based on Released Gelatinase Activity.* Medical and Veterinary Entomology, 2017. 31(2): pp. 200–206, https://doi.org/10.1111/mve.12220.

79. Stadler, F., R.Z. Shaban, and P. Tatham, *Maggot Debridement Therapy in Disaster Medicine.* Prehospital and Disaster Medicine, 2016. 31(1): pp. 79–84, https://doi.org/10.1017/s1049023x15005427.

80. Amorim, P., et al., *Managing Perishability in Production-distribution Planning: A Discussion and Review.* Flexible Services and Manufacturing Journal, 2013. 25(3): pp. 389–413, https://doi.org/10.1007/s10696-011-9122-3.

81. BioMonde. *BioBag Ordering Guide.* http://biomonde.com/images/US_Linked_Docs/BM029_US_02_0215.pdf.

82. Bohac, M., et al., *Maggot Therapy in Treatment of a Complex Hand Injury Complicated by Mycotic Infection.* Bratislava Medical Journal, 2015. 116(11): pp. 671–673, https://doi.org/10.4149/bll_2015_128.

83. Stadler, F., *Distribution Logistics*, in *A Complete Guide to Maggot Therapy: Clinical Practice, Therapeutic Principles, Production, Distribution, and Ethics*, F. Stadler (ed.). 2022, Cambridge: Open Book Publishers, pp. 363–382, https://doi.org/10.11647/OBP.0300.17.

84. Stadler, F., *Supply Chain Management for Maggot Debridement Therapy in Compromised Healthcare Settings.* 2018. Unpublished doctoral dissertation, Griffith University, Queensland, https://doi.org/10.25904/1912/3170.

85. ISO. *ISO 13485:2003 Medical Devices — Quality Management Systems — Requirements for Regulatory Purposes.* https://www.iso.org/standard/36786.html.

86. Hamimi Abdul Razak, I., et al., *ISO 13485:2003: Implementation Reference Model from the Malaysian SMEs Medical Device Industry.* The TQM Journal, 2009. 21(1): pp. 6–19, https://doi.org/10.1108/17542730910924718.

87. Robitaille, D.E. and I. ebrary, *ISO 9001:2008 for Small and Medium-sized Businesses.* Vol. 2nd. 2010, Milwaukee: ASQ Quality Press.

88. Blackburn, J.K., et al., *The Necrophagous Fly Anthrax Transmission Pathway: Empirical and Genetic Evidence from Wildlife Epizootics.* Vector-Borne and Zoonotic Diseases, 2014. 14(8): pp. 576–583, https://doi.org/10.1089/vbz.2013.1538.

89. Böhnel, H., *Household Biowaste Containers (Bio-bins) — Potential Incubators for Clostridium botulinum and Botulinum Neurotoxins.* Water, Air, and Soil Pollution, 2002. 140(1–4): pp. 335–341, https://doi.org/10.1023/A:1020169520369.

90. Fischer, O.A., et al., *Blowflies Calliphora vicina and Lucilia sericata as Passive Vectors of Mycobacterium avium subsp. avium, M. a. paratuberculosis and M. a.*

hominissuis. Medical and Veterinary Entomology, 2004. 18(2): pp. 116–122, http://dx.doi.org/10.1111/j.0269-283X.2004.00477.x.

91.   Laurie, R., *Larval Therapy: Is It Effective against MRSA?* Journal of Community Nursing, 2010. 24(4): pp. 10–12.

92.   WHO. *Safe Management of Wastes from Health-care Activities — 2nd edition.* 2014; 2nd: http://apps.who.int/iris/bitstream/10665/85349/1/9789241548564_eng.pdf?ua=1.

93.   Stadler, F., et al., *Maggot Menageries: High School Student Contributions to Medicinal Maggot Production in Compromised Healthcare Settings.* Citizen Science: Theory and Practice, 2021. 6(1): 36, p. 1–16, http://doi.org/10.5334/cstp.401.

15. Establishment of a Medical Maggot Rearing Facility and Maggot Therapy Programme for Human and Veterinary Medicine in Kenya[1]

Peter Takáč, Milan Kozánek, Grace A. Murilla, Phoebe Mukiria, Bernard Wanyonyi Kinyosi, Judith K. Chemuliti, J. Kimani Wanjerie, Christopher K. Kibiwott, and Frank Stadler

This case study describes the process and experience of establishing a maggot therapy programme in Kenya. Initially, the programme included a technology- and knowledge-transfer initiative which successfully developed production capacity and clinical skills among the surgical and nursing workforce at Kenyatta National Hospital. This work was followed by a pilot study that demonstrated the positive impact mainstreaming of maggot therapy can have on the treatment of patients with chronic and infected wounds. The project highlights the importance of regulatory and supply-chain barriers that need to be addressed from the outset when introducing maggot therapy to new markets.

1 This work was funded by the Operational Program of Research and Development and co-financed by the European Fund for Regional Development (EFRD). Grant: ITMS 26240220030: Research and development of new biotherapeutic methods and its application in the treatment of some illnesses; and by Slovak Aid, Grant: SAMRS/2010/03/06; The introduction of sterile larval therapy into clinical practice for human and veterinary medicine in the Republic of Kenya.

https://doi.org/10.11647/OBP.0300.15

Introduction

Maggot therapy is the treatment of non-healing or infected wounds with disinfected fly larvae also called maggots. When placed on a wound, medicinal maggots remove dead tissue, fight infection, and promote wound healing [1–3]. Maggot therapy has been used to treat all kinds of chronic wounds including diabetic ulcers, pressure ulcers, burns, gangrene, and osteomyelitis, to name a few [4]. There are two ways medicinal maggots may be applied to a wound—free-range or contained within a mesh bag [5]. During free-range maggot therapy, maggots are placed directly onto the wound and held in place with a cage-like dressing made of a fabric material that allows maggots to breathe and wound exudate to drain off. Alternatively, maggots can be applied within a mesh bag similar to a tea bag. This is possible because maggots do not consume solids but liquefy their food in the wound environment. Digestive secretions and liquefied food easily pass through the mesh material.

Most maggot therapy around the world employs the greenbottle blowfly *Lucilia sericata* or the closely related *L. cuprina*, but other blowfly species such as Cochliomyia macellaria [6], Chrysomya putoria [7], and Sarconesiopsis magellanica [8] are also used or explored for potential use. As every medicinal fly should, *L. sericata* feeds only on dead and devitalised tissue and not on living cells, which does not impede healing. The competitive feeding of *L. sericata* larvae quickly removes dead tissue and slough and thus the source of nutrition for bacteria. Besides, bacteria are consumed and digested in the process. The removal of dead tissue also allows better diffusion of oxygen into the healthy tissues, which prevents the proliferation of anaerobic bacteria. However, the digestive excretions and secretions of maggots convey therapeutic benefits far beyond debridement. Not only do they contain compounds efficacious against fungal and bacterial pathogens, they also actively promote wound healing through a range of physiological mechanisms and pathways. These multiple therapeutic benefits of maggot therapy are discussed in great detail in Chapters 8 to 10 of this book [1–3].

The biological and life-history characteristics of green bottle maggots make them particularly suitable for biosurgery. They are easily cultured under insectary conditions, have a fast life-cycle and complete metamorphosis. The larvae feed preferentially on decomposing flesh and their performance in the wound is generally unaffected by illicit or therapeutic drugs [9], but topical wound care products must be removed prior to maggot therapy [10]. It is also helpful that medicinal maggots can be stored for a couple of days at cool temperatures as low as 6°C, which arrests their activity and slows down growth. This helps with production scheduling and allows for delivery times of up to 48 hours [11]. All in all, maggot therapy is a highly efficacious wound care modality and well-suited to high-resource and compromised healthcare settings alike.

Maggot Therapy in Kenya

The introduction of a maggot therapy treatment programme in a new jurisdiction requires the establishment of medicinal maggot production facilities and capabilities among the local workforce. This chapter presents the activities and outcomes of a programme that sought to introduce maggot therapy in the Kenyan healthcare system. Transfer of the necessary technology and know-how to the Kenyan setting was achieved via a partnership between Scientica Ltd, the Institute of Zoology at the Slovak Academy of Sciences, and the Kenyan Agriculture & Research Institute (KARI) with financial support from SlovakAid, and diplomatic support from the Ministry of Foreign and European Affairs of the Slovak Republic. Activities included building a laboratory for the production of medicinal maggots and the training of medical and veterinary staff in the clinical aspects and use of maggot therapy. Because maggot therapy had been a new therapy to the Kenyan health system, it was also necessary to demonstrate its benefit via a clinical study. This is why the initial establishment of medicinal maggot production capacity and the training of wound care practitioners was followed by a pilot study at Kenyatta National Hospital which is also described below. The chapter concludes with an update on the current status of maggot therapy in Kenya and some reflections on the Kenyan experience.

Maggot Therapy Technology Transfer and Training

Pre-project assessment of healthcare provider acceptance. In the first instance, it had to be established whether the local healthcare workforce involved in wound care would be accepting of maggot therapy because the buy-in of healthcare providers is critical to the successful introduction of maggot therapy. The Kenyan partners conducted a cross-sectional survey of staff from Kenyatta National Hospital that are involved in wound care. The survey did not find any deep-seated rejection of maggot therapy among the workforce and any concerns raised could be easily addressed with an education and sensitisation programme.

Activities carried out by the Slovak partners during the first half-year of the project, from December 2010 to the end of May 2011, were intended to create conditions for the effective launch of the project. A tender was issued for the supply of instrumentation and other supplies. A draft plan was developed for reconstruction work, which was subsequently discussed in detail with KARI and implementation work begun for breeding and laboratory facilities. Detailed technical specifications of breeding technology were developed, the manufacturer was selected and the first insect-rearing cage built, which was tested at the Institute of Zoology in Bratislava. After some adjustments, the remaining cages were built. In May 2011, the Slovak team completed the first mission to KARI. The trip focussed on the monitoring and assessment of the construction and refurbishment of the laboratory and insectary facilities, evaluation of activities, and the planning of activities for the next period including the required laboratory furniture, appliances, and equipment.

An important aspect of the project was joint awareness raising and stakeholder engagement with KARI Director Dr Ephraim A. Mukusira via publicity, workshops, and project presentations:

- Meeting with the Kenyan State Secretary of the Ministry of Livestock Development, Kennet M. Lusaka EBS.

- Preparation of a training programme for technical staff of KARI.

- Visits to healthcare facilities that were identified as likely early adopters of maggot therapy.

- Project presentation at a business lunch with the Ambassador of the Slovak Republic, Milan Zachar, in Nairobi.

- Interviews with local media representatives concerning the objectives of the project and its potential contribution to society in Kenya.

Project activities during the second six-month period, from June 2011 to December 2011, focussed on finalising the refurbishment works at KARI to create facilities for medicinal maggot production and related research activities. In this period, the Slovak team also finalised the standard operating procedures for the production of *L. sericata* medicinal maggots and other species that may be utilised for maggot therapy purposes. Finally, the Slovak team coordinated the shipment of purchased insectary and laboratory equipment, furniture, and supplies. Unfortunately, late delivery of the shipping container to Bratislava postponed shipment of equipment by 3 months.

Activities implemented during the six-month period from December 2011 until the end of May 2012 focussed on fine-tuning of the laboratory and insectary refurbishment at KARI (Figure 15.1). This included the shipment of laboratory equipment, furniture, and supplies to Mombasa and then on to KARI. The release of the laboratory equipment was delayed a further six months due to bureaucratic processes regarding tax exemption for imported donated goods. We continuously informed the project manager of Slovak Aid about this unforeseen delay. The installation of equipment and furniture was finally carried out in May 2012.

In addition to the technology transfer, it was necessary to ensure that Kenyan laboratory technicians and wound care providers were trained in the rearing of medicinal flies and the treatment of wounds with maggot therapy. To that end, two technicians (Phoebe Mukiria and Bernard Wanyoyi) were trained in the mass rearing of the greenbottle blowfly *L. sericata* and medicinal maggot production at Scientica Ltd in Bratislava. The Kenyan clinician Dr Saratian Nyabera Lugia, MD (Chairman of the Diagnostics Division and Head of Accident and Emergency at Moi Teaching and Referral Hospital) also travelled to Slovakia for maggot therapy training at the First Department of Surgery of the Faculty of Medicine in Bratislava, and at the hospital of Čadca and a hospital in the town of Liptovský Mikuláš.

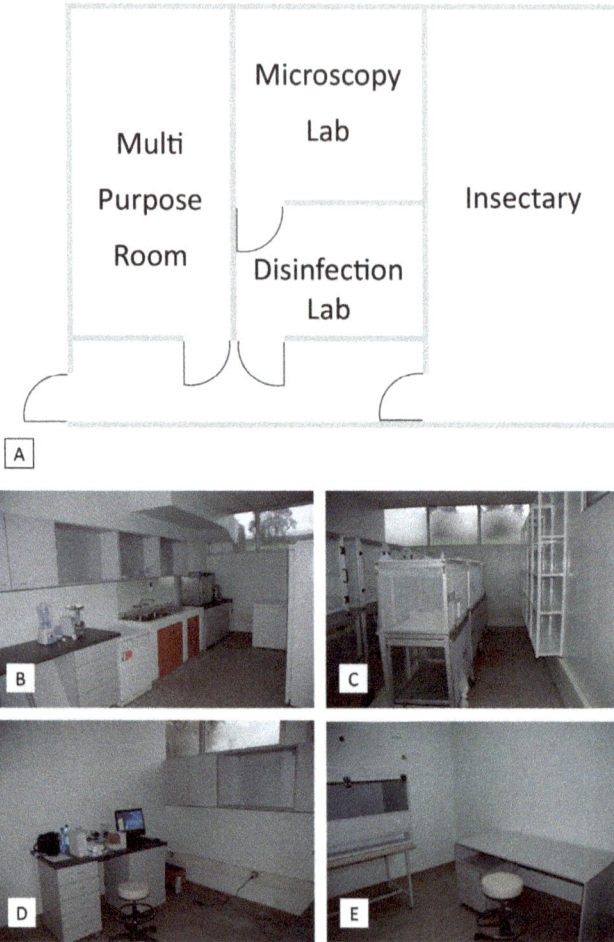

Figure 15.1 Medicinal maggot production and research laboratory facilities established at KARI (now KALRO). A) Plan drawing of the facility layout. An under-utilised building was refurbished to house B) a multipurpose room for washing up, diet preparation, and cool storage of dietary ingredients, C) an insectary, D) a microscopy research laboratory, and E) a dedicated room furnished with a laminar flow cabinet for the disinfection of fly eggs, and the preparation and packaging of medicinal maggots. Photos by P. Takáč, Scientica Ltd and Slovak Academy of Sciences, CC BY-NC.

Activities implemented during the six-month period from June to November 2012 focussed on the successful introduction of maggot therapy to human and veterinary clinical practice in Kenya. Marek Čambal MD, PhD from the First Surgical Clinic of the University Hospital, Comenius

University of Bratislava, visited Kenya in July 2012 and trained medical doctors and nursing staff. In addition to these activities, we organised a public lecture at the hospital on the topic of "Maggot debridement therapy—A modality for chronic wound treatment". There was great interest in the lecture, which was attended by more than 70 doctors and medical staff.

The most important result of this project was the Kenyatta National Hospital (KNH) research and ethics approval for a clinical study entitled "Maggot therapy as a method of treatment of chronic non-healing wounds". The Slovak and KARI project teams partnered with Dr A Wanjeri and Christopher Kibiwott to pilot maggot therapy at KNH. The ethics and research approval also authorised the KNH group to administer maggot therapy anywhere in Kenya.

Slovak technology transfer activities concluded with the dissemination of project outcomes:

- Presentation and exhibition of project outcomes at the University Library in Bratislava (17 October 2012), attended by 100 participants. The event was organised by the Platform of Development NGOs.

- Presentation of project outcomes at the first Slovak Development Forum in Nairobi (19–21 November 2012). This inaugural forum was organised by the Slovak Embassy in Nairobi with the aim of assessing the almost 17-year history of support provided by Slovak non-governmental and not-for-profit organisations, and the aid contributions to Kenya made by the Slovak government over almost 10 years.

First Clinical Study of Maggot Therapy in Kenya

Study Type and Ethical Clearance

On 26 October 2012, the Kenyatta National Hospital, University of Nairobi (UoN) Ethics and Research Committee (KNH-UoN ERC) approved a pilot study entitled "Maggot Debridement Therapy: The Biotherapeutic Method of Healing Chronic Wounds in Kenya". The pilot study was conducted between August and December 2013 at KNH. 24 patients were treated with a total of 30 maggot applications.

Repeat applications were necessary for some wounds due to the amount of necrotic tissue present. Maggot therapy was carried out by two nurses headed by Dr Wanjeri, a plastic surgeon, and Christopher Kibiwott, a senior nurse.

The Study Site Selection

Two hospitals, Kenyatta National Referral Hospital in Nairobi and Tenwek Mission Hospital in Bomet, were initially selected as study sites due to their high numbers of wound patients. Subsequently, the study was conducted solely at KNH for ease of access and availability of patients. Negotiating the study across two sites with logistical difficulties in the transport of medicinal maggots to Bomet proved too difficult.

Patient Selection and Inclusion Criteria

24 patients were recruited for the pilot study after assessing their wounds and obtaining signed consent. Patients were drawn from the entire in-patient population at KNH. Criteria for selection included the presence of one or more infected wounds that had been debrided more than once without success. Patients and their wounds were excluded from the study for the following reasons:

- Wounds exhibited granulation tissue without necrosis
- Wounds involved a major blood vessel
- Wounds were covered with eschar that required surgical debridement
- Ischemic wounds or presence of arterial insufficiency
- Wounds with significant *Pseudomonas aeruginosa* infection
- Osteomyelitis
- Patients had severe life-threatening infections
- Patients had an allergy to egg yolk (a component of the maggot-rearing process)
- Patients who had had surgery in the previous 24 to 48 hours
- Patients who refused the therapy

Medicinal Maggot Preparation

Adult *L. sericata* flies were maintained in the insectary at KARI, Muguga, at 26±2°C, 40–50% relative humidity, and 12 hours of daylight. Newly eclosed flies started producing eggs after 7–10 days. Eggs were collected with an oviposition bait made of minced bovine liver and wheat bran that was offered to flies for two hours. The bait was covered with a plastic container fitted with holes to make a darkened oviposition chamber while providing flies with access. Egg masses were placed into 10 mL Falcon® tubes and disinfected with 1% sodium hypochlorite solution. The number of eggs disinfected depended on the number of patients to be treated. The disinfected eggs were then incubated overnight at 27±2°C for larvae to emerge and grow sufficiently for medical application. The larvae were washed and packed aseptically into appropriate-size biobags or directly into plastic containers for free-range application. The medicinal maggots were then delivered to KNH.

Maggot Therapy Treatment

A total of 24 patients between 21 and 78 years old with a mean age of 32 years were recruited to the study from the KNH in-patient cohort. Of these, 12 were male and eight females. The aetiologies of the wounds treated included road traffic accidents (31%) including degloving injuries, pressure ulcers, diabetic foot ulcers (42%), fractures, arteriovenous insufficiency, and burns. Biobags were used on only 6 (25%) patients who then needed a repeat treatment with free-range application of maggots. 23 patients completed maggot therapy treatment and one participant chose not to continue after the first application of medicinal maggots. Aseptic technique was strictly observed and the usual wound management protocols followed. The wounds were rinsed with sterile saline and excess moisture was removed with gauze. Where eschar was present, incisions were made to make it easier for maggots to access the necrotic tissue. Maggot therapy was performed using biobags that contained maggots, or free-range (loose) maggots directly into the wound. The mode chosen depended on the patients' preference and the size and extent of the wound. After placement of maggots the wounds were covered lightly with a gauze bandage and left for 48 hours. Thereafter, the wound was assessed.

Study Outcome

In 16 patients (67%), complete debridement was achieved with only one application of maggots. In seven patients, maggot therapy achieved 70% debridement after the first application and complete debridement after the second application. The wound of the patient who decided to discontinue the therapy after 12 hours was 50% debrided after that short time. The wounds of 18 patients (75%) received regular care after maggot therapy and healed uneventfully without a need for any other intervention. The remaining patients had to undergo procedures such as flap closure and skin grafting. In all patients, maggot therapy successfully controlled infection without additional antibiotic therapy. Case examples are presented in Figure 15.2.

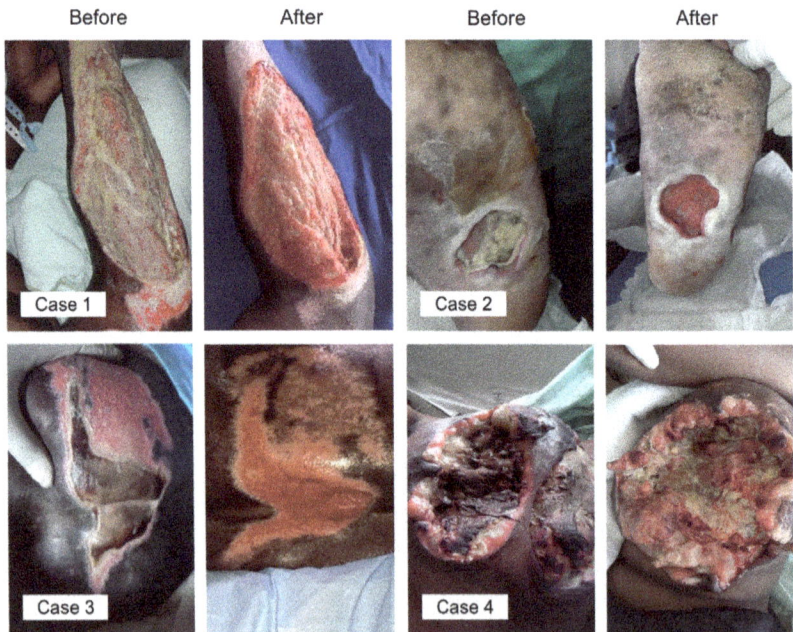

Figure 15.2 Examples of successful maggot therapy treatments during the pilot study. **Case 1**) Female, age 38, retrovirus disease under treatment, degloving injury of the head and right arm, road traffic accident. History: One day post-admission she was taken to theatre for surgical debridement and closure of the head wound. Due to its size, it was not closed. The degloving injury on the right hand was not debrided. Wound: 15 cm x 8 cm, 80% necrotic tissue with moderate infection. Maggot therapy: 1 treatment, 48 hours. Result: 100% debridement, patient was scheduled for skin grafting the following week, wound fully closed

within ten days. **Case 2**) Female, age 55, diabetic foot ulcer on sole of the left foot. History: Surgical debridement was not successful, patient was scheduled for below knee amputation, antibiotic treatment included Augmentin, Cefuroxime and Meropenem. Wound: 5 cm x 6cm, 4 cm deep, communicating from the small toe to the mid-foot area, edematous to the level of the knee, exudating and filled with slough, odorous, osteomylitis. Maggot therapy: 50% debridement after 1st and 100% after 2nd treatment, no further antibiotic treatment. Discharged one week later with much-improved wound. **Case 3**) Male, age 72, sacral pressure ulcer. History: Diabetic patient, high blood pressure, prostate cancer. Wound: Stage 3, septic, exudating purulent discharge, slough, odorous. Maggot therapy: 1 treatment, 95% debridement, followed up with negative pressure therapy and conventional dressings. **Case 4**) Female, age 42, ulcerated tumour on left breast. History: No co-morbidities. Wound: Very large mass, ulcerated, necrotic, filled with thick sloughy tissue, bled easily, odorous. Maggot therapy: 40% debridement after 1st treatment, 80% debridement after 2nd treatment. Antibiotic treatment: Ceftriaxone and metronidazole injection. Photos © Kenyatta National Hospital, Nairobi.

Current Status of Maggot Therapy

Medicinal maggot production capacity. In 2013, KARI was renamed the Kenya Agricultural and Livestock Research Organization. The KALRO insectary houses on average only 3,000 to 4,000 adult flies at any one time. Due to a lack of demand, there is not daily medicinal maggot production, and production occurs only when orders are received. It takes between two to three days to prepare an order depending on the time and date of order placement. However, the facility has the capacity (including equipment, materials, and personnel) to maintain more fly colonies and to produce medicinal maggots on a regular basis.

Nevertheless, strict adherence to established standard operating procedures has led to a shortage of egg yolk powder for medicinal maggot production. However, this does not seriously jeopardise production because egg yolk powder can easily be substituted with fresh poultry egg yolk and albumin. Larger production volumes may lead to stock-outs of net fabric for the construction of maggot confinement and containment dressings, as it has to be sourced from overseas. It, too, is not essential for maggot therapy. Free-range treatment using alternative retention systems could proceed while the netting is sourced. For example, free guidance on maggot therapy in compromised healthcare settings can be accessed via www.medmaglabs.com, which explains the use of ordinary clothing items to construct maggot confinement dressings, including two step-by-step videos describing free-range maggot therapy.

Medicinal maggot supply. KALRO supplies medicinal maggots confined in a biobag or loose maggots in a container for free-range application. The biobag is packaged in a sterile plastic container with a perforated lid for ventilation. The packaged medicinal maggots are placed in a cool box with ice packs and transported immediately to the hospital. The delivery is done through the informal transport system. Delivery to Nairobi-based hospitals or homecare patients is relatively fast but timely and affordable delivery to other parts of Kenya is a challenge.

Demand for medicinal maggots and maggot therapy. Although there is a growing interest in maggot therapy across Kenya, it is still a much under-utilised wound care intervention limited to a few patients. Under current medicinal maggot supply chain arrangements, the reasons for the slow uptake of maggot therapy include i) the outstanding regulatory approval by the Pharmacy and Poisons Board, ii) the high cost of delivery to hospitals outside of Nairobi, and iii) the overall cost of maggot therapy to poor patients. A consignment of medicinal maggots to hospitals or homecare settings around Nairobi costs from USD40 to USD60 for an average treatment. The cost is per application, irrespective of the size of the wound, and is made up of around USD20 for the medicinal maggots and USD20 for delivery [12].

Approval of Maggot Therapy in Kenya. The findings of the pilot study "Maggot Debridement Therapy: The Biotherapeutic Method of Healing Chronic Wounds in Kenya" were presented to the KNH-UoN ERC on 6 August 2014 along with a report. After careful assessment, the KNH-UoN ERC provided a favourable opinion on 20 July 2016, recognising the benefits of maggot therapy for patients with chronic wounds, especially when antibiotics fail. Despite this favourable finding, maggot therapy has not yet been approved by the Kenyan Pharmacy and Poisons Board because there is uncertainty as to whether medicinal maggots are best governed by human therapeutics regulation or livestock production regulation. The original ethics and research approval first granted for the pilot study in 2013 has been renewed on an annual basis to support treatment of patients by the KNH team. This means that as of 2021, seven years after the presentation of their findings, maggot therapy in Kenya is still limited to the KNH team, with a national rollout of the treatment still not possible.

Patients treated and national reach. Between 2013 and 2020, a total of 140 patients were treated by Christopher Kibiwott and Dr Wanjeri at KNH and other hospitals such as Aga Khan Hospital, Texas Cancer Centre, Nyeri Hospital, Oyugis District Hospital in Homa Bay County (about 400 km from Nairobi), Kiambu District Hospital, and patients in home care as far afield as Kisumu, Nyahururu, and Machakos.

Summary

Over ten years later, the introduction of maggot therapy to the Kenyan healthcare system is still an ongoing process. The initial technology and knowledge transfer initiative successfully developed production capacity at KARI/KALRO and clinical skills among the surgical and nursing workforce at KNH. The subsequent pilot study was also a success as it convinced the KNH-UoN ERC of the positive impact that mainstreaming of maggot therapy can have on the treatment of patients with chronic and infected wounds. However, medicinal maggot production and the number of patients treated in 2021 is well below capacity. Without full regulatory approval by the Pharmacy and Poisons Board, this is unlikely to change, which means that hundreds or even thousands of patients each year will miss out on efficacious maggot-assisted wound care. Moreover, what has not yet been addressed is the development of sustainable and affordable distribution logistics and supply chain management solutions for medicinal maggot therapy in Kenya. While good things always take time and the groundwork for a thriving maggot therapy programme has been laid, there is the danger that chronic under-utilisation of the production facility and a lack of funding and sales cashflow will erode institutional commitment to the programme and lead to the closure of the insectary and laboratory.

There are important lessons to be learned. Entrepreneurs and medical professionals wanting to establish a maggot therapy programme in their country or region must invest considerable time and effort to collaborate with and lobby medical regulators to secure approval of maggot therapy. At the same time, it is not enough to establish medicinal maggot production capacity and clinical skills. Medicinal maggots must also reach patients across the country, including in provincial, rural and remote locations, and not only near the production facility. It therefore pays to involve medical supply chain logistics experts and formal as well as informal transport service providers early on. Please refer to Chapter 17 for guidance on distribution logistics [13], and Chapter 18 for drone-assisted distribution of medicinal maggots [14].

References

1. Nigam, Y. and M.R. Wilson, *Maggot Debridement*, in *A Complete Guide to Maggot Therapy: Clinical Practice, Therapeutic Principles, Production, Distribution, and Ethics*, F. Stadler (ed.). 2022, Cambridge: Open Book Publishers, pp. 143–152, https://doi.org/10.11647/OBP.0300.08.

2. Nigam, Y. and M.R. Wilson, *The Antimicrobial Activity of Medicinal Maggots*, in *A Complete Guide to Maggot Therapy: Clinical Practice, Therapeutic Principles, Production, Distribution, and Ethics*, F. Stadler (ed.). 2022, Cambridge: Open Book Publishers, pp. 153–174, https://doi.org/10.11647/OBP.0300.09.

3. Nigam, Y. and M.R. Wilson, *Maggot-assisted Wound Healing*, in *A Complete Guide to Maggot Therapy: Clinical Practice, Therapeutic Principles, Production, Distribution, and Ethics*, F. Stadler (ed.). 2022, Cambridge: Open Book Publishers, pp. 175–194, https://doi.org/10.11647/OBP.0300.10.

4. Sherman, R., *Indications, Contraindications, Interactions, and Side-effects of Maggot Therapy*, in *A Complete Guide to Maggot Therapy: Clinical Practice, Therapeutic Principles, Production, Distribution, and Ethics*, F. Stadler (ed.). 2022, Cambridge: Open Book Publishers, pp. 63–78, https://doi.org/10.11647/OBP.0300.04.

5. Sherman, R., *Medicinal Maggot Application and Maggot Therapy Dressing Technology*, in *A Complete Guide to Maggot Therapy: Clinical Practice, Therapeutic Principles, Production, Distribution, and Ethics*, F. Stadler (ed.). 2022, Cambridge: Open Book Publishers, pp. 79–96, https://doi.org/10.11647/OBP.0300.05.

6. Masiero, F.S., et al., *Histological Patterns in Healing Chronic Wounds Using Cochliomyia macellaria (Diptera: Calliphoridae) Larvae and Other Therapeutic Measures*. Parasitology Research, 2015. 114(8): pp. 2865–2872, https://doi.org/10.1007/s00436-015-4487-y.

7. Dallavecchia, D.L., R.G. da Silva Filho, and V.M. Aguiar, *Sterilization of Chrysomya putoria (Insecta: Diptera: Calliphoridae) Eggs for Use in Biotherapy*. Journal of Insect Science (Online), 2014. 14, https://doi.org/10.1093/jisesa/ieu022.

8.   Diaz-Roa, A., et al., *Evaluating Sarconesiopsis magellanica Blowfly-derived Larval Therapy and Comparing It to Lucilia sericata-derived Therapy in an Animal Model*. Acta Tropica, 2016. 154: pp. 34–41, https://doi.org/10.1016/j.actatropica.2015.10.024.

9.   Sherman, R.A. and E.A. Pechter, *Maggot Therapy: A Review of the Therapeutic Applications of Fly Larvae in Human Medicine, Especially for Treating Osteomyelitis*. Medical and Veterinary Entomology, 1988. 2(3): pp. 225–230.

10.   Sherman, R.A., *Maggot Therapy for Foot and Leg Wounds*. International Journal of Lower Extremity Wounds, 2002. 1(2): pp. 135–142, https://doi.org/10.1177/1534734602001002009.

11.   Čičková, H., et al., *Growth and Survival of Bagged Lucilia sericata Maggots in Wounds of Patients Undergoing Maggot Debridement therapy*. Evidence-based Complementary and Alternative Medicine, 2013. 29(4): pp. 416–424, https://doi.org/10.1155/2013/192149.

12.   Stadler, F., *Supply Chain Management for Maggot Debridement Therapy in Compromised Healthcare Settings*. 2018. Unpublished doctoral dissertation, Griffith University, Queensland, https://doi.org/10.25904/1912/3170.

13.   Stadler, F., *Distribution Logistics*, in *A Complete Guide to Maggot Therapy: Clinical Practice, Therapeutic Principles, Production, Distribution, and Ethics*, F. Stadler (ed.). 2022, Cambridge: Open Book Publishers, pp. 363–382, https://doi.org/10.11647/OBP.0300.17.

14.   Stadler, F. and P. Tatham, *Drone-assisted Medicinal Maggot Distribution in Compromised Healthcare Settings*, in *A Complete Guide to Maggot Therapy: Clinical Practice, Therapeutic Principles, Production, Distribution, and Ethics*, F. Stadler (ed.). 2022, Cambridge: Open Book Publishers, pp. 383–402, https://doi.org/10.11647/OBP.0300.18.

PART 4

LOGISTICS

16. Packaging Technology

Frank Stadler

This chapter is concerned with the packaging of medicinal maggots for sale and transport. After fly eggs have been disinfected, incubated, and the microbial safety of eggs and maggots has been confirmed, medicinal maggots are counted and transferred to primary packaging for safe transit to the point of care. This primary packaging may then be further packaged within a cardboard box that forms the secondary packaging along with package inserts that specify vital product and use information. In addition, when medicinal maggots are transported over greater distances or under unfavourable climatic conditions, insulated transport packaging is essential.

Introduction

This chapter is concerned with the packaging of medicinal maggots post-production and in preparation for transport to the wound care provider. After the eggs are disinfected and incubated, and after the microbial safety of eggs and maggots has been confirmed, medicinal maggots are counted into treatment units—usually in multiples of 50 maggots per unit (e.g. 100, 250, 500). For safe transit to the point of care, they need to be placed into a suitable container that holds a single medicinal maggot unit. Because this container is in direct contact with the product, it is called the primary packaging. In the case of ordinary pharmaceuticals (e.g. tablets) the primary packaging is then further

    https://doi.org/10.11647/OBP.0300.16

packaged, for example inside a cardboard box, which is referred to as the secondary packaging [1]. For medicinal maggots that are produced at the point of care, for example at a hospital, such secondary packaging may not be necessary, provided that the primary packaging is labelled with all the information that would ordinarily be on both the primary and secondary packaging. However, if a producer supplies medicinal maggots on a commercial basis to customers, then appropriate secondary packaging is desirable to convey essential product information, and to protect the product. In addition, transport of medicinal maggots to care providers that are not located in the same institution where the maggots are produced requires insulated cool-chain packaging. Distribution logistics is covered in Chapter 17 of this book [2].

This chapter follows guidance on the essential requirements for primary and secondary packaging as well as temperature-controlled transport packaging for medicinal maggots. The chapter provides only an overview of the aspects that must be considered when packaging maggots. It is critical that producers confirm with their own national regulators the specific local requirements for the packaging and labelling of therapeutic goods.

Primary and Secondary Packaging

The primary packaging must provide adequate humidity, ventilation and a secure enclosure so that the small, young maggots cannot escape. In addition, the primary packaging must be sterile at the time of packaging and protect medicinal maggots from microbial contamination for the duration of transport until they are applied to the wound. The primary packaging may hold maggots that are either i) provided for free-range application, which means that they are directly placed into the container—with or without a moistened gauze pad, or ii) they are sealed first in a teabag-like net pouch and then placed into the primary packaging [3].

Producers may package medicinal maggots in sterile, hard-shelled pathology sample jars made of plastic, or various other types of laboratory-grade plastic containers of similar volume (Figure 16.1). There is no hard and fast rule, so long as the above-mentioned conditions are provided. The larger the volume of the jar the less need there is for ventilation and tightly sealed containers can be used for primary packaging purposes—but only if there is fast delivery of the maggots at cool temperatures, which slows down maggot metabolism and oxygen consumption. Medicinal maggots die if not adequately ventilated. In addition, larger volume containers result in parcel space being wasted with thin air. Therefore, smaller-volume, slender tissue culture vials or tubes that are fitted with a filter lid, and thereby allow gas exchange, may be used to reduce the volume of packaging, and consequently healthcare waste (Figure 16.1). The primary packaging system may then be packed either directly into a transport box or further placed inside branded secondary packaging that does not inhibit ventilation of the primary packaging.

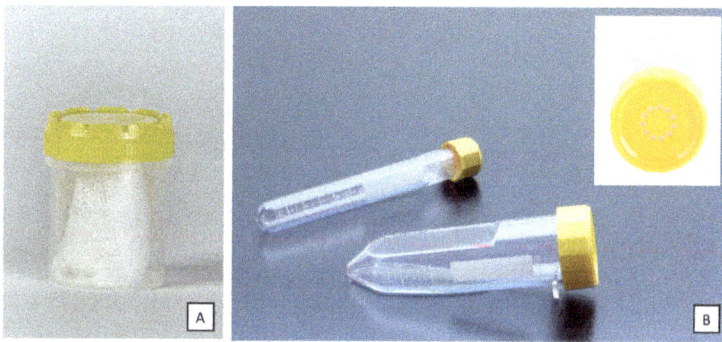

Figure 16.1 Primary packaging containers that may be used for the transport of medicinal maggots: A) Sterile 70 mL pathology specimen jar suitable only for rapid delivery at cool temperatures, unless modified to permit air exchange, B) Tissue culture tubes fitted with a filter lid that permits air exchange while maintaining sterility. Photos by (A) F. Stadler, MedMagLabs and Creating Hope in Conflict: A Humanitarian Grand Challenge, CC BY-ND and (B) © TPP, www.tpp.ch).

Consumer safety is a major concern in healthcare and therefore providers of therapeutic goods need to ensure that their goods cannot be tampered with prior to reaching the patient. In the case of medicinal maggot packaging, this may be achieved with

- a tape seal, a heat shrink band, or a perforated wrapper applied to the primary packaging that will need to be broken in the process of opening the container [4]; and/or

- a tape seal on the secondary packaging box which also reveals any access to the packaging content when broken [4].

Air-tight plastic wrapping around the secondary packaging box must be avoided because it would restrict airflow and ventilation of the primary packaging container and its living content.

As alluded to earlier, the primary or secondary packaging (if used) for medicinal maggots will need to be labelled according to best practice. The World Health Organization (WHO) guidelines on packaging for pharmaceutical products [1] say that the labels on primary/secondary packaging should at least provide the following information:

- the name of the drug product;
- a list of the active ingredients and their amounts;
- a statement of the net contents (number of dosage units, mass or volume)
- the batch number assigned by the manufacturer;
- the expiry date in an uncoded form;
- any special storage conditions or handling precautions that may be necessary;
- the directions for use, and any warnings and precautions that may be necessary;
- the name and address of the manufacturer or the company or person responsible for placing the product on the market.

Ideally, wound care practitioners should be familiar with maggot therapy prior to ordering and receiving medicinal maggots from the producer. A package insert should nevertheless be forwarded with each medicinal maggot consignment or inserted into the secondary packaging boxes. Information provided on the package insert should complement information printed on labels. It must explain to the healthcare practitioner what medicinal maggots are, how to use them, what the indications and contraindications for maggot therapy are, and what potential side-effects to look out for. With the rise in mobile telephony especially in low- and middle-income countries, the package label and package insert may also refer to a website or mobile device application that provide i) helpful treatment information, ii) answer frequently asked questions, and iii) contact details for a helpline in case practitioners require additional guidance.

Counterfeiting. Counterfeit medicines are a growing problem, particularly in developing countries [5]. They imitate the original product and apart from being an intellectual property infringement, counterfeit medicines may be of poorer quality and potency. Because flies are relatively easy to produce, maggot therapy will be vulnerable to counterfeiting in low- and middle-income countries.

The food and pharmaceutical industries seek to prevent counterfeiting with radio frequency identification and one- and two-dimensional barcode technologies, which in turn allow track-and-trace monitoring of batches throughout the supply chain [6]. The Guidelines for Bar Coding in the Pharmaceutical Supply Chain [7, 8] set out best-practice barcode use in the pharmaceutical supply chain. In addition to authentication of products, such bar coding can facilitate the back-tracing of production batches in case of an adverse event during treatment. For example, the Australian Red Cross Blood Service is a bio-medical product supply chain that successfully uses bar code identification and tracking of blood products from collection to transfusion [9]. However, radio frequency identification and other tracking technologies come at an extra cost, which must be borne by the supply chain and, ultimately, the customer [10].

In Nigeria, mobile phone solutions are available for patients to detect counterfeit drugs. A short code found on the packaging is sent via text message to the service provider who then verifies authenticity of the medicine [11]. In addition, the packaging technology itself can assist with the identification of authentic medication. Solutions include packaging design features, security labels, coding, printing and graphics, holograms and forensic markers [12].

Irrespective of these measures, poor patients receiving care from unqualified healthcare providers will be the most likely targets for counterfeit medicinal maggots. Heavy discounting of maggot therapy through a means-tested payment schedule or other financial support from governments and NGOs may be more effective than the above-mentioned counterfeit prevention measures because if the poor are given access to affordable, high-quality maggot therapy products and services, there is little incentive for them to use risky, illegal alternatives.

Having discussed the dangers of counterfeit medicinal maggots and options to guard against fraudulent supply, it must be mentioned that there are situations when such informal entrepreneurial activity might be welcome. For example, modern warfare and conflict increasingly target and affect civilian communities which are consequently impacted by violence, isolation and lack of resources. In such cases, it would be beneficial for isolated, conflict-affected communities to rear their own medicinal maggots to care for casualties and those patients with chronic wounds [13].

Transport Packaging

Temperature Control

Medicinal maggots are temperature-sensitive products. For example, *Lucilia sericata* maggots will die at temperatures over 47°C [14], which are easily reached during the summer in vehicles that are not equipped with appropriate air conditioning. At the other extreme, prolonged exposure to cold temperatures below 6°C can also harm medicinal maggots. Under no circumstance must they be cooled below 0°C as freezing will kill these fragile organisms. However, cool temperatures at and above 6°C can be exploited to slow down the maggots' metabolism in order to arrest their development and extend the period they can be kept without food. Some producers have stored *L. sericata* maggots at temperatures as low as 4°C for up to 5 days [15, 16] without unsustainable mortality, but it is now generally accepted that medicinal maggots in transit should be maintained at temperatures between 6°C and 25°C and that they should be administered within 24 to 48 hours from dispatch [17, 18].

As Figure 16.2 illustrates, the acceptable temperature range for medicinal maggots in transit and short-term storage ahead of maggot therapy appears to overlap with that of many heat- and freeze-sensitive vaccines, which must be stored at all times between 2°C and 8°C [19], and red blood cell products which must be stored between 1°C and 10°C [20]. Thus, the management of vaccine and blood supply chains faces the same challenges as medicinal maggot distribution, and this provides opportunities for supply chain collaboration and integration, as well as mutual learning [21].

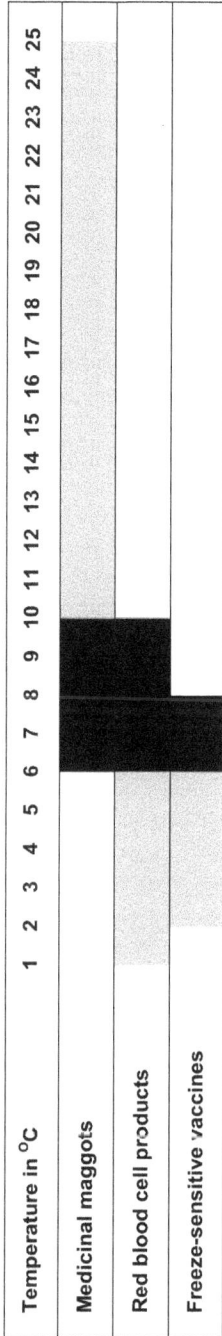

Figure 16.2 Safe temperature ranges for heat-sensitive medical products, including medicinal maggots. The safe temperature range that medicinal maggots share with the other two products is shown in solid shading.

Ineffective cooling with temperatures rising beyond recommended levels has been observed for blood product shipping containers [20, 22]. In the vaccine cold chain, however, it is the accidental freezing of vaccines that leads to frequent and significant vaccine wastage. It appears that vaccine cold chains fail because healthcare workers are insufficiently trained, cold storage and transport equipment is inadequate, and there is an unreliable power supply or other disruptions to refrigeration equipment [23]. In compromised healthcare settings these conditions may be the result of socio-economic disadvantage or armed conflict [24], but they are also encountered in high-income healthcare settings. It is a common observation that there are significant awareness and training gaps in health workers and cold chain system inadequacies in high-, low-, and middle-income countries, and that these put vaccine potency at risk [25, 26]. Consequently, improved training and education, implementation of equipment upgrades, and improved systems and standards can lead to significant improvements in cold-chain management [27–29]. It follows that the performance of medicinal maggot cool chains will also benefit from such measures, especially in compromised healthcare settings.

Cool- and Cold-Chain Packaging Solutions

Heat sensitive pharmaceuticals, chemicals and biologics are generally shipped using disposable cold-chain packaging [30]. These containers are made of highly insulating materials such as polystyrene and cool elements are used to lower the internal temperature to the desired range. Commercial medicinal maggot suppliers in Europe and the United States use such disposable packaging. However, in recent times, multi-use cold-chain packaging solutions have come on the market that are able to maintain the 6–25°C temperature range necessary for medicinal maggot transport [30]. Moreover, multi-use new vaccine transport container designs also utilise passive cold storage which employs sophisticated insulation, phase-change cooling elements, and precise temperature monitoring [31].

There are economic and environmental considerations when deciding on the best packaging solution for medicinal maggots. Reusable packaging systems have been shown to save money and significantly reduce waste and carbon emissions when compared to disposable packaging [30, 32].

These are important issues to consider when establishing a supply chain, particularly in low- and middle-income countries, because distribution inefficiencies and the need to provide affordable wound care may require more cost-effective distribution solutions. Furthermore, pharmaceutical waste is a significant environmental issue and should be reduced if possible [33–35]. The benefit of reusable packaging in the cold and cool chain has been demonstrated by Eli Lilly who implemented the Credo system of reusable packaging [36] and closed-loop reverse logistics for cold chain shipments using four sizes of shippers. As a result, they reduced the number of shippers per order, achieved a shipper return rate of 96%, reduced waste by 192,505 kg in the first year, and saved $2 million annually [37].

What type of packaging medicinal maggot producers choose will depend ultimately on the transport distance, the environmental conditions encountered in transit and at the point of care, and the number of primary packaging units to be shipped. For example, if a producer only supplies a few local hospitals that are nearby and can be reached by courier or personal delivery within an hour, only very basic packaging is required to keep temperatures at or below 25°C. If the aim is to maintain ideal conditions for 24 to 48 hours because of distribution distance or transport inefficiencies, then more sophisticated cool-chain packaging is required. Packaging systems will also need to be selected to match the volume of shipments. Fortunately, cool-chain packaging comes in a variety of sizes. In practice, wound care providers order one or a few medicinal maggot units at a time, which means that producers require mostly small-volume cool-chain packaging solutions.

Temperature Monitoring and Field Testing of Packaging

Producers are advised to test the performance of their selected packaging before routine use and bulk purchase. This can be done easily and inexpensively with multi-use temperature data loggers [38]. Testing is as simple as sending parcels to customers using the preferred cool-chain packaging that contains i) typical consignments of medicinal maggots, ii) cool elements, and iii) a small electronic data logger that measures and records the internal temperature of the package at intervals. It is important that the data logger is not stored directly next to the cool elements but instead in close proximity to the medicinal maggot primary packaging units. Upon receipt of the consignment, the customer records the date and time of delivery, checks whether the shipped maggots are alive and active at room temperature, and returns the data logger to the producer for analysis. Such testing should be repeated periodically, especially if the producer receives complaints regarding poor-quality maggots or the therapeutic efficacy of supplied medicinal maggots.

Summary

Like most therapeutic products, medicinal maggots will need to be transported from the lab where they are produced to the point of care. If the point of care is located in the same organisation or place, demands on packaging are not so great and simple, sterile primary packaging with WHO-compliant labelling will suffice.

However, for commercial producers shipping medicinal maggots over great distances to their customers, primary packaging that permits ventilation and gas exchange while still protecting medicinal maggots from microbial contamination is required. In addition, high-performing insulated packaging is required to maintain the fragile payload at a temperature range between 6–25°C. Fortunately, there is an ever-increasing array of cool- and cold-chain packaging solutions to choose from. Commercial producers may also like to brand their products with secondary packaging which must not obstruct primary packaging air exchange. Every shipment of medicinal maggots should also be accompanied by a package insert that complements primary packaging labels with vital information about the producer and product such as indications, contraindications, treatment advice, and side-effects.

The establishment of a black market for counterfeit medicinal maggots must be avoided when maggot therapy is introduced to low- and middle-income healthcare systems. Various technologies can be adopted from the pharmaceutical industry, including tamper-proof packaging, radio frequency identification, and phone-based verification systems. Appropriate packaging technology that ensures not only product viability and safety, but also safe use of medicinal maggots once they arrive at the point of care, is a critical part of the maggot therapy supply chain. Importantly, the available packaging technology options determine which distribution systems for medicinal maggots can be established.

References

1. WHO Expert Committee on Specifications for Pharmaceutical Preparations. *Annex 9 — Guidelines on Packaging for Pharmaceutical Products.* WHO Technical Report Series, No. 902 — Thirty-sixth Report. 2002. https:// apps.who.int/iris/bitstream/handle/10665/42424/WHO_TRS_902. pdf;sequence=1.

2. Stadler, F., *Distribution Logistics*, in *A Complete Guide to Maggot Therapy: Clinical Practice, Therapeutic Principles, Production, Distribution, and Ethics*, F. Stadler (ed.). 2022, Cambridge: Open Book Publishers, pp. 363–382. https://doi.org/10.11647/OBP.0300.17.

3. Sherman, R., *Medicinal Maggot Application and Maggot Therapy Dressing Technology*, in *A Complete Guide to Maggot Therapy: Clinical Practice, Therapeutic Principles, Production, Distribution, and Ethics*, F. Stadler (ed.). 2022, Cambridge: Open Book Publishers, pp. 79–96, https://doi. org/10.11647/OBP.0300.05.

4. TGA. *Code of Practice for Tamper-evident Packaging of Therapeutic Goods. Version 2.0, May 2017.* https://www.tga.gov.au/sites/default/files/code-practice-tamper-evident-packaging-therapeutic-goods.pdf.

5. Hollein, L., et al., *Routine Quality Control of Medicines in Developing Countries: Analytical Challenges, Regulatory Infrastructures and the Prevalence of Counterfeit Medicines in Tanzania.* TrAC Trends in Analytical Chemistry 2016. 76: pp. 60–70, https://doi.org/10.1016/j.trac.2015.11.009.

6. Rotunno, R., et al., *Impact of Track and Trace Integration on Pharmaceutical Production Systems.* International Journal of Engineering Business Management, 2014. 6, 25: pp. 1–11, https://doi.org/10.5772/58934.

7. GS1, *GS1 General Specifications. The Foundational GS1 Standard that Defines How Identification Keys, Data Attributes and Barcodes Must Be Used in Business Applications. Release 17.0.1.* 2017, GS1. https://gs1it.org/content/public/58/ d7/58d73d56-ebc1-4372-b6f0-e5d7d0a5abcc/gs1_general_specifications_ v17.pdf.

8. HDMA, *HDMA Guidelines for Bar Coding in the Pharmaceutical Supply Chain.* 2011.

9. Australian Red Cross Blood Service, *The Australian Guidelines for the Labelling of Blood Components Using ISBT 128.* 2020, Australian Red Cross Blood Service. https://www.lifeblood.com.au/sites/default/

files/resource-library/2021-12/94.-ISBT128-Australian-Guidelines-V9-final-30032020.pdf.

10.   Schapranow, M.-P., et al., *Costs of Authentic Pharmaceuticals: Research on Qualitative and Quantitative Aspects of Enabling Anti-counterfeiting in RFID-aided Supply Chains*. Personal and Ubiquitous Computing, 2012. 16(3): pp. 271–289, https://doi.org/10.1007/s00779-011-0390-4.

11.   Taylor, N. *Sproxil & Orange Fight for Anti-counterfeiting Market in Kenya*. 2011.   https://www.outsourcing-pharma.com/Article/2011/10/13/Sproxil-Orange-fight-for-anti-counterfeiting-market-in-Kenya.

12.   Zadbuke, N., et al., *Recent Trends and Future of Pharmaceutical Packaging Technology*. Journal of Pharmacy & Bioallied Sciences, 2013. 5(2): pp. 98–110, https://doi.org/10.4103/0975-7406.111820.

13.   MedMagLabs. *Creating Hope in Conflict: A Humanitarian Grand Challenge*. http://medmaglabs.com/creating-hope-in-conflict/.

14.   Richards, C.S., B.W. Price, and M.H. Villet, *Thermal Ecophysiology of Seven Carrion-feeding Blowflies in Southern Africa*. Entomologia Experimentalis et Applicata, 2009. 131(1): pp. 11–19, https://doi.org/10.1111/j.1570-7458.2009.00824.x.

15.   Baer, W.S., *The Treatment of Chronic Osteomyelitis with the Maggot (Larva of the Blow Fly)*. The Journal of Bone and Joint Surgery. American Volume, 1931. 13: pp. 438–475, https://doi.org/10.1007/s11999-010-1416-3.

16.   Sherman, R.A. and F.A. Wyle, *Low-cost, Low-maintenance Rearing of Maggots in Hospitals, Clinics, and Schools*. American Journal of Tropical Medicine and Hygiene, 1996. 54(1): pp. 38–41, https://doi.org/10.4269/ajtmh.1996.54.38.

17.   Čičková, H., M. Kozánek, and P. Takáč, *Growth and Survival of Blowfly Lucilia sericata Larvae under Simulated Wound Conditions: Implications for Maggot Debridement Therapy*. Medical and Veterinary Entomology, 2015. 29(4): pp. 416–424, https://doi.org/10.1111/mve.12135.

18.   BioMonde. *Application Guide and Daily Care Plan*. 2015. http://biomonde.com/attachments/article/7/BM197_EN_03_0115.pdf.

19.   Lloyd, J., et al., *Reducing the Loss of Vaccines from Accidental Freezing in the Cold Chain: The Experience of Continuous Temperature Monitoring in Tunisia*. Vaccine, 2015. 33(7): pp. 902–907, https://doi.org/10.1016/j.vaccine.2014.10.080.

20.   Webster, J., I.M. Croteau, and J.P. Acker, *Evaluation Of The Canadian Blood Services Red Blood Cell Shipping Container*. Canadian Journal of Medical Laboratory Science, 2008. 70(5): pp. 167–176.

21.   Stadler, F. *Supply Chain Management for Maggot Debridement Therapy in Compromised Healthcare Settings*. 2018. Unpublished doctoral dissertation, Griffith University, Queensland, https://doi.org/10.25904/1912/3170.

22. Lippi, G., et al., *Suitability of a Transport Box for Blood Sample Shipment over a Long Period*. Clinical Biochemistry, 2011. 44(12): pp. 1028–1029, https://doi.org/10.1016/j.clinbiochem.2011.05.028.

23. Samant, Y., et al., *Evaluation of the Cold-chain for Oral Polio Vaccine in a Rural District of India*. Public Health Reports, 2007. 122(1): pp. 112–121, https://doi.org/10.1177/003335490712200116.

24. Obradovic, Z., et al., *The Impact of War on Vaccine Preventable Diseases*. Materia Socio-Medica, 2014. 26(6): pp. 382–384, https://doi.org/10.5455/msm.2014.26.382-384.

25. Rogie, B., Y. Berhane, and F. Bisrat, *Assessment of Cold Chain Status for Immunization in Central Ethiopia*. Ethiopian Medical Journal, 2013. 51 Suppl 1: pp. 21–29.

26. Yakum, M.N., et al., *Vaccine Storage and Cold Chain Monitoring in the North West Region of Cameroon: A Cross Sectional Study*. BMC Research Notes, 2015. 8, 145: pp. 1–7, https://doi.org/10.1186/s13104-015-1109-9.

27. Fernando, M., *An Analysis of Clinical Risks in Vaccine Transportation*. British Journal of Community Nursing, 2004. 9(10): pp. 411–415, https://dx.doi.org/10.12968/bjcn.2004.9.10.16111.

28. Mallik, S., et al., *Assessing Cold Chain Status in a Metro City of India: An Intervention Study*. African Health Sciences, 2011. 11(1): pp. 128–133 https://www.ncbi.nlm.nih.gov/pmc/articles/PMC3092313/.

29. Turner, N., A. Laws, and L. Roberts, *Assessing the Effectiveness of Cold Chain Management for Childhood Vaccines*. Journal of Primary Health Care, 2011. 3(4): pp. 278–282.

30. Forcinio, H., *Packaging Addresses Cold-Chain Requirements*. Pharmaceutical Technology Europe, 2014. 26(10): p. 54.

31. Chen, S.-I., et al., *Passive Cold Devices for Vaccine Supply Chains*. Annals of Operations Research, 2015. 230(1): pp. 87–104, https://doi.org/10.1007/s10479-013-1502-5.

32. Hartman, L.R., *Pharma Packs Sustain Temperatures and the Environment: Walmart Specialty Pharmacy's Thermal-management Shippers Maintain Temperatures, Regardless of the Weather, Are Sustainable and Cut Shipping Costs by 50 percent*, in *Packaging Digest*. 2008, UBM Canon LLC. p. 50.

33. Oke, I.A., *Management of Immunization Solid Wastes in Kano State, Nigeria*. Waste Management, 2008. 28(12): pp. 2512–2521, https://doi.org/10.1016/j.wasman.2007.11.008.

34. Patwary, M.A., W.T. O'Hare, and M.H. Sarker, *An Illicit Economy: Scavenging and Recycling of Medical Waste*. Journal of Environmental Management, 2011. 92(11): pp. 2900–2906, http://dx.doi.org/10.1016/j.jenvman.2011.06.051.

35. Sartaj, M. and R. Arabgol. *Quantitative Assessment and Statistical Analysis of Medical Waste Generation in Developing Countries: A Case Study in Ifahan*

(*Iran*). Iranian Journal of Science and Technology-Transactions of Civil Engineering 38: C2, 409–420, 2014. http://ijstc.shirazu.ac.ir/pdf_2418_92 16d0a563d024c0edad2e847dd29774.html.

36. Pelican. *Credo — Reusable Passive Thermal Packaging.* http://www.pelicanbiothermal.com/products/credo.

37. Mohan, A.M. *Study: Reusable Pharma Packs 'Greener' than Single Use.* 2013. https://www.healthcarepackaging.com/article/sustainability/reusability/study-reusable-pharma-packs-greener-single-use.

38. PATH. *Temperature Monitoring Devices: An Overview.* 2013. http://www.path.org/publications/files/TS_opt_handout_tmd_overview.pdf.

17. Distribution Logistics

Frank Stadler

Speedy delivery to the point of care and application to the wound should occur within 24–48 hours of dispatch from the production facility. Consequently, there is a need for reliable and efficient logistics infrastructure and a diversity of distribution models tailored to regional and local conditions. This chapter describes supply chain architectures and logistics solutions that can be adopted for medicinal maggots. In particular, it explores the case of a small Kenyan medicinal maggot supply chain and the wider Kenyan transport logistics infrastructure for medical commodities with similar characteristics.

Introduction

Medicinal maggots should be delivered at a transit temperature of between 6–25°C and application to the wound should occur within 24–48 hours of dispatch from the production facility [1]. These requisite conditions significantly limit the number of healthcare providers and patients that can be reached, especially in low- and middle-income countries with poor infrastructure [2]. Consequently, under current supply chain models around the world, medicinal maggots are either produced centrally and shipped to locations that can be reached within 24–48 hours with available courier services [3], or produced very close to or at the point of care, for example at a hospital or research organisation [4]. For maggot therapy to be considered a viable

https://doi.org/10.11647/OBP.0300.17

alternative to conventional wound care options and for it to become available to patients worldwide, there is a need for reliable and efficient logistics infrastructure and a diversity of distribution models tailored to regional and local conditions [2]. This chapter first describes supply chain architectures that can be adopted by medicinal maggot producers and transport service or healthcare providers to achieve this end. Key is the placement of production facilities relative to the points of care and the utilisation of technological advances from portable healthcare infrastructure to drone delivery—which is further elaborated in Chapter 18 of this book [5]. The second part of this chapter explores the case of a small Kenyan medicinal maggot supply chain and the wider Kenyan transport logistics infrastructure for medical commodities with similar characteristics. Since there is little information on maggot therapy supply chain management in the public domain [6], the Kenyan case study provides a suitable lens through which to view medicinal maggot distribution, particularly in low- and middle-income countries. Note that Chapter 15 of this book describes the establishment of a maggot therapy service in Kenya from the vantage point of the implementation team [7].

Medicinal Maggot Distribution Models

Hub-and-spokes Model

The hub-and-spokes model for distribution of goods is tried and tested. Production facilities are strategically located and supply customers that surround them. The distance over which supply takes place depends on the perishability of the goods and the logistics infrastructure that supports distribution. When visualising the geographic map of a production and distribution system as a bicycle tyre, the production facility is located at the centre (hub), connected by spokes to all the customers. These may be end-users of the supplies or wholesalers or retailers who in turn distribute the goods further. However, there are many factors that influence the location of fixed production facilities, for example, i) the distribution of customers, ii) the volume of sales per individual customer, iii) proximity to natural resources and suppliers, iv) freight costs, or v) workforce requirements. In the case of medicinal maggot production and the tight time window in which the maggots must be transported, it makes sense to co-locate with the largest market and thereby reduce distribution time and costs while increasing supply reliability.

Importantly, however, in the maggot therapy supply-chain context, it should be noted that such population centres are not necessarily the geographic centre of the serviced country or region. For example, Dar es Salaam is the most populous city in Tanzania but is located in the far-east of the country, on the shores of the Indian Ocean. Therefore, this model of medicinal maggot production and distribution relies heavily on sophisticated producer coordination, reliable logistics infrastructure, and highly efficient third-party transport service providers. For example, producers need to have convenient communication channels for customers to place orders and make enquiries. This may happen via phone, fax, email, online order forms, or e-commerce shop fronts. It is important that producers also communicate clearly to customers i) the geographic areas that can be serviced, ii) how fast deliveries can be made to a particular location, and iii) what the order placement deadlines are. Once an order has been placed, its details need to be shared with the production laboratory, which will prepare and package the requested medicinal maggots and dressing products, if they are also offered by the supplier. A third-party transport provider (courier service) is usually used to deliver the consignment to the customer. The producer has the choice to either deliver the parcels to the nearest courier service centre or let the courier come to the production facility for pickup. It is generally the responsibility of the producer to ensure that during transit the content (in this case medicinal maggots) is adequately ventilated and protected from excessive heat or cold. Couriers only take responsibility for timely and accurate delivery of the consignment.

A good example of such a functioning hub-and-spokes distribution system that is supported by advanced logistics infrastructure and third-party transport providers is that operated by Monarch Labs based in Irvine, California, USA [3]. Customers can choose from

- standard overnight (arrival by 3:30pm),

- priority overnight (arrival by 10:30am),

- first overnight (arrival by 8:30am), and

- immediate delivery via Midnight Express.

While overnight delivery using air and land transport is the standard for medicinal maggot distribution in the US and Europe, this may not be logistically feasible or financially viable for remote low- and middle-income country communities. However, it should be noted that research at the Walter Reed Army Institute of Research demonstrated that medicinal maggots can withstand vibrations and pressure changes due to airlift in rotary or fixed-wing military aircraft [8] and that 'Golden Hour Containers' for military use [9] successfully maintained red blood cells at 1–10°C during shipment and protected this payload during airlift to above 1000 ft altitude and on airdrops [10]. This suggests that medicinal maggots could also be delivered via airdrop to remote, inaccessible locations in humanitarian aid and disaster response, or in rural and remote care situations. Moreover, emergent remotely piloted aircraft systems, otherwise known as 'drones', may offer an additional flexible and cost-competitive alternative for medicinal maggot shipment to rural and remote healthcare centres and during disaster response [11]. Chapter 18 of this book is dedicated to the logistics of drone-assisted medicinal maggot delivery [5].

Airdrops and drone delivery aside, when certain regions with a demand for maggot therapy cannot be reached in a timely or economical manner, it may be necessary to set up production hubs closer to customers to ensure reliable supply (Figure 17.1). Alternatively, if remote care needs are highly localised, there is the option to co-locate small-scale production facilities at the point of care (see Point-of-care Production below).

Point-of-care Production

Production in existing clinical laboratories. Maggot therapy programmes often start out in research or clinical laboratories [12]. Commercial large-scale production only becomes viable when regulatory approvals have been obtained, health insurance reimbursement is in place, and markets for maggot therapy have been established. Non-commercial medicinal maggot production in existing research and clinical settings is mainly for in-house use or to meet limited demand from healthcare providers further afield [13].

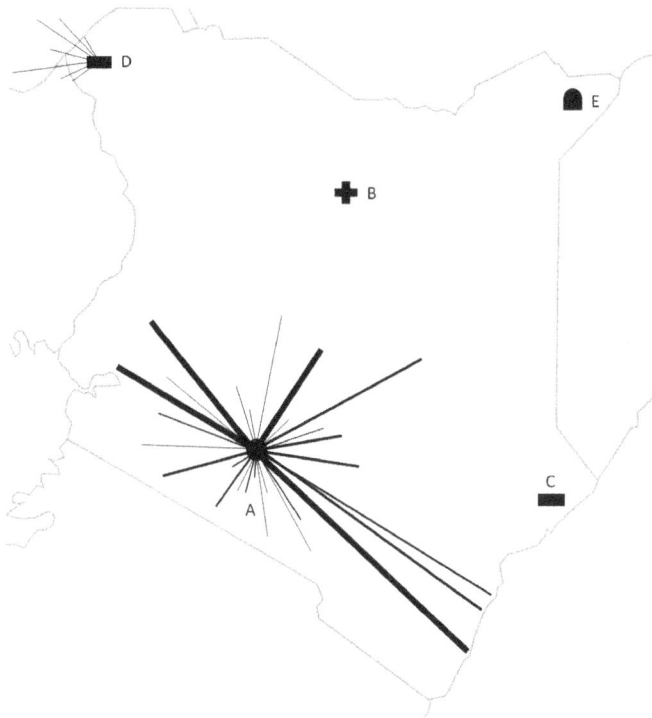

Figure 17.1 Simplified representation of medicinal maggot supply and distribution models. Kenya has been chosen for illustration purposes only. The Kenyan medicinal maggot supply chain is still in its infancy and has not progressed significantly beyond supply to few healthcare providers across greater Nairobi [7]. **A**) Hub-and-spokes model supplying medicinal maggots from Nairobi. The varying thickness of lines indicates that there would be differences in supply volume. **B**) Point-of-care supply with production integrated in healthcare facility operations. **C**) Relocatable medicinal maggot facility deployed in response to a natural disaster or other temporary healthcare crisis. **D**) Relocatable production facility supplying medicinal maggots on and off the battlefield. **E**) Isolated community operating a do-it-yourself (DIY) medicinal maggot laboratory.

Mobile production facilities. Remote locations may be serviced by means of transportable production facilities consisting of stand-alone or combined insectary and laboratory modules. For example, MedMagLabs at Griffith University, Australia have designed and built the first version of a mobile medicinal maggot laboratory (Figure 17.2). For this prototype, a standard, 20-ft-high cube shipping container was modified to house an insectary for the maintenance of medicinal fly colonies and a laboratory space for disinfection and incubation of eggs, quality control work, and packaging [14].

Mobile (relocatable) production laboratories would also facilitate maggot therapy in times of disaster and conflict when logistics infrastructure is damaged and access to the point of care is dangerous. However, the deployment of sophisticated mobile production facilities still requires initial access to the point of care. This can be achieved by pre-positioning ready-to-operate mobile systems in regions that are prone to conflict. Alternatively, mobile production facilities can be transported to the point of care via land or air, only when needed, but potentially at great cost and/or security risk. Along with the physical laboratory infrastructure, personnel will also need to be deployed, either permanently, or temporarily to train the local operators of the production facility.

Informal do-it-yourself production. There will always be communities that are too hard to reach in the aftermath of disasters, during war, or simply because of their extreme remoteness. Under austere conditions and when wound care needs are great, it is quite feasible to source medicinal fly eggs and maggots from the wild for the purpose of maggot therapy without breeding flies and producing medicinal maggots [15, 16]. However, it is better to provide isolated communities with the guidance to establish and permanently run small-scale medicinal maggot production laboratories with local resources. This would ensure a greater level of quality control and supply security. Such guidance has been developed by MedMagLabs. The research group translated evidence-based treatment guidance and medicinal maggot production know-how from the literature into easy-to-understand, highly illustrated, multilingual, and user-tested Treatment and Production Manuals [14]. The aim was to ensure the performance, safety, and user-friendliness of solutions. While DIY medicinal maggot production has its place, there remains the risk of adverse outcomes due to poor operation or treatment by lay-producers and -carers. Therefore, it is important that DIY medicinal maggot production and maggot therapy is reserved for austere environments and collapsed healthcare systems. In healthcare settings with adequate resources and functioning governance, medicinal maggots must be produced and maggot therapy performed under regulatory and expert clinical supervision.

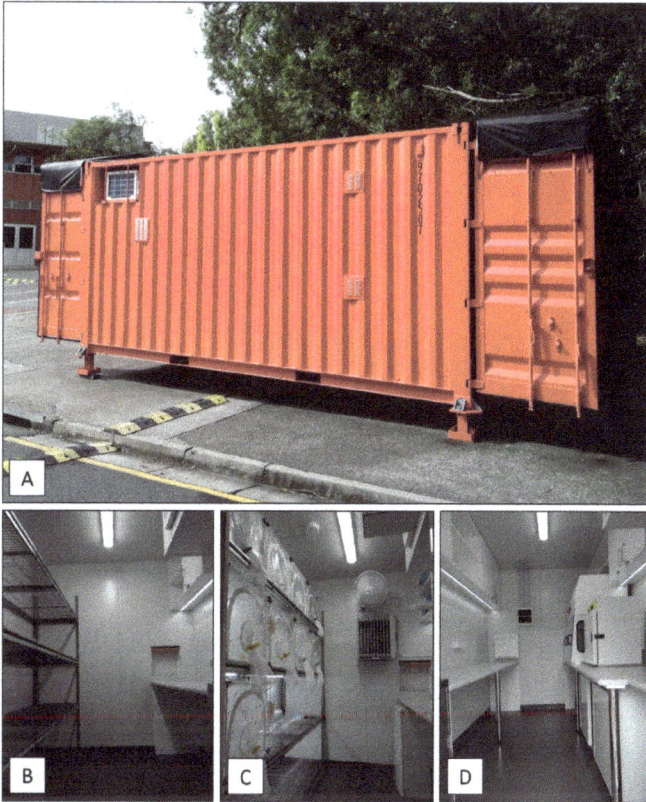

Figure 17.2 A converted shipping container laboratory for the production of medicinal maggots. A) Full side view of laboratory at Griffith University, Australia. B) Insectary room with separate access door and a pass-through hatch for transfer of specimens to the lab. C) Modified insectary, partially stocked with fly cages. D) Laboratory room equipped with a laminar flow cabinet, an incubator, fridge, freezer and sink. Photos by F. Stadler, MedMagLabs and Creating Hope in Conflict: A Humanitarian Grand Challenge, CC BY-ND.

Lessons from Kenya and Other Low- and Middle-income Countries

Thanks to modern logistics infrastructure and sophisticated third-party transport providers, the distribution of medicinal maggots in high-income countries is relatively straightforward and reliable. However, even for developed economies with a large land mass and remote communities like Australia, timely distribution to all parts of the country is still not technically or economically feasible. Therefore, operational and reliable distribution logistics are of critical importance to producers and wound care practitioners in low- and middle-income countries, or those wanting to service rural or remote communities at the margins of advanced economies. Learnings from a fledgling maggot therapy programme in Kenya provide some helpful insights regarding the management of medicinal maggot distribution in low- and middle-income country settings. This Kenyan case study is based on the findings of a qualitative research study which, for privacy reasons, was required to anonymise participants and relevant organisations [4]. What is important, however, is the overall picture of the distribution logistics environment in relation to medicinal maggots.

The logistics landscape in Kenya and other low- and middle-income countries is far more diverse than in high-income countries. For example, in Kenya, there are a multitude of operators from multinationals such as DHL to larger local companies like Fargo Couriers, and last-mile delivery is often provided by owner-driver motorbike taxis or coach and town bus services. The challenge for medicinal maggot producers will be to partner with a few larger reliable service providers for day-to-day transfers to the main distribution nodes in major population centres, but then to utilise unconventional providers of transport and courier services for last-mile delivery where the larger players cannot or will not deliver for technical or security reasons.

Kenyan courier service operators have become highly sophisticated in fleet management, network planning, contingency management, and consignment tracking. For example, one local courier company specialises in overnight and same-day delivery services covering all major towns. The product range offered includes Overnight Courier Service, Priority Overnight Courier Service, Same Day Express Delivery Service, One Hour Delivery Service, insurance, warehousing and distribution, and document archiving. About 200 vehicles are in service including motorbikes, closed pickups and two- to ten-ton cargo trucks. As of 2016, the company employed 950 trained staff in 176 locations across 38 Kenyan counties. Each location has its own workforce and fleet. Regional management consists of an area manager, branch managers, supervisors, hub managers, and courier drivers or riders.

A sign of progress made in transport service provision in Kenya is the presence of an advanced online marketplace. Kenya has well-developed Internet shopping supported by M-Pesa, a phone-based money transfer technology. An online search revealed that there are numerous online retailers operating in Kenya such as Jumia, Kilimall, Mimi, Jumia Market, Cheki, Chinabuy, VituMob, etc. Many also access international United Kingdom, United States, and Chinese online retail offerings [17]. To support this Internet shopping, there is a system of fast courier services in place that reach the remotest communities.

In the healthcare space, consumers who can afford it can order medicines remotely from a chemist and have them couriered to their home. The order is placed by phone then the chemist rings back with the price including cost of courier transport. The customer pays via M-Pesa, after which the chemist sends the package per overnight courier for arrival the next day.

When asked to envisage the delivery of a medicinal maggot consignment from Nairobi to a healthcare facility in Siaya County, the abovementioned courier company described the following schedule:

- The medicinal maggot producer books a courier on the day of pickup and collection takes place before 5 p.m.

- Usually, a waybill is raised and the customer pays for delivery in cash at pick-up. However, contract customers receive an invoice and pay within 30 days.

- The courier takes the consignment to the main hub in Nairobi. There, further verification and documentation takes place.

- Dispatch to Kisumu, a regional hub, occurs the same night and the consignment arrives at 5:30 am the next morning.

- Sorting of consignments and loading onto trucks destined for Siaya takes about 30 to 45 minutes from arrival in Kisumu.

- From Siaya office, last mile delivery to the healthcare provider takes place within one hour and, at worst, by 1:30 pm.

- The receiving healthcare provider signs Proof of Delivery.

The same courier company also provides reverse logistics services, which is relevant to maggot therapy supply chains because producers may decide to use reusable cool chain shipping boxes for environmental and economic reasons as discussed in Chapter 16 [18]. In the case of medicinal maggot distribution, the reverse logistics service would play out as follows:

- A courier collects a medicinal maggot consignment packaged in a reusable shipper and delivers it to a healthcare facility as described above.

- Once the goods have been delivered, there are three alternatives for collection and return of reusable packaging items.

  - If the consignment is processed within 15 minutes, it is feasible for the courier to wait for the return freight.

  - If it takes longer than 15 minutes to unpack the medicinal maggots, the courier drops off the consignment in the morning and picks up the packaging in the afternoon.

  - Alternatively, the courier delivers the medicinal maggot consignment one day and picks up the packaging another day after notification by the client.

It appears that the Kenyan medicinal maggot producer has not yet utilised these courier distribution options but an example of already practiced reverse logistics in healthcare is the pathology supply chain. Specimens are collected from hospitals and clinics and transported to a hub where they are placed in multi-use cooler boxes. These specimens are then shipped either by bus or courier to a pathology laboratory. The cooler boxes are then sent back to the collection hub.

In 2016, the Communications Authority of Kenya published guidelines for courier and postal operators to improve and promote e-commerce [19]. These guidelines require measures such as tracking and insurance for high-risk items like lab samples, specimens, and medicines [20]. Companies who adopted such systems benefit from improved efficiency and customer confidence. The automated tracking of shipments provides accurate performance details which means that deviations are captured, followed up and corrective action can be taken. Medicinal maggot producers seeking to engage courier companies in low- and middle-income countries should also enquire whether the courier has a Business Continuity Plan in place that outlines the measures to be taken in the event of service failure (e.g. blocked roads due to rains and floods, or riots and civil unrest).

Transport costs can be as much or more than the actual costs of medicinal maggots. Therefore, it is important to patients who pay out of pocket (in the absence of health insurance cover for maggot therapy) that cost effective transport options are provided that also satisfy safety and reliability expectations. The courier delivery of a medicinal maggot consignment weighing no more than 5 kg from Nairobi to a hospital in Siaya County would cost in the order of KES850 (USD8.40) plus Value Added Tax (16%). According to a healthcare consumer living in Gilgil, 120 km from Nairobi, an overnight courier delivery of medicines costs KES230 (USD2.30). For high-income healthcare consumers these costs appear negligible, but they are prohibitive for many Kenyans living on less than the average yearly income (2018) of around KES727,000 or USD7,197 [21].

Formal Healthcare Supply Chains

The vaccine and blood supply chain. The acceptable temperature range for medicinal maggots in transit, and short-term storage ahead of maggot therapy, overlaps with that of many heat- and freeze-sensitive vaccines, which must be stored at all times between 2°C and 8°C [22], and red blood cell products which must be stored between 1°C and 10°C [23]. Thus, the management of vaccine and blood supply chains faces the same challenges as medicinal maggot distribution, and it may well be possible to utilise these existing cold and cool chains for the distribution of medicinal maggots. For example, the Kenya National Blood Transfusion Service collects, tests, processes, and distributes blood to all transfusing healthcare facilities across Kenya. They use a range of transport options for blood and blood products that are shipped between 21 satellite blood collection centres, the 6 Regional Blood Transfusion Centres and the transfusing hospitals, including ambulances, motorcycles, and public transport. Their cold chain utilises modern equipment such as reliable fridges and cooler boxes and is capable of maintaining a safe cool chain for blood products [24].

It is important to note that the vaccine and blood supply chains have more distribution points than the maggot therapy supply chain can afford because both commodities can be stored for longer than medicinal maggots [25] which must be delivered directly from producer to treating health centre within 24 to 48 hours. Moreover, temperature control in vaccine and blood supply chains can be unreliable in both developed and developing regions [e.g. 26]. Ineffective refrigeration with temperatures rising beyond recommended levels has been observed for blood product shipping containers [23]. However, this would not be a significant issue for medicinal maggots with a tolerable temperature range of up to 25°C in transit. Accidental freezing of vaccines, however, is a serious problem and such temperature extremes would be lethal to medicinal maggots. It appears that temperature management in vaccine supply chains fails because i) healthcare workers are insufficiently trained, and/or ii) storage and transport equipment is inadequate, and/or iii) there is an unreliable power supply, or other disruptions to refrigeration equipment [27]. Improved training, education, systems and standards, and implementation of equipment upgrades can lead to significant improvements in cold/cool chain management [28]. In summary, there is much to be learned from the management of vaccine and blood supply chains. Indeed, there is scope for medicinal maggot supply integration provided that the supply chain infrastructure and services that are used meet, or can be modified to meet, medicinal maggot distribution requirements.

Medical goods suppliers. Both faith-based (operated by religious groups) and public health supply organisations, such as the Mission for Essential Drugs and Supplies (MEDS) in Kenya or the Kenya Medical Supplies Authority (KEMSA), respectively, may offer unique distribution partnership opportunities for medicinal maggot producers in low- and middle-income countries. A typical pharmaceutical purchase from MEDS by a faith-based hospital takes place as follows:

- The pharmacist orders via email.
- MEDS provides a quotation.
- The hospital confirms the purchase and pays with bank cheque. Account processing takes three days and hospitals follow up on payment by phone. While M-Pesa payments would speed up orders, this is usually reserved for small purchases. Larger-volume and higher-value purchases are made with a bank cheque.

- It takes one week from order to delivery by MEDS or a courier.

This is how the procurement process with KEMSA works [29]:

- The healthcare facility orders online using the KEMSA Logistics Management Information System.

- Transport is coordinated and Expected Time of Arrival determined.

- Customer Service representatives communicate shipment status and Expected Time of Arrival to the facility.

- Upon delivery the completeness of the delivery is checked, and Proof of Delivery is confirmed.

- Invoicing occurs after Proof of Delivery is confirmed.

It is important to note that for immediate or next-day needs, both faith-based and public healthcare providers buy from private pharmacies that are often located close to healthcare facilities. Moreover, in the event of stockouts and if medical products recommended by doctors are not typically stocked by the facility, patients routinely purchase these items themselves from a nearby pharmacy. This indicates that the public and faith-based health systems permit the procurement of medicinal maggots directly from private suppliers. Of course, this assumes affordability of the treatment.

Whether faith-based, government, or private pharma suppliers and their medical supply-chain logistics are suitable for the distribution of medicinal maggots remains to be explored and tested. The necessity for rapid distribution of highly perishable medicinal maggots is likely to prohibit wholesale supply of medicinal maggots to pharma distributors.

Informal Supply Chains

The informal sector in Kenya and other low and middle income countries exhibits some of the most inventive supply-chain solutions and these should not be ignored when designing and managing last-mile delivery of medicinal maggots. In Kenya, matatu minibus drivers are happy to deliver parcels at the cost of a bus fare. The driver rings the recipient of the delivery shortly before passing by a convenient stop where she then waits for the bus to pick up the parcel. Although cheaper than ordinary courier services, safe delivery is not guaranteed by either the sender or the matatu driver, and the loss of a consignment is not reimbursed. The motorbike taxi is a common sight in Kenya and across the developing world. Although dangerous, it is a cheap and convenient way to transport people and goods especially where road infrastructure is poor and urban streets are chaotically congested. Where road infrastructure is poor, delivery of consignments is locally subcontracted to motorbike taxis, and goods may even be delivered by boat and oxen- or donkey-pulled carts.

There is one informal supply chain that illustrates more than any other the capacity of transport operators in low- and middle-income countries to deliver highly perishable goods in a timely manner. Miraa is a plant whose leaves have narcotic properties and are chewed recreationally across the region. The leaves need to be kept fresh, not too cold and not too hot, and consumed within 24 to 48 hours from harvest, and therefore the supply-chain demands are similar to those for medicinal maggots. Miraa is grown in central Kenya but a speedy supply network extends across East Africa, into troubled Somalia, and even across the sea to Europe, the United States, and Australia [30]. Delivering Miraa is not for the faint-hearted as it involves risky driving, speeding, and frequent accidents. While this makes the Miraa supply chain unsuitable for medicinal maggot distribution, it illustrates that, if operators are sufficiently motivated, supply chains can be highly effective even under the most trying circumstances. The challenge is to learn from reliable formal and informal transport service providers when designing and operating medicinal maggot supply chains in Kenya and other low- and middle-income countries.

Regulations and Guidelines

Activities related to the distribution of medicinal maggots may well be regulated in a particular jurisdiction and this needs to be considered. For example, the production, trade, transport, and use of medicines and other medical products in Kenya is governed by the Ministry of Health. The Pharmacy and Poisons Board is the regulatory and licencing authority for producers, traders, distributors, and prescribers of medicines, as well as for practitioners. Licenced distributors are expected to comply with the Guidelines for Good Distribution Practice, which specifies fleet characteristics, as well as the effective, efficient and safe handling, storage and distribution of such products [31]. Given that medicinal maggots are medicinal goods, their distribution will need to comply with these and other relevant Pharmacy and Poisons Board rules, regulations, and guidelines.

The presence of a seemingly comprehensive regulatory framework is not a guarantee of compliance by transport service providers. Maggot therapy supply chain coordinators (usually the producer organisation) must, therefore, monitor the delivery progress and the environmental conditions during delivery to be certain of the safety and efficacy of medicinal maggots destined for treatment. Producers should only engage third-party transport providers that offer parcel tracking, which means that the delivery progress can be followed online by both the customer and producer, and problems with delivery can be quickly identified, investigated, and rectified. Critical to safe delivery of medicinal maggots is not only the speed of delivery but also the temperature during transit. The ideal transit temperature range of between 6–25°C for the period of shipment should be tested at least for frequent and representative delivery routes and during different seasons (e.g. summer/winter or dry/wet). It is possible to monitor transport temperatures inside cool- and cold-chain shippers either routinely or sporadically with modern temperature monitoring systems such as electronic data loggers. These are highly accurate and can record the payload temperature throughout the shipment period [32]. This is particularly necessary where last-mile service providers need to be engaged and regular parcel tracking may or may not be facilitated. See also Chapter 16 for guidance on temperature monitoring [18].

Summary

Medicinal maggots require distribution logistics solutions that consider the fragility of the medical commodity being transported and the transport infrastructure connecting the producer and healthcare providers. Physical distance between them is of secondary importance. Consignments may be delivered faster across continents thanks to air transport than over the last mile to much closer healthcare clinics. It is therefore important that the supply chain for maggot therapy adapts to the circumstances, and supply models are developed that ensure reliable and timely delivery of medicinal maggots to where there is demand for maggot therapy.

In the hub-and-spokes model producers supply medicinal maggots to many healthcare providers within timely and economical reach depending on the distribution options available. If reliable distribution to healthcare facilities cannot be achieved but demand exists, production can be geographically or indeed institutionally co-located with these healthcare settings. Point-of-care production facilities have generally been established and operated out of existing laboratories in research organisations and hospitals. However, in the case of severely compromised healthcare settings, such as when disasters strike or during war, there is also an opportunity to support maggot therapy with relocatable production facilities and with guidance for isolated communities to establish and operate their own small-scale medicinal-maggot and maggot-therapy programme with local resources.

Finally, the exploration of a Kenyan fledgling maggot therapy supply chain and the wider Kenyan supply chain for similar medical goods gives reason for optimism. Third-party transport providers continuously improve their capacity and capability due to governmental guidance and the rapid growth of phone-based payment and e-commerce. Although last-mile and remote-area delivery of goods remains a challenge, producers should consider utilising the informal transport sector where it exists. There are also opportunities for medicinal maggot producers to partner with other public health supply chains such as vaccination programmes or blood transfusion services as they share the need for reliable and safe temperature-controlled transport of medical commodities.

References

1.　Čičková, H., M. Kozánek, and P. Takáč, *Growth and Survival of Blowfly Lucilia sericata Larvae under Simulated Wound Conditions: Implications for Maggot Debridement Therapy*. Medical and Veterinary Entomology, 2015. 29(4): pp. 416–424, https://doi.org/10.1111/mve.12135.

2. Roy, D. and R. Sherman, *Commnetary: Why Is Maggot Therapy Not More Commonly Practiced in India?* Medical Journal of Dr. D.Y. Patil University, 2014. 7(5): pp. 642–643.

3. Monarch Labs. *Order Form*. 2019. https://www.monarchlabs.com/Monarch-Labs-Order-Form.pdf.

4. Stadler, F. *Supply Chain Management for Maggot Debridement Therapy in Compromised Healthcare Settings*. 2018. Unpublished doctoral dissertation, Griffith University, Queensland, https://doi.org/10.25904/1912/3170.

5. Stadler, F. and P. Tatham, *Drone-assisted Medicinal Maggot Distribution in Compromised Healthcare Settings*, in *A Complete Guide to Maggot Therapy: Clinical Practice, Therapeutic Principles, Production, Distribution, and Ethics*, F. Stadler (ed.). 2022, Cambridge: Open Book Publishers, pp. 383–402, https://doi.org/10.11647/OBP.0300.18.

6. Stadler, F., *The Maggot Therapy Supply Chain: A Review of the Literature and Practice*. Med Vet Entomol, 2020. 34(1): pp. 1–9, https://doi.org/10.1111/mve.12397.

7. Takáč, P., F. Stadler, et al., *Establishment of a Medicinal Maggot Production Facility and Treatment Programme in Kenya*, in *A Complete Guide to Maggot Therapy: Clinical Practice, Therapeutic Principles, Production, Distribution, and Ethics*, F. Stadler (ed.). 2022, Cambridge: Open Book Publishers, pp. 289–330, https://doi.org/10.11647/OBP.0300.14.

8. Peck, G., et al., *Airworthiness Testing of Mecial Maggots*. Military Medicine, 2015. 180(5): pp. 591–596, https://doi.org/10.7205/MILMED-D-14-00548.

9. Pelican BioThermal. *CRĒDO™ Medic Pack Military/Government Solutions — Original Golden Hour® Container*. 2015. http://pelicanbiothermal.com/products/credo-medic-pack-militarygovernment-solutions-original-golden-hour-container.

10. Macdonald, V.W., et al., *New Containers Allow Shipment and Precision Airdrop Delivery of Viable Red Blood Cells*. Transfusion, 2005. 45(3): p. 79A.

11. Tatham, P., et al., *Flying Maggots: A Smart Logistic Solution to an Enduring Medical Challenge*. Journal of Humanitarian Logistics and Supply Chain Management, 2017. 7(2): pp. 172–193, https://dx.doi.org/10.1108/JHLSCM-02-2017-0003.

12. Kruglikova, A.A., and S.I. Chernysh, *Surgical Maggots and the History of Their Medical Use*. Entomological Review, 2013. 93(6): pp. 667–674, https://doi.org/10.1134/S0013873813060018.

13. Geary, M.J., A. Smith, and R.C. Russell, *Maggots Down Under*. Wound Practice & Research, 2009. 17(1): pp. 36–42, https://www.awma.com.au/files/journal/1701_04.pdf.

14. MedMagLabs. *Creating Hope in Conflict: A Humanitarian Grand Challenge*. 2021. http://medmaglabs.com/creating-hope-in-conflict/.

15. Sherman, R.A. and M.R. Hetzler, *Maggot Therapy for Wound Care in Austere Environments*. Journal of Special Operations Medicine, 2017. 17(2): pp. 154–162.

16. US Army, *ST 31–91B US Army Special Forces Medical Handbook*. 1982: United States Army Institute for Military Assistance.

17. kiqwaireset. *20+ Online Shopping Sites in Kenya*. 2016. https://theazania.com/list-online-shopping-sites-kenya/.

18. Stadler, F., *Packaging Technology*, in *A Complete Guide to Maggot Therapy: Clinical Practice, Therapeutic Principles, Production, Distribution, and Ethics*, F. Stadler (ed.). 2022, Cambridge: Open Book Publishers, pp. 349–362, https://doi.org/10.11647/OBP.0300.16.

19. Ochieng', L. *Communications Authority Sets New Guidelines for Courier Firms*. 2016. https://www.nation.co.ke/business/-CA-orders-courier-and-postal-firms/996-3056714-f2a0fh/index.html.

20. Communications Authority of Kenya. *Guidelines For Postal And Courier Licensees On Promotion Of E-Commerce*. 2015. https://ca.go.ke/wp-content/uploads/2018/02/Guidelines-For-Postal-And-Courier-Licensees-On-Promotion-Of-E-Commerce-1.pdf.

21. CEIC. *Kenya Average Wage Earnings*. https://www.ceicdata.com/en/kenya/average-wage-earnings-by-sector-and-industry-international-standard-of-industrial-classification-rev-4/average-wage-earnings.

22. Lloyd, J., et al., *Reducing the Loss of Vaccines from Accidental Freezing in the Cold Chain: The Experience of Continuous Temperature Monitoring in Tunisia*. Vaccine, 2015. 33(7): pp. 902–907, https://doi.org/10.1016/j.vaccine.2014.10.080.

23. Webster, J., I.M. Croteau, and J.P. Acker, *Evaluation Of The Canadian Blood Services Red Blood Cell Shipping Container*. Canadian Journal of Medical Laboratory Science, 2008. 70(5): pp. 167–176.

24. KNBTS. *Who We Are*. https://nbtskenya.or.ke/about-us/.

25. Yadav, P., et al., *Integration of Vaccine Supply Chains with Other Health Commodity Supply Chains: A Framework for Decision Making*. Vaccine, 2014. 32(50): pp. 6725–6732, https://doi.org/10.1016/j.vaccine.2014.10.001.

26. Murhekar, M.V., et al., *Frequent Exposure to Suboptimal Temperatures in Vaccine Cold-chain System in India: Results of Temperature Monitoring in 10 States*. Bulletin Of The World Health Organization, 2013. 91(12): pp. 906–913, https://doi.org/10.2471/BLT.13.119974.

27. Samant, Y., et al., *Evaluation of the Cold-chain for Oral Polio Vaccine in a Rural District of India*. Public Health Reports, 2007. 122(1): pp. 112–121, https://doi.org/10.1177/003335490712200116.

28. Turner, N., A. Laws, and L. Roberts, *Assessing the Effectiveness of Cold Chain Management for Childhood Vaccines.* Journal of Primary Health Care, 2011. 3(4): pp. 278–282.

29. KEMSA. *Distribution.* http://www.kemsa.co.ke/distribution/.

30. Carrier, N.C.M., *Kenyan Khat: The Social Life of a Stimulant.* 2007, Boston; Leiden: Brill.

31. Pharmacy and Poisons Board, *Guidelines for Good Distribution Practices for Medical Products and Health Technologies in Kenya.* 2022, Republic of Kenya. https://web.pharmacyboardkenya.org/download/guidelines-for-good-distribution-practices-for-medical-products-and-health-technologies-in-kenya/.

32. McColloster, P. and C. Vallbona, *Graphic-output Temperature Data Loggers for Monitoring Vaccine Refrigeration: Implications for Pertussis.* American Journal of Public Health, 2011. 101(1): pp. 46–47, https://doi.org/10.2105/AJPH.2009.179853.

18. Drone-assisted Medicinal Maggot Distribution in Compromised Healthcare Settings

Frank Stadler and Peter Tatham

Timely delivery of medicinal maggots is challenging when logistics infrastructure is poor due to underinvestment or disaster-related destruction of roads, bridges and railway lines. Unmanned Aerial Vehicles, commonly known as 'drones', are much cheaper to procure and operate than planes and helicopters and can overfly the areas where roads or railway lines are impassable. This chapter provides a brief profile of current drone technology, and explores drone service design considerations in relation to medicinal maggot distribution. It also presents case examples of drone technologies that could be used for medicinal maggot distribution, and provides guidance for the implementation of drone-assisted medicinal maggot distribution.

Introduction

There is a particular logistic challenge in the administration of maggot therapy because medicinal maggots need to be transferred from the laboratory in which they are produced to the patient within 24–48 hours. In addition, they need to be kept at a temperature of between 6 and 25°C to maintain their health and vigour and, therefore, their therapeutic efficacy [1]. With these constraints in mind, Chapter 17 discusses

https://doi.org/10.11647/OBP.0300.18

various options that exist for the distribution of medicinal maggots in compromised healthcare settings [2]. The concept of drone-assisted transport was briefly mentioned but it warrants greater attention in this dedicated chapter in light of the ever-increasing application of drone technology in the humanitarian setting.

In low- and middle-income countries or in the aftermath of a disaster, distribution of perishable medical goods can present a significant challenge when fast distribution of goods is hindered by poor infrastructure due to underinvestment or disaster-related destruction of roads, bridges and railway lines, and associated communication systems. Although these distribution challenges can often be overcome with aerial transport using helicopters or aeroplanes, these are expensive to procure and operate, especially if they were to be employed to distribute only medicinal maggots. Furthermore, during disasters there are multiple competing demands for helicopters and planes and it is therefore unlikely that the transport of medicinal maggots will be considered a high priority. By contrast, 'drones'—also known as Remotely Piloted Aircraft Systems (RPAS) or Unmanned Aerial Vehicles (UAVs)—are much cheaper to procure and operate and, like planes and helicopters, can overfly the areas where roads or railway lines are impassable. Drones are frequently used by military forces for both surveillance or attack but are increasingly employed in non-military contexts including: the structural evaluation of buildings [3], the provision of aerial surveillance and mapping [4], and fire detection [5]. There is also a growing realisation in the military and civilian context that drones can deliver rapid pre-hospital medical care and medical supplies from a distance whether that be in war, in times of disaster, or to provide development aid [6, 7]. Pre-hospital applications of drone technology are being developed for i) search and rescue, ii) resuscitation and telemedicine, iii) damage assessment and response coordination, iv) medical evacuation, and v) medical supplies delivery [6, 8, 9]. Thus, although there is great potential for the use of drones to transport medicinal maggots to inaccessible healthcare settings, to date this mode of transport has not been utilised. This chapter therefore aims to encourage maggot therapy supply chain managers to consider drone-assisted distribution of medicinal maggots. In doing so it offers:

1. a brief profile of current drone technology,

2. an exploration of drone service design considerations and how they apply to medicinal maggot distribution,

3. case examples of drone technologies that could be used for medicinal maggot distribution, and

4. points to bear in mind when considering implementation of drone-assisted medicinal maggot distribution.

Please note that the information provided in this chapter may well be out of date by the time it is published. Such is the speed of development in this field of transport logistics. However, the main aim of this introduction to drone-assisted medicinal maggot distribution is to convey an appreciation for the opportunities of drone transport and to sensitise supply chain partners to the issues that need to be considered.

Drones and Their Capabilities

According to the United Nations Office for the Coordination of Humanitarian Affairs [10] (UNOCHA) drones are becoming relatively commonplace, with 270 companies in 57 countries reported as manufacturing such aircraft in 2014 [10], figures that have undoubtedly increased since then. Furthermore, it has been estimated that annual sales of drones will surpass US$12 billion in 2021, which reflects a compound annual growth rate of 7.6% from the US$8.5 billion recorded in 2016 [11]. Having said this, it must be appreciated that there are significant capability differences between various classes of drones—in particular in respect of their endurance, speed, payload and normal operating altitude.

In essence, drones range from small rotary-wing platforms that cost around USD4,000 [12] to high-end aeroplanes such as the USAF Global Hawk, which is the size of a small executive jet and has a unit cost of USD130M [13]. However, their generic features include the ability to be flown by an operator who remains on the ground at a distance from the aircraft itself, together with a payload that can include video or still cameras, or items such as equipment or medicines (for example, medicinal maggots). Such drones can use either fixed or rotary wings and are powered by battery or fuel-driven engines—as a result their endurance varies from minutes to hours.

Short Range

The most prevalent type of drones (both in terms of numbers sold and the quantity of different platforms available) is the relatively short-range aircraft that is battery-powered and utilises four rotor blades to provide the vertical and horizontal movement. Such quadcopters are perceived to have particular promise in the context of providing a transport medium for medicinal maggots as they are extremely easily moved to the desired operational location and can carry a respectable payload given (as will be discussed further below) the relatively light weight of maggots and their associated packaging. They are able to fly Beyond Visual Line of Sight (BVLOS), and also represent an area where significant research and development is being undertaken. For example, between them, Amazon and Walmart have registered 153 new drone patents in the period July 2018–June 2019, whilst over 9,000 patents exist across the world as of June 2019. Examples of such drones are to be found in Table 18.1.

Table 18.1 Examples of the payload/endurance of short-range drones [14, 15].

Model	Maximum Payload	Endurance
DJI MATRICE 100	3.6 kg	40 min
DJI MATRICE 600	6.0 kg	16 min
DJI S1000	6.8 kg	15 min
Tarot-T18	8.0 kg	20 min
DJI S900	8.2 kg	18 min
FREEFLY ALTA 8	9.0 kg	16 min
DJI Agras MG-1	10.0 kg	24 min
ONYXSTAR HYDRA-12	12.0 kg	30 min
AZ 4K UHD	20.0 kg	20 min

Short-range drones for humanitarian missions. The Humanitarian UAV Network (UAViators, www.uaviators.org) is a community of practitioners with the mission to promote the safe, coordinated and effective use of drones for data collection and cargo delivery in humanitarian and development settings. They have collated information on drone trials for humanitarian missions which mainly used short range aircraft to provide commodities to either remote communities or those impacted by disasters [16]. What is particularly beneficial to humanitarian operations is the ability of these drones to fly in the aftermath of floods (for example those which devastated Mozambique in 2019) or earthquakes (as was the case in the 2015 disaster in Nepal), directly from their base to the location of need. However, the relatively short range of these small, low-cost aircraft is a challenge, albeit one that is slowly being overcome by a general increase in endurance found in the most recent drones emerging on the market.

Medium-/long-range drones. In contrast to the short-range drones described above, some longer-range platforms are also available. These carry a similar payload to the short-range variants but have a considerably longer endurance. This can be utilised either by flying significantly greater distances or by 'loitering' in an area until it is appropriate to transfer their payload. Some examples of such drones are offered in Table 18.2, and it will be noted that these can launch/land either in a similar way to a regular aircraft (fixed-wing models) or vertically (hybrid fixed-wing/rotary mimicking a helicopter). The former requires the drone to be launched either by a mechanical catapult or from the roof of a specially modified moving vehicle, and to land either on a relatively flat surface of several hundred metres in length or be caught by a net or line-and-hook system as employed by Zipline (www.flyzipline.com). Thus, both the land and launch systems needed for such drones require pre-positioning of the necessary equipment.

Zipline drones are launched by a catapult system which reduces the drain on the drone's battery in the initial phase and results in an operational radius of some 80 km with a payload of up to 1.8 kg. On reaching the destination, the payload is despatched to the ground by means of a parachute. On return from a delivery, the drones are snagged by a wire stretched between two masts and physically land on a large inflatable mattress or come to rest suspended on the wire system. This is a unidirectional distribution strategy which results in a hub-and-spokes transport network structure where drone distribution centres (launch and landing facilities) are co-located with medical warehouses.

It does not permit bi-directional transport of cargo. Nevertheless, at its maximum capacity, a 30-drone system as has been deployed in Ghana is capable of moving up to 1,000 kg/day [17].

By contrast, drones that operate using vertical take-off and landing mechanisms typically have a reduced flying speed (and, hence, range) but are less constrained in terms of their operations as they require only a launch/land zone of 5 m in diameter. The Wingcopter (www.wingcopter.com) and Swoop Aero (www.swoop.aero) drone models have been developed for medical supply-chain applications among other uses [18, 19, 20]. Both have rotor systems that allow the drones to launch vertically and fly in forward motion. For delivery purposes, the Wingcopter 198 can deliver three separate packages with a total weight of 5 kg to different locations within a range of 75 km per flight [19]. The latest Swoop Aero platform Kite™ (Figure 18.1) can transport 3 kg of supplies over a distance of 175 km, or 5 kgs over a distance of 130 km, all at a speed of up to 200 km per hour [21].

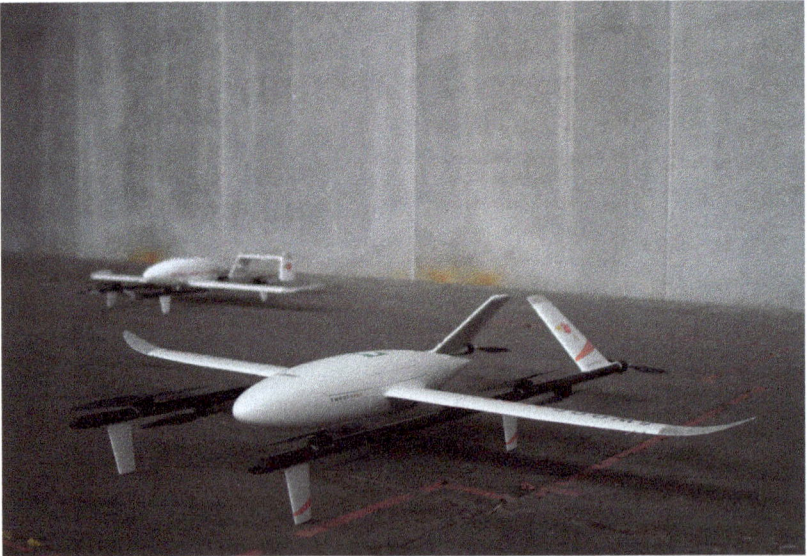

Figure 18.1 The Kite™ drone from Swoop Aero for medium-range deliveries. Photo: © Swoop Aero.

Table 18.2 Exemplar Medium-/Long Range Drone Key Performance
Data [19, 22–24].

	Wingcopter	Latitude HQ 160B	Aerosonde Mk 4.7	Boeing Insitu Scaneagle
Endurance	2.5 hrs	15 hrs	14+ hrs	24+ hours
Cruising Speed	40 km/h	65 km/h	90–110 km/h	90–110 km/h
Ceiling	5,000 m	6,200 m	4,570 m	4,500 m
Wingspan	1.78 m	3.81 m	3.6 m	3.11 m
Overall Length	1.32 m	2.44 m	1.7 m	1.7 m
Max. Gross Take-Off Weight	17 kg	53 kg	36.4 kg	22 kg
Max. Payload Weight	6.0 kg	9.97 kg	9.1 kg	3.4 kg

Longer-range drones would appear to be particularly suited to deployment in the aftermath of disasters such as the two major cyclones that struck Vanuatu in 2015 and Fiji in 2016. For example, they can capture video or photographs of the impacted regions, fly geo-stationary and mimic the action of a cell phone tower, and survey resupply routes to see if these have been compromised by fallen trees, broken bridges, etc. In addition, they can deliver cargo payloads to the disaster-affected area [25].

In summary, drones are highly-suited to the delivery of medical supplies because of their ability to fly directly to the point of care such as a remote healthcare clinic or a field hospital, and because of their relative cheapness when compared to helicopters/fixed-wing aircraft. In addition, as unmanned modes of transport, they do not endanger logistic workers if isolated communities affected by unrest and armed conflict require medical supplies.

However, if it is envisaged that drones will be employed to transport materiel to those in in need, a key decision that needs to be addressed is whether to operate with a short-range drone that costs in the order of US$4,000 versus a long-range drone such as the Aerosonde Mk4.7 (see Table 18.2) which in 2014 cost some US$100,000 [26]. Applied to the delivery of medicinal maggots for maggot therapy, the response to this question will depend on the locations of the medical facilities and the presence/absence of alternatives that would allow the timely and cost-effective provision of medical supplies [27].

In practice, however, the use of drones in a medical delivery role has, to date, been largely limited to short-range micro or mini variants. Whilst such micro/mini drones can provide significant benefit to the responding agencies (and, hence, the affected populations), their endurance is typically less than 30–40 minutes with a payload, in most cases, of less than 10 kg (see Table 18.1). Thus, such systems have a limited capability when required to transit significant distances from their base to the patient. Consequently, consideration should be given to the potential benefits in terms of reach and cost savings of long-endurance drones. In particular, it should be noted that whilst the payload of such drones is similar to their smaller counterparts, their range is in excess of 1,000 km thus allowing them to cover significant distances from their base station without refuelling.

Drone Service Design Considerations Specifically for Medicinal Maggot Distribution

Although drone technology has enormous potential to ease the medicinal maggot distribution challenge, it will be important to select the particular combination of aircraft and service infrastructure with the appropriate capabilities to meet the circumstances in which the supply chain is operating. To illustrate this challenge, it follows a brief discussion of drone service design considerations [28] and how they might apply to drone-assisted medicinal maggot distribution.

What Level of Autonomy and Automation is Required? It is unrealistic to expect that drone operators and technicians can be located at every remote healthcare facility that requires medicinal maggots for wound care and other medicines. Likewise, a comprehensive rollout of training programmes for lay operators in these facilities may also be hard to implement. Therefore, it is desirable that drone technology is as autonomous and automated as possible. Ideally it should require no, or very little, intervention from staff at the receiving end.

What Are the Ground- and Flight-support Requirements Regarding Technology, Staffing, and Training Needs? Drone service operation and monitoring of the drone fleet in transit is not trivial and requires adequate financial investment, access to technical support, and staff that are appropriately skilled. While it is unlikely that medicinal maggot producers will run drone delivery services themselves, they will want to be assured that their consignments of highly perishable medicinal maggots will be reliably delivered in good condition, to the right place, at the right time, and all this at a low cost. Therefore, they and other customers will have a vested interest in the drone systems established and their overall operational requirements. Ideally, these customers should be consulted and have a say in the process of identifying the drone technology that best suits their needs.

What Is the Regulatory Environment for the Operation of Drone Services? Drone service providers must operate within the laws and regulations given by the air safety regulators of the relevant country. These regulators have been caught off-guard by the fast pace of research and development in the aerial robotics field but are now beginning to regulate for the wide-spread use of drones. However, there will be a transition period where the global regulatory landscape for drone operations will be in flux and drone service providers must therefore work closely with these agencies when establishing operations in a new jurisdiction. Regulatory matters are further discussed under 'Ethical and Regulatory Considerations'.

How Much Space Is Available to Launch and Land the Drone? Different drone technologies require different launch and landing or drop-off infrastructure. Short-range helicopter-style drones can land and take off vertically, as do some fixed-wing drones with a vertical take-off and landing capability. Other fixed-wing drones require small runways for landing, whilst Zipline drones (discussed in more detail below) do not land to deliver their cargo but drop it by parachute above the destination healthcare facility. For healthcare facilities receiving medicinal maggots it would be most convenient if the drone landing and launch pad i) had a small footprint, ii) was physically close to the receiving department such as the hospital pharmacy, and iii) was cheap to construct and maintain.

What Is the Desired Range for the Drone? Are Stopovers for Delivery or Refuelling/Battery Change Intended or Possible? It is foreseeable that there is a constant but dispersed need for maggot therapy in hard-to-reach areas, meaning that medicinal maggots for only one or two patients will need to be delivered to several healthcare facilities in a given geographic area. Therefore, it would be convenient for the drone to visit more than one facility on a single trip to fully utilise its cargo capacity. For battery-powered drones with a limited flight range this might make recharging or a battery change necessary. Likewise, hybrid vertical take-off and landing drones such as the Latitude HQ160B use battery power to run the rotors that enable them to land and take-off vertically, which imposes a limit on how many times this can be done before recharging or battery changes become necessary [23]. If drones were required to regularly operate beyond their battery range, then infrastructure at designated stop-over points would need to be in place.

What Delivery Network Structure Is Possible or Desirable? The primary concern to a medicinal maggot producer and the customer healthcare facilities is the reliability of delivery and the condition in which the highly perishable medicinal maggots arrive at the point of care. From this perspective, the producer is likely to be only interested in a hub-and-spoke distribution network where the hub is the producer location and the spokes are the trips to the remote healthcare centres. Whether the drone operator chooses to fly the drone back to the producer location or sends it on to another location is of no consequence to the medicinal maggot producer.

What Is the Nature of the Payload? What Is Its Relative Density (Mass-to-Volume Ratio)? Is the Primary Packaging Rigid or Plastic? Does It Require Temperature Control? Is It Fragile, or Hazardous? Medicinal maggots prepared for maggot therapy are minute and have negligible weight and so are normally packaged in light but rigid small plastic containers (primary packaging). The perishability of the product also demands temperature-controlled parcel packaging. It follows that a key concern when sending medicinal maggots via drone is the consignment volume and the need to maintain the acceptable temperature range of 6–25°C [1]. Producers wanting to utilise drone transport will have to work with drone service providers to develop packaging and payload compartment solutions that ensure efficient use of payload capacity and maintain temperature control. Recently developed short-range drones and the medium-range Wingcopter and Swoop Aero drones have been developed with a focus on the transport of general medicines and blood products [18, 19]. They are likely to meet the general requirements for medicinal maggots, but it appears that the use of long-endurance drones for cargo transport (including medicinal maggots) may still require some more research and development.

Case Examples of Drone Technology that Could Meet Medicinal Maggot Distribution Needs

Short-range Quadcopter Drones

Matternet (https://www.mttr.net/) is a drone technology company focussing on the development of drone logistics networks for the transport of goods. For example, Swiss Post is using Matternet quadcopter technology for the delivery of blood and other pathology specimens in the Swiss cities of Lugano, Bern and Zurich [29], whilst the feasibility of their short-range drone systems has also been demonstrated in several LMIC settings. For example, in Bhutan Matternet collaborated with the World Health Organization (WHO) to trial the transport of medical supplies across difficult Himalayan terrain to provide hard-to-reach communities with access to healthcare [30].

The effectiveness of this form of quadcopter technology has also been demonstrated in a collaboration with Médecins Sans Frontières (MSF) who, in 2014, trialled the use of a battery-operated drone to transport tuberculosis samples from a remote health clinic to a main hospital laboratory in Papua New Guinea [31]. Whilst the clinic was 43 km by air from the hospital, by road the distance was 63 km. Under normal conditions the road trip took four hours but in bad weather the road was impassable. The US$5,000 drone employed had a range of 28km, and so had to stop over at a village for a battery change. Even so, the transit time with a 0.5 kg payload was under one hour compared with the (at least) four-hour regular journey by road [31].

Medium-range Fixed-wing Drones

The challenge of limited endurance of drones has been overcome by a number of drone developers with varying technological approaches. For example, Zipline has been providing a core transport service for medical supplies initially from two locations in Rwanda, and more recently (2019) in Ghana, where 30 drones have been operated from four distribution centres [17].

In 2016 WeRobotics conducted test flights with various fixed-wing drone systems in the Peruvian Amazon, where poor infrastructure and remoteness prevents timely distribution of life-saving medicine [32]. Drones were used to transport snake bite anti-venom, blood samples and various other essential medical and non-medical items between a local health hub and remote villages. For one such village, drone delivery took only 35 minutes compared to the six-hour river-boat trip that would normally be necessary to access the remote community.

Wingcopter medical delivery drones have been successfully tested in Tanzania and Malawi. In Tanzania the drone was used to deliver medicines over a 60 km distance to the 400,000 residents of Ukerewe Island, Lake Victoria. Over the six-month pilot project, the drone performed more than 180 take-offs and landings and spent a total of 2,000 minutes flying 2,200 km to and from the island [33].

Implementation of Drone-assisted Medicinal Maggot Distribution

Packaging requirements. Medicinal maggots are a highly perishable commodity which must be protected from extreme heat, cold and mechanical stress. The rotary drone systems developed for transport of medical and other goods are designed to carry their payload in generous payload compartments that may be part of the fuselage or a separate payload pod. The long-endurance drones typically carry cargo within the fuselage which imposes limitations on the volume of the payload as well as its shape which must align with that of the fuselage. However, it appears there has been less focus on the design and development of long-endurance cargo drones to maximise payload capacity and convenient loading and unloading of cargo, and so this is likely to be an area that will benefit from further investigation. Medical goods such as blood products, vaccines, and medicinal maggots also require protection from adverse temperature conditions, especially when flying for many hours in all kinds of weather. Given that medicinal maggots have not, as yet, been distributed by drone, it is clear that trials would need to be conducted under different climatic conditions to test whether medicinal maggots can be safely delivered without suffering loss of vigour.

Training. There would need to be a robust training programme that ensures the safe and ethical operation of drone services. Depending on the mode of drone technology employed, staff at healthcare facilities receiving medicinal maggots would need to be able to safely oversee the landing of the drone, or the retrieval of a parachuted parcel as in the case of Zipline services. Regarding the former, staff will almost certainly need to be able to report to the controlling agency that the landing area is clear and that it is safe to land the drone. They would then need to remove the medicinal maggot consignment and re-launch the craft safely. For fully autonomous drones this would simply involve securing the launch area and giving remote operators permission to launch. For less sophisticated drone models, it might involve catapulting the drone by hand. However, the emerging generation of cargo drone services are moving towards complete automation, with customers requiring no training whatsoever to dispatch or receive deliveries [34, 35].

Ethical and regulatory considerations. Drones were originally developed as weapons of war. It is therefore important to consider the ethics of using drones to transport medical supplies such as medicinal maggots. Fortunately, recent studies on the perception and application of drones in medical and humanitarian contexts [27, 36] suggest that most stakeholders endorse drone technology because it can strengthen humanitarian responses, enable rapid needs assessment, and fast delivery of vital medical goods. Nevertheless, a sizeable minority still have doubts and view the deployment of drones in humanitarian work unfavourably. The prevalent attitude toward drones will differ from community to community and depend on the humanitarian situation. For example, it can be expected that conflict-affected communities who have experienced military drone attacks would be apprehensive about humanitarian drone use, while hard-to reach and natural disaster-affected communities are more likely to embrace the use of drones. In this regard it would be important to ensure that all stakeholders involved in the operation of drones are comfortable with this technology ahead of its implementation. This could, for example, involve community and business consultations explaining the benefits of drone technology and discussing any potential downsides, actual or perceived.

Irrespective of community buy-in, drone services cannot be implemented without regulatory approval. The key issue is the development of a suitable regime that ensures the safety of those involved in the use of drones as well as those with whom they may interact, such as regular commercial aircraft flights or ad hoc operations by fixed or rotary aircraft. Multiple national and transnational aviation agencies across the globe are actively engaged in developing regulations that provide an appropriate balance between safety and privacy concerns and the potential benefits of drone operations [37]. Unsurprisingly, rapid progress in drone technology and a push by industry to operationalise civil drone services in both high- and low-income countries is resulting in a complex mix of regulatory responses depending on geographic location and jurisdiction. Given this fluid regulatory landscape, a detailed discussion in the context of maggot therapy supply-chain management is best postponed because it would be quickly out of date. Nevertheless, three key areas will need to be considered as part of the overall approach adopted.

- *Airspace management.* Drone operations occur under the International Civil Aviation Organisation (ICAO) rules which state that the lower ceiling for commercial aircraft operations is 500 feet (or 1,000 feet over buildings, towns or cities). Under this ceiling, countries set their own rules and these would generally apply to drone operations. This division is aimed at de-conflicting the airspace and thereby allowing room for industry to work with local civil aviation authorities to develop a suitable regulatory regime to oversee what is sometimes described as Unmanned Traffic Management (UTM). As an example, in the aftermath of Typhoon Haiyan (locally known as Yolanda), which struck the Philippines in 2013, the mayor of the affected region banned the operation of all aircraft (including rescue helicopters) for a period in order to allow the use of drones to provide maps of the region for subsequent use by the responding agencies and non-government organisations (NGOs) [38]. It follows, therefore, that this aspect should be considered as part of the distribution network design, selection of drone capabilities, and actual operations.

- *Privacy issues.* Each country sets its own rules around the issues of privacy. For example, in some countries a drone operator should obtain express permission from all individuals and landowners within the proposed flight path, and this also applies to members of the public overflown in public spaces such as parks, etc. Such laws are routinely flouted by amateur operators, but compliance with local regulations such as this would be a major consideration for any medicinal maggot drone operators—although the local authorities may be able to provide specific authority for drone flights in the event of a disaster or an emergency response.

- *Licencing of operators.* In most countries the operation of drones requires the individual 'pilot' to possess an appropriate licence. Obtaining such licences and maintaining the required continuation training has the potential to create further challenges as there is no guarantee that a pilot who is certified in Country A will be permitted to operate in Country B. Thus, it will be important to ensure that the drone operators do, indeed, hold the required operating licences. Given the areas of challenge summarised above, it is relevant to note that the previously mentioned UAViators Network has led the development of a Humanitarian UAV Code of Conduct (https://www.uavcode.org/code-of-conduct/) and accompanying guidelines which were developed via an extensive process of expert consultations including a UAV Experts Meeting in 2015, co-organised with the UNOCHA, the World Humanitarian Summit (WHS) and Massachusetts Institute of Technology (MIT) [39].

- *Outsourcing to third-party service providers.* The proliferation of drone systems and services to provide transport for medical supplies provides ample opportunity to collaborate with other organisations wanting to distribute medical commodities such as vaccines, blood products, and pathology samples. For instance, a medicinal maggot production laboratory might sensibly share drone services with a pathology laboratory. In such a scenario (that is similar to the case study in PNG described earlier) medicinal maggots would be flown one way to remote communities, and instead of returning empty, the drone could deliver pathology specimens from those communities to the local pathology lab for analysis. This would lead to better utilisation and fewer empty trips, and thus more cost-effective operations. From this it could be argued that drone-services are best provided by a third-party service provider who coordinates and operates transport services for a host of customers and commodities. This would ensure better utilisation of drone capacity by more customers, which is essential for the financial sustainability of the service [40].

Summary

Medicinal maggots are highly perishable and need to be delivered within 24–48 hours to the point of care. In most instances this can be achieved with third-party transport providers using regular air- and land-based transport networks. However, where such transport infrastructure does not exist, or where it is interrupted due to war or disaster, it will become necessary to utilise alternative technologies such as cargo drones. Rapid improvements in endurance, range, payload capacity and automation are already making drones a viable alternative to traditional high-speed courier services in cities as well as in compromised healthcare settings. Consequently, maggot therapy supply-chain managers are encouraged to consider drone-assisted distribution of medicinal maggots and related consumables where other forms of transport would not guarantee timely delivery.

Medicinal maggot transport with drones has not been tested yet. Particularly long-duration flight may expose medicinal maggot payloads to detrimental environmental conditions, e.g. high or sub-zero temperatures, or excessive vibration. Therefore, implementation research and development trials are required to test the capacity of various drone technologies to safely deliver medicinal maggots, and to make improvements to drone design and medicinal maggot packaging if necessary.

It is unlikely that medicinal maggot producers will have the volume of deliveries required to make the operation of a drone fleet financially viable. Rather, with the growing uptake of drone technology in the development and humanitarian sector, it makes more sense to take advantage of commercially operating drone service providers.

To conclude, cargo drone technology has the potential to bring maggot therapy to patients in healthcare settings previously considered unsuitable for this therapy because effective, efficient and timely supply chains were impossible to maintain.

References

1. Čičková, H., et al., *Growth and Survival of Bagged Lucilia sericata Maggots in Wounds of Patients Undergoing Maggot Debridement Therapy*. Evidence-based Complementary and Alternative Medicine, 2013. https://doi.org/10.1155/2013/192149.

2. Stadler, F., *Distribution Logistics*, in *A Complete Guide to Maggot Therapy: Clinical Practice, Therapeutic Principles, Production, Distribution, and Ethics*, F. Stadler (ed.). 2022, Cambridge: Open Book Publishers, pp. 363–382, https://doi.org/10.11647/OBP.0300.17.

3. Artemenko, O., et al., *Validation and Evaluation of the Chosen Path Planning Algorithm for Localization of Nodes Using an Unmanned Aerial Vehicle in Disaster Scenario*. Lecture Notes of the Institute for Computer Sciences, Social-Informatics and Telecommunications Engineering (LNICST), 2016. 140: pp. 192–203.

4. Nex, F. and F. Remondino, *UAV for 3D Mapping Applications: A Review*. Applied Geomatics, 2014. 6(1): pp. 1–15, https://dx.doi.org/10.1007/s12518-013-0120-x.

5. Huang, Y., S. Yi, and Z. Li, *Design of Highway Landslide Warning and Emergency Response Systems Based on UAV*, in *Proceedings SPIE 8203, Remote Sensing of the Environment: The 17th China Conference on Remote Sensing*, 820317, 15 August 2011. https://doi.org/10.1117/12.910424.

6. Braun, J., et al., *The Promising Future of Drones in Prehospital Medical Care and Its Application to Battlefield Medicine*. The Journal of Trauma and Acute Care Surgery, 2019. 87(1S): pp. S28-S34, https://doi.org/10.1097/TA.0000000000002221.

7.   Holtz, R.L. *In Rwanda Drones Deliver Medical Supplies to Remote Areas*. 2018, 3 July. https://www.wsj.com/articles/in-rwanda-drones-deliver-medical-supplies-to-remote-areas-1512124200.

8.   Ling, G. and N. Draghic, *Aerial Drones for Blood Delivery*. Transfusion, 2019. 59(S2): pp. 1608–1611, https://doi.org/10.1111/trf.15195.

9.   Thiels, C.A.D.O., et al., *Use of Unmanned Aerial Vehicles for Medical Product Transport*. Air Medical Journal, 2015. 34(2): pp. 104–108, https://doi.org/10.1016/j.amj.2014.10.011.

10. UNOCHA, *Unmanned Aerial Vehicles in Humanitarian Response*. UNOCHA Policy and Studies Series, 2013 (Occasional Paper No 10).

11. Joshi, D. *Commercial Unmanned Aerial Vehicle (UAV) Market Analysis — Industry Trends, Companies and What You Should Know*. 2017, 8 August. http://www.businessinsider.com/commercial-uav-market-analysis-2017-8/?r=AU&IR=T.

12. DJI. *Inspire 2, DJI Official Website*. 2019. https://www.dji.com/fi/inspire-2.

13. United States Government Accountability Office. *Defense Acquisitions: Assessments of Selected Weapon Programs*. 2013. http://www.gao.gov/assets/660/653379.pdf.

14. Brown, L. *Top 10 Heavy Lift Drones 2019*. 2019. https://filmora.wondershare.com/drones/top-heavy-lift-drones.html.

15. DronesGlobe. *7 Drones that Can Lift Heavy Weights*. 2017. http://www.dronesglobe.com/guide/heavy-lift-drones/.

16. UAViators. *Case Studies of Drones Deployed for Humanitarian Purposes*. 2019. https://docs.google.com/document/d/1KlJyxGLIhGaCmaA8ehzOaS9Yue8zj2PcR3TlxAQME3o/edit.

17. Bright, J., *Drone Delivery Startup Zipline Launches UAV Medical Program in Ghana — TechCrunch*. 2019, AOL Inc: New York.

18. McNabb, M. *Swoop Aero Medical Drone Delivery in Australia: Eliminating a 3 Hour Drive to the Pharmacy*. 2021. https://dronelife.com/2021/02/22/swoop-aero-medical-drone-delivery-in-australia-eliminating-a-3-hour-drive-to-the-pharmacy/.

19. Wingcopter. *Wingcopter 198*. https://wingcopter.com/wingcopter-198#specs.

20. Davitt, L. *Long-Range Drones Deliver Medical Supplies To Remote Areas Of Malawi*. 2019, 19 June. https://www.forbes.com/sites/unicefusa/2019/06/19/long-range-drones-deliver-medical-supplies-to-remote-areas-of-malawi/#6fdee8316add.

21. Swoop Aero. *Say Hello to Kite*. https://swoop.aero/kite.

22. Insitu. *Scaneagle — The Industry-leading UAS that Invented and Continues to Define the Agile ISR Category.* 2015. https://pdf.directindustry.com/pdf/insitu-inc/scaneagle/101665-287663.html.

23. L3HARRIS. *Hybrid Quadrotor(TM) Technology.* https://www.l3harris.com/all-capabilities/hybrid-quadrotortm-technology.

24. Textron Systems. *Aerosonde(TM) SUAS.* 2016.

25. Tatham, P., et al., *Long-endurance Remotely Piloted Aircraft Systems (LE-RPAS) Support for Humanitarian Logistic Operations: The Current Position and the Proposed Way Ahead.* Journal of Humanitarian Logistics and Supply Chain Management, 2017. 7(1): pp. 2–25, https://doi.org/10.1108/JHLSCM-05-2016-0018.

26. Corcoran, M. *Drone Journalism: Newsgathering Applications of Unmanned Aerial Vehicles (UAVs) in Covering Conflict, Civil Unrest and Disaster.* 2014. https://cryptome.org/2014/03/drone-journalism.pdf.

27. Tatham, P., et al., *Flying Maggots: A Smart Logistic Solution to an Enduring Medical Challenge.* Journal of Humanitarian Logistics and Supply Chain Management, 2017. 7(2): pp. 172–193, https://dx.doi.org/10.1108/JHLSCM-02-2017-0003.

28. Safi'I, I., et al., *The Development of Operational Concept and Design Requirements and Objectives (DRO) of Medical Transport Drone in Liukang Tangaya Archipelago.* 2018. Journal of Physics: Conference Series 1130: 012034, https://doi.org/10.1088/1742-6596/1130/1/012034.

29. Swiss Post. *Drones — A Vision Has Become Reality.* https://www.post.ch/en/about-us/company/innovation/swiss-post-s-innovations-for-you/drones.

30. iRevolutions. *WHO Using UAVs to Transport Medical Supplies (Updated).* 2014. https://irevolutions.org/2014/08/27/who-using-uavs/.

31. Fondation Suisse de Déminage. *Using Drones for Medical Payload Delivery in Papua New Guinea.* 2016.

32. WeRobotics. *First Ever Cargo Drone Deliveries in Amazon Rainforest.* 2016. https://irevolutions.org/2016/12/21/amazon-rainforest-cargo-drones/.

33. McNabb, M. *Watch DHL and Wingcopter Deliver the Future in Tanzania.* 2018, 9 October. https://dronelife.com/2018/10/09/watch-dhl-and-wingcopter-deliver-the-future-in-tanzania/.

34. Anonymous, *Google Patents Drone Delivery of Medical Devices.* Biomedical Instrumentation and Technology, 2016. 50(3): p. 150, https://meridian.allenpress.com/bit/article/50/3/148/142146/The-RoundupA-compilation-of-items-about-healthcare.

35. Dickey, M.R. *UPS Partners with Drone Startup Matternet for Medical Sample Deliveries.* 2019. https://techcrunch.com/2019/03/26/ups-partners-with-drone-startup-matternet-for-medical-sample-deliveries/.

36. Soeliso, D. and K.B. Sandvik. *Drones in Humanitarian Action — A Survey on Perceptions and Applications*. Foundation Suisse De Déminage, 2016.

37. Balasingam, M., *Drones in Medicine—The Rise of the Machines*. International Journal of Clinical Practice, 2017. 71(9): e12989-n/a, https://doi.org/10.1111/ijcp.12989.

38. Fondation Suisse de Déminage. *Testing the Utility of Mapping Drones for Early Recovery in the Philippines*. 2016. https://reliefweb.int/report/philippines/drones-humanitarian-action-case-study-no5-testing-utility-mapping-drones-early.

39. UAViators. *Humanitarian UAV Code of Conduct & Guidelines*. 2017. https://humanitariandronecode.files.wordpress.com/2017/12/uaviators-code-and-guidelines.pdf.

40. Haidari, L.A., et al., *The Economic and Operational Value of Using Drones to Transport Vaccines*. Vaccine, 2016. 34(34): pp. 4062–4067, https://doi.org/10.1016/j.vaccine.2016.06.022.

PART 5

ETHICS

19. The Ethics of Maggot Therapy

Frank Stadler

Maggot therapy needs a social licence, which means that regulators, healthcare administrators, doctors, nurses, allied health providers, and patients must accept and support the treatment. Therefore, medicinal maggot production and maggot therapy must be informed and guided by strong animal and healthcare ethics. The first part of this chapter explores the animal ethics of rearing flies in laboratories and using medicinal maggots for wound care. The second part is dedicated to the biomedical and healthcare ethics of maggot therapy. Rather than a definitive treatise, this chapter should be understood as a first-pass examination of ethical issues related to maggot therapy.

Introduction

Maggot therapy is the treatment of wounds that require debridement and infection control with living fly larvae (maggots). Medicinal maggots are generally produced under strict quality control in medical laboratories and insectaries. Maggot therapy has great potential to be simple, affordable and highly efficacious in both high- and low-resource healthcare settings alike. Apart from supply-chain barriers hindering global supply, there is also the need for a social licence, which means that regulators, healthcare administrators, doctors, nurses, allied health providers, and patients must accept and support the treatment. Therefore, medicinal maggot production and maggot therapy must be

https://doi.org/10.11647/OBP.0300.19

informed and guided by strong animal and healthcare ethics, but any meaningful discussion of the ethical questions emerging from the use of medicinal maggots for healthcare purposes has not taken place, yet.

This paucity of work may be seen as a reflection of the status of invertebrates before the law as well as in public perception, and the fact that maggot therapy is just one of many healthcare interventions guided by ethical norms and local rules and regulations. In other words, biomedical ethicists and maggot therapy researchers may consider it already covered by discussions in general medical ethics. In addition, workers in the field of maggot-assisted wound care have been preoccupied with the biological-, biomedical-, and clinical issues that maggot therapy presents and may not have felt the need to engage on a scholarly basis with relevant ethical considerations. Moreover, foundational ethical principles in healthcare such as 'do no harm' are implicitly adopted in maggot therapy treatment guidelines that, for example, explain indications, contra-indications, side-effects, and risks [1]. Similarly, a discussion of maggot therapy in the context of humanitarian ethics has not been necessary because maggot therapy has not been part of any humanitarian response to disaster or war, yet.

This chapter is divided into two parts. The first explores the animal ethics of rearing flies in laboratories and using medicinal maggots for wound care. The second part is dedicated to the human ethics of maggot therapy within the context of biomedical and healthcare ethics. In most jurisdictions, flies and other invertebrates are not considered animals capable of suffering to the same extent as vertebrate animals. This has implications for the care and treatment of flies during mass rearing and maggot therapy, and particularly the disposal of maggots after therapy. From a healthcare ethics standpoint, the treatment of patients with maggot therapy should always be in line with international medical codes and declarations [2] and the four principles of biomedical ethics: autonomy, beneficence, nonmaleficence, and justice [3].

Rather than a definitive treatise on the ethics of maggot therapy, this chapter should be understood as a first-pass examination of ethical considerations as they apply to maggot therapy.

Animal Ethics and the Humane Treatment of Medicinal Maggots

Very little is known about an insect's inner life, its ability to feel pain and distress, and whether this can be compared with our own human experiences of pain and distress. There is also very little information on methods for euthanasia of invertebrate animals and what method is the most humane for insects. There is, however, no doubt that medicinal maggot producers and maggot therapists have a moral obligation to minimise the potential suffering of these animals during production, distribution, and therapy.

Animal Ethics and Invertebrates: Are Flies Animals before the Law?

It is incumbent on anyone who utilises animals, for example for food, fibre, research, or companionship, to ensure the wellbeing of these animals. Medicinal flies are vulnerable to ill treatment from the time they are collected in the field to the time they are disposed of in the insectary, laboratory, or the clinical setting. It is therefore regrettable that insects are not considered animals before the law in Australia, the United States [4, 5], and other jurisdictions. The 8th edition of the Australian code for the care and use of animals for scientific purposes [5] defines animals as "any live non-human vertebrate (that is, fish, amphibians, reptiles, birds and mammals encompassing domestic animals, purpose-bred animals, livestock, wildlife) and cephalopods" (p. 3). The U.S. Animal Welfare Act, 1966, is even more restrictive regarding the animals falling under its purview. The ARRIVE guidelines [6], however, consider laboratory animals as "any species of animal undergoing an experimental procedure in a research laboratory or formal test setting." (p. 258). An excellent and comprehensive review of ethical considerations regarding the use of insects in research has been prepared by Freelance [7]. It has been used to inform and structure the animal ethics discussion in this chapter.

Considering the healing benefits derived from medicinal maggots, it is fair to demand that their production, use, and eventual disposal should be guided by ethical principles that align with those applied to the treatment of vertebrates. Given the special ecological, anatomical, and physiological differences between vertebrates and calliphorid flies, some concessions will be reasonable, but there is very little literature on appropriate and humane treatment of invertebrate animals [8].

What Does the Ethical Utilisation of Medicinal Flies Look Like?

Freelance [7] made recommendations for ethical research with insects which also apply to medicinal maggot production, maggot therapy research, and maggot therapy itself (Table 19.1). It appears prudent to use these recommendations as the scaffold for the discussion of what humane and ethical utilisation of medicinal flies may look like.

Table 19.1 Recommendations by Freelance [7] for the ethical treatment of insects in research, applied to medicinal maggot production and maggot therapy.

Recommendation (abbreviated)	Recommendation applied to the treatment of medicinal flies
Responsible research design	Experimentation with live medicinal flies of all life stages should be designed and conducted to optimise data quality and minimise the impact on the experimental animals. This intersects with the reduction and refinement recommendations below.
Beneficence	The benefit of treating wounds with medicinal maggots should outweigh the harm done to flies during production and to medicinal maggots in maggot therapy.
3Rs — Replacement	Medicinal maggots should be replaced, where possible, with other wound care therapies that do not use living animals.
3Rs — Reduction	The number of flies kept to maintain colonies and to produce medicinal maggots should be minimised to the amount that is necessary and overproduction should be avoided. This also applies to the production of medicinal maggots for therapy.

Recommendation (abbreviated)	Recommendation applied to the treatment of medicinal flies
3Rs — Refinement	Husbandry practices, medicinal maggot production methods, and therapy procedures should be developed and refined so that they minimise the potential suffering of flies and maggots.
Support for natural behaviours in captive specimens	Conditions for natural behaviour of flies and maggots should be provided in the insectary, e.g. sufficiently large cages for flight.
Responsible and sustainable live animal capture	Medicinal flies for the establishment or genetic replenishment of fly colonies in the laboratory should be collected in a way that minimises harm to the collected flies, non-target species, or the ecosystem. Moreover, meat bait for attracting flies should be sourced from already butchered animals or road kill.

Responsible research design. Much of what is known of medicinal maggots regarding their ecological, life-history, and physiological characteristics, and clinical performance has been learned from experiments and trials. Such research should be designed and executed so it produces high-quality data, minimises the number of flies used (all life stages), and minimises the negative impact of experimental treatments on the animals.

The idea of responsible design can also be extended to the design of the maggot-therapy supply chain. For most aspects of fly colony maintenance, medicinal maggot production, distribution, and therapy, the objectives of animal welfare align with the objective to produce high-quality, healthy medicinal maggots. For flies to produce large numbers of eggs for the production of medicinal maggots, they need to be in good health and receive optimal nutrition. At the distribution stage of the maggot therapy supply chain the producer is obliged to package medicinal maggots in protective primary and secondary packaging and then to transport the consignment in insulated transport shippers, which minimises mortality and ensures that healthy, viable maggots reach the point of care [9, 10]. The dressing technology for the application and retention of maggots to the wound, as well as patient instructions and care directives during treatment, all ensure that maggots find conditions for rapid and optimal debridement and thus growth [11]. It is only at the end of treatment that the maggots will need to be disposed of in the clinical waste stream, as will be discussed in more detail later.

Beneficence. The ethical principle of beneficence says that on balance any intervention should be beneficial by maximising the benefit and minimising harm as much as is possible [3]. This principle can be applied to both animal ethics and human ethics, as will be discussed later. Here, the focus is on the benefit of maggot therapy to the patient versus the harm it causes to medicinal flies. Maggot therapy is a highly efficacious wound care therapy and its clinical benefits [12, 13] as well as its therapeutic principles [14–16], have been presented in this book. With this in mind, it can be argued that the sacrifice of flies that have been sustainably reared in the insectary rather than collected from the wild is justified.

It also helps to consider the ecological and evolutionary strategy calliphorid flies pursue. They are an r-selected species and their reproductive strategy is such that they produce large numbers of eggs in order to capitalise on ephemeral resources and high mortality of offspring [17]. Each female may lay 1000 to 2000 eggs in her lifetime [18, 19]. If all offspring survive, they would exponentially multiply. However, the world is not drowning in flies, owing to high mortality of flies during all life stages. Indeed, the vast majority of offspring succumb to unfavourable climatic conditions, disease, or become prey before they can reproduce. This ecological strategy provides a strong ethical rationale for the sustainable utilisation of a species such as the greenbottle blowfly, *Lucilia sericata*, whose evolutionary destination is to naturally sacrifice most of its offspring to predation and other misfortune. Some may suggest that the ecologically-determined and habitually-experienced misfortune of flies in the wild should not be justification for equal treatment in captivity. The difference here is that the domestication and exploitation of flies may well be justified on ecological grounds, but not their ill treatment. As will be discussed later under 'Refinement', it is imperative that any potential suffering of medicinal flies is minimised or avoided altogether.

3Rs — Replacement. Over the past decade, there has been considerable interest in the excretions and secretions of medicinal maggots. This research has revealed that the therapeutic benefits of debridement, infection control, and wound healing are brought about by enzymes and other biochemical factors secreted or excreted by the maggots [14–16]. For example, in 2017 the company SolasCure was founded to develop and commercialise a hydrogel dressing containing an enzyme found in medicinal maggot excretions and secretions [20]. While this is in principle a welcome step from an animal ethics standpoint, it is not certain whether a drug based on one enzyme only has the same therapeutic effect as is provided by the whole organism. This means the benefit derived from maggot therapy may continue to outweigh the harm caused to the few medicinal maggots used for treatment. Secondly, drug development is expensive and developers want to recoup these costs plus profit. Therefore, it is unlikely that disadvantaged and impoverished populations around the world will be able to afford such innovative cures until generic versions become available after the patent has expired. In the meantime, there is a strong argument for the use of affordable maggot therapy to treat wounds, particularly in low- and middle-income countries.

3Rs — Reduction. The best way to minimise potential suffering is to avoid it altogether. Flies are prolific breeders with each female laying up to 2000 eggs over her lifetime. This means that there is the potential to breed enormous numbers of flies. However, producers should only maintain enough flies to be able to meet unforeseen demand for medicinal maggots, to maintain genetically diverse colonies, and perhaps for research purposes. Producers will also be inclined to maintain only necessary fly stock for financial reasons, i.e. to reduce variable costs such as labour and consumables. To conclude, by maintaining a stable population of flies with excess individuals produced being diverted to medicinal maggot production, the producer mimics natural population-limiting ecological dynamics.

3Rs — Refinement. Pain, distress, and general suffering should be minimised when collecting, transporting, captive breeding, and euthanising animals. The objectives for each are very similar but it is instructive to review those for euthanasia in more detail. According to Close and colleagues [21] the method for killing an animal should be

- painless
- quick

- minimally distressing to the animal
- reliable
- reproducible
- irreversible
- simple to administer
- safe for the operator
- aesthetically acceptable.

The knowledge base for humane treatment of invertebrates in zoos, research, and elsewhere is still poor and there is, as yet, an absence of reliable knowledge as to whether invertebrate animals perceive pain the same way vertebrate animals and humans do [22], let alone what their psychological states might be under certain circumstances. Nonetheless, mounting evidence reviewed by Freelance [7] suggests that some insects, for example, may experience emotive states similar to vertebrate animals. As for euthanasia and analgesia of invertebrate animals, the Institute for Laboratory Animal Research has published a special edition dedicated to invertebrate animals. It recommends anaesthesia for terrestrial invertebrates using isoflurane (5–10%), sevoflurane, halothane (5–10%), or carbon dioxide (CO_2; 10–20%), and for aquatic invertebrates tricaine (Sigma) and benzocaine [22, 23].

- *Euthanasia in the fly insectary.* The health of flies that reach the end of their productive lifetime may slowly decline in the absence of predators who would ordinarily put a swift end to any unfit prey. When productivity declines and age-related mortality increases, it is time to terminate the colony. Current practice (author's) is to euthanise adult flies still in their cage (assembled or collapsed) at -20°C. When harvesting eggs, any surplus not used for medicinal maggot production and colony propagation should also be placed in the freezer while still at the egg stage.

- *Euthanasia in the laboratory.* Surplus disinfected maggots and pre-packaged maggots for shipment that are not sent out to clinicians should also be euthanised as soon as feasible by freezing.

- *Disposal after therapy.* It is at the point of care where animal welfare considerations are hardest to observe because healthcare providers are time-poor, must prioritise the welfare of patients, and observe infection control practices. The Joanna Briggs Institute [24] recognised in their report, *Recommended Practice: Wound Debridement–Larval Therapy*, the need for humane treatment of medicinal maggots and suggested that practitioners should place used medicinal maggots in the freezer to kill them prior to disposal. Whether healthcare providers are willing to put soiled dressings and maggots into shared clinic freezers, double-bagged or not, is another matter.

When studying the development times of forensically important blowflies, some researchers use alcohol to kill the maggots ahead of measurement [25] and others kill maggots swiftly by immersion in hot water [26]. When considering the speed with which each of the currently practiced euthanasia methods work, immersion in hot water is by far the fastest, resulting in instant death, followed by freezing, which may take a few minutes depending on how exposed the eggs, maggots, and adult flies are. Cooling slows down cold-blooded animals' metabolism until sub-zero temperatures cause tissue freezing and death. This is a fairly rapid process in small animals with a large surface area such as maggots. Immersion in 70% ethanol is by far the slowest method and maggots may still be alive after an hour of immersion (author's observation), which suggests that it is the lack of oxygen that kills the maggots eventually rather than the alcohol. It must be stressed that immersion in hot water or pouring boiling water over soiled dressings and maggots after treatment is impractical and can be quite dangerous. Handling boiling water is dangerous in and of itself but in addition, germs and toxins may become airborne with the steam that is generated and may lead to serious health problems when breathed in—a phenomenon that has been documented for aquarists who used boiling water to sterilise marine rocks [27].

For now, given insufficient research and practical solutions for euthanasia of maggots, the safest bet is to freeze medicinal maggots prior to disposal. If maggots are disposed of in the clinical waste stream, they will end up being incinerated or otherwise treated with heat, chemicals, or irradiation [28]. Industrial clinical-waste incineration facilities operate at very high temperatures and death should come almost instantaneously to disposed maggots. Incinerators used in low- and middle-income country healthcare settings are often less efficient and operate at lower temperatures. In such cases, it can be assumed that the burning of waste and therefore the euthanasia of maggots is a slower process leading to a more gradual heating of maggots among other clinical waste. Of course, maggots may also succumb long before incineration due to crushing during handling, a build-up of CO_2 in the waste bag, and contact with other healthcare chemicals in the same waste bag.

Support for natural behaviours in captive specimens. There is a trade-off between production efficiency and practicality on one hand, and environmental enrichment for the benefit of flies on the other. It is unrealistic to provide life-like vegetated aviary enclosures for flies that would simulate the natural environment. A suitable compromise is to provide roomy insect cages. In the author's experience, cages of 450 x 450 x 450 mm provide ample room for flight. It is also advisable to illuminate the insectary with daylight-spectrum lighting for optimal fly health. Adult flies are usually dispersed in the ecosystem and congregate in large numbers only when feeding and laying eggs on cadavers or as larvae feeding on such cadavers. Although high density of flies can lead to aggression, particularly by males toward females, it is in the interest of the producer to maximise efficiency and therefore the stocking rate of flies in insectary cages. Producers are encouraged to monitor colony performance and health regularly and adjust stocking rates as necessary. In the author's experience, stocking rates of up to 1 fly per 110 cm^3 are sustainable and do not lead to high or premature mortality, provided all other environmental requirements are met. Please refer to Chapter 14 for a comprehensive discussion of medicinal fly husbandry [29].

Optimising fly wellbeing through the provision of optimal environmental conditions that stimulate natural behaviour is not only an ethical imperative but it also makes good business sense. Any practice that improves the wellbeing of flies in the production system will translate into a better product, i.e. medicinal maggots for clinical treatment. In addition, if the humane treatment of flies can be demonstrated to clients it may also increase consumer acceptance, as is the case in the poultry industry, where free-range and barn-laid eggs are preferred by ethically-minded consumers.

Responsible and sustainable live animal capture. Producers and researchers may collect flies to establish colonies or to replenish genetic material after longer periods of captive breeding. All life stages may be collected. The recommendation for responsible and sustainable live animal capture (Table 19.1) requires collectors to reduce bycatch when traps are used. This may be difficult as a range of fly species in addition to the target species may be trapped. Bycatch might be reduced by monitoring catch rate and not leaving the trap set up for longer than necessary. Fortunately, the aim is to capture live flies so when sorting takes place, non-target species can be released if practical. Bycatch of adult flies can be altogether avoided if immature life stages (eggs and maggots) are collected from cadavers or putrid meat bait is offered to attract flies for oviposition. When transporting captured specimens to the insectary, it is in the interest of the collector to store them in an insulated transport container to avoid overheating. Finally, there is generally no need to purposely kill a domestic or other livestock to attract flies. Road kill is usually not hard to find and inexpensive meat waste from butchers is also suitable for attracting flies. Chapter 13 provides guidance on the establishment of laboratory colonies including the collection of fly breeding stock.

The Healthcare Ethics of Maggot Therapy

Having reviewed the ethics of medicinal maggot production and maggot therapy from an animal ethics standpoint, we now shift to investigate the human ethics of maggot therapy, particularly in compromised healthcare settings such as in war, disaster, poverty, or extreme geographic isolation. Here, the focus shifts from medicinal flies to the relationship between care provider and patient—before, during, and after maggot therapy. The ethical foundations for this relationship have already been laid. There are a plethora of ethical codes and declarations relevant to healthcare delivery. Amnesty International has compiled most of them in the 5th edition of *Codes of Ethics and Declarations Relevant to the Health Professions* [2]. Some of these are of particular interest to medical practitioners who provide wound care in ordinary times and during war, disaster, and development:

- The Hippocratic Oath
- WMA Declaration of Geneva
- International Code of Medical Ethics
- Declaration of Helsinki: Ethical Principles for Research Involving Human Subjects
- Regulations in Time of Armed Conflict
- Geneva Conventions
  - Common Article 3 of the Geneva Conventions
  - Convention I For the Amelioration of the Condition of the Wounded and Sick in Armed Forces in the Field. Geneva, 12 August 1949.
  - Convention II For the Amelioration of the Condition of the Wounded and Sick and Shipwrecked Members of Armed Forces at Sea. Geneva, 12 August 1949.

The field of medical and healthcare ethics has been greatly influenced by Beauchamp and Childress' seminal work on the principles of biomedical ethics, now in its 5th edition [3]. The four principles are autonomy, beneficence, nonmaleficence, and justice. Autonomy refers to the patients' ability to make their own decisions in healthcare which includes the ability to give informed consent or refuse a particular intervention. Beneficence requires healthcare to be of benefit to the patient. In this respect there can be conflict between the interests of the individual patient and the larger patient cohort, especially when healthcare resources are limited and utilitarian decisions have to be made to maximise the benefit to all patients. The principle of nonmaleficence asks the care provider to do no harm, while justice calls for the fair, appropriate, and equitable treatment of patients. Much of the discussion in this chapter is informed by Beauchamp and Childress [3] but this does not mean that the other codes of ethics listed in the Amnesty International compendium [2] can be ignored. Fortunately, they greatly overlap and align with the ethical notions encapsulated in the four principles while tailored to a particular healthcare setting, as the Geneva Conventions are tailored to armed conflict. A detailed discussion of the ethics of maggot therapy in all these contexts is beyond the scope of this chapter.

Autonomy

For clinicians who understand the therapeutic benefits of medicinal maggots and have successfully treated many wounds with maggot therapy, it may become somewhat tedious to sensitise and educate each new patient whose wounds are amenable to maggot therapy. However, there is no escaping this obligation. The principle of autonomy demands that patients have control over their bodies and are in the position to make treatment decisions.

Beauchamp and Childress propose a stepwise process by which the practitioner ensures that the patient understands what the treatment entails, consents to a treatment plan, and authorises this treatment plan [3, p. 80]:

I. Threshold Elements (Preconditions)
    1. Competence (to understand and decide)
    2. Voluntariness (in deciding)

II. Information Elements
    3. Disclosure (of material information)
    4. Recommendation (of a plan)
    5. Understanding (of 3. and 4.)

III. Consent Elements
    6. Decision (in favor of a plan)
    7. Authorization (of the chosen plan)

Competence and voluntariness. In the first instance, the patient must be able to understand care information given by the practitioner and then able to make care decisions. If patients can't make their own decisions (i.e. they are not autonomous), their interests need to be faithfully represented. Consider the following scenarios. A patient with a pressure ulcer might also have advanced dementia, as was the case with the author's own grandfather, which means he is no longer able to make his own decisions. Another example might be found in a conflict or disaster setting, where the blast wound of a comatose civilian casualty has become severely infected with methicillin-resistant *Staphylococcus aureus*. In such cases when patients are unable to make their own decisions, Beauchamp and Childress [3] suggest that an advanced care directive by the patient is preferable. Advanced care planning seeks to clarify and capture how the patient would want to be treated, what treatments the patient would refuse, and who might be vested with the power of attorney to represent the patient's wishes [30]. Such care directives may be of a general nature or more specific but it seems unlikely that patients would give directives explicitly on maggot therapy, perhaps unless they already face chronic wound care challenges. In the absence of advanced care plans, the decision should be made by a person who knows the patient well. This person should be able to make a decision that reflects the patient's opinions and attitudes, in other words, a decision the patient would most likely have made. In cases where the patient was never autonomous or there is no representative such as a next of kin, and it is therefore impossible to get a sense of the patient's wishes, a surrogate must decide in the patient's best interest:

> a surrogate decision maker must determine the highest net benefit among the available options, assigning different weights to interests the patient has in each option and discounting or subtracting inherent risks or costs. The term best is used because the surrogate's obligation is to maximize benefit through a comparative assessment that locates the highest net benefit. The best-interests standard protects another's well-being by assessing risks and benefits of various treatments and alternatives to treatment, by considering pain and suffering, and by evaluating restoration or loss of functioning. [3, p. 102]

Of course, the decision to accept or refuse maggot therapy must be voluntary and neither the practitioner nor other third parties must exert undue influence over the patient's decision [31]. Given the unusual and for some people disconcerting nature of maggot therapy, there is always the danger that patients are unduly encouraged or dissuaded by their loved ones. Likewise, a practitioner who is passionate about maggot therapy may be tempted to pressure the patient to consent. Therefore, the role of objective sensitisation and education in maggot therapy cannot be overemphasised.

Disclosure, recommendation, and understanding. Practitioners need to consider what a reasonable person would want and need to know about maggot therapy. This typically includes information about the wound and its prognosis, the benefits of maggot therapy, alternative treatments, side-effects, risks, and how maggot therapy may limit daily life (e.g. bathing and showering, off-loading, etc.), and a treatment plan [32]. Fortunately, the general concept of maggot therapy and its three main therapeutic principles is easily understood especially when explained in simple, non-technical terms, and the same is true for the dressings used to apply and keep maggots in place. However, clinicians will need to tailor the information to the individual needs of the patient [3], especially because maggot therapy is still considered an unusual treatment. It is important to also take the patient's attitude toward flies, maggots, and other invertebrate animals ('creepy crawlies') into account. While mere dislike of maggots and repulsion are not reliable predictors of non-consent, Petherick and colleagues suggest the use of positive language and phrases to describe the maggots' therapeutic benefits [33]. Depending on the patient, it may also be helpful to explain the biology of maggots and how their evolutionary history and adaptation to unhygienic environments has given rise to the multiple therapeutic properties of maggot therapy.

Decision and authorisation. As the patient receives appropriate and easily understood information about maggot therapy and the treatment plan, the clinician needs to encourage patient feedback through open dialogue, and deduce whether the patient has understood maggot therapy, and what the consequences of consenting or declining the treatment would be [3]. Clinicians generally seek only verbal consent for relatively minor non-surgical procedures, which would include maggot therapy. However, depending on local rules and regulations and the patient's capacity to make a decision, clinicians may need to obtain written consent or refusal of consent from the patient or surrogate [34].

Beneficence and Nonmaleficence

Medical treatments, including maggot therapy, must be performed with the primary objective to benefit the patient. At the same time, the treatment should not harm the patient. In practice, there are many treatments with varying efficacy and varyingly harmful side-effects. Thus, in order to align with the principles of beneficence and nonmaleficence it is necessary to maximise the net-benefit of any treatment regimen [35].

Chronic and infected wounds have been recognised as a major healthcare challenge in both high-resource and low-resource care settings such as disasters, conflict, and poverty [36–39]. Patients or their insurers in high-resource healthcare systems can afford advanced therapies and wound dressings but these are out of reach for people with wounds in low- and middle-income countries where a chronic wound can incur catastrophic healthcare expenditure for patients and their families [40]. Moreover, when limbs need to be amputated due to life-threatening infection this results in prolonged incapacity or even disability which greatly diminishes the patient's ability to care for their families and contribute to society.

Maggot therapy is widely applicable and generally indicated for non-healing wounds with necrotic tissue and slough including infected wounds [41]. Maggot therapy can improve wound care particularly in low-resource healthcare settings because it not only removes necrotic tissue but also controls infection and promotes wound healing. This means that wound care with maggot therapy is less reliant on surgical expertise, antibiotic use, and advanced wound dressings [42]. It follows that on the health system- and societal level, the use of maggot therapy aligns with the principle of beneficence. As far as treatment decision making for individual patients is concerned, practitioners have to consider a range of factors that determine whether maggot therapy will on balance benefit the patient: i) wound aetiology and condition, ii) general patient characteristics and comorbidities, iii) treatment alternatives, iv) contraindications and treatment risks, and v) cost of treatment and the patient's capacity to pay. As with all therapies and medicines, there are contraindications that increase the risk of adverse outcomes for the patient, such as allergic reaction, pain, or bleeding [1]. However, most of these contraindications can be carefully monitored and managed or circumvented, especially if the benefits of maggot therapy outweigh the risk of adverse events.

While informed consent of the patient is always necessary, the ultimate responsibility regarding patient safety still rests with the practitioner. This is not to say, though, that the producers and suppliers of medicinal maggots are absolved of responsibility. Indeed, in well-regulated healthcare systems the manufacturers of medical goods are required to adhere to stringent quality control standards and Good Manufacturing Practices [43]. If medicinal maggots are produced in low- and middle-income countries the sophistication of producers may vary greatly, especially because medicinal flies are very easy to keep and breed. In such circumstances it may be difficult to hold producers accountable for poor-quality medicinal maggots and adverse outcomes. However, there have been efforts by the author and colleagues to provide lay producers of medicinal maggots and healthcare providers in compromised healthcare settings with easy-to-understand visual, multi-lingual, and multimedia instructions to ensure production of high-quality medicinal maggots and safe maggot therapy (http://www. medmaglabs.com/creating-hope-in-conflict). Fortunately, adverse outcomes due to poor production practice is probably a rather small risk because of the extraordinary capacity of medicinal maggots to control infection even in cases of myiasis, the unintended wild colonisation of wounds with fly maggots [44]. In other words, as long as appropriate fly species are used to produce medicinal maggots, the risk to patients is limited. Nevertheless, it is incumbent on the treating practitioners to ensure that they procure medicinal maggots from reputable and proficient producers irrespective of the level of regulatory oversight in that healthcare system.

Justice

Maggot therapy in a resource-constrained healthcare setting. The moral obligation on healthcare providers to provide optimal care to every patient is at odds with the utilitarian imperative as it applies to resource-constrained healthcare settings. Under such circumstances, the aim is to provide the best possible wound care to the greatest possible number of patients, rather than prioritising optimal care to only a few patients [3]. This means that compromises need to be made in the care that can be provided (Figure 19.1). However, in care settings where low-cost medicinal maggots are made available, maggot therapy can ensure highly efficacious wound care for a large number of patients even if other wound care modalities, antibiotics, and medical personnel are in short supply. This is because maggot therapy i) can be performed by nurses rather than physicians, ii) can replace costly conventional wound dressings, iii) can replace, or reduce dependence on, the use of antibiotics, iv) can replace surgical debridement, and v) can promote wound healing and thus prepare wounds for surgical closure while patients in immediate and urgent need of care are looked after [45].

Lack of access to limb- and life-saving treatment. Having pointed out that maggot therapy can make a meaningful contribution to fair healthcare provision in compromised healthcare settings, it is regrettable that maggot therapy has not yet been used in disaster settings and is unavailable in all but a few low- and middle-income countries. Despite the deep history of tribal and ancient use of maggot therapy in many regions of the world [47], maggot therapy is mainly offered to patients in North America, Europe and to a lesser extent elsewhere such as in Iran, Malaysia, Singapore, Japan, and Australia. With exceptions, these countries are generally high- or middle-income countries with excellent to reasonable access to healthcare and advanced wound care. In compromised healthcare settings, where maggot therapy could make a real difference, it is rarely used. There have been a number of attempts to introduce maggot therapy to Sub-Saharan Africa but such efforts have failed or are hampered by regulatory and bureaucratic barriers. For example, a recent programme supported by a grant from the Slovak government established a medicinal maggot production laboratory in Kenya and supported the training of the local workforce [48, 49]. Despite documented positive outcomes and improvements to the care of intractable wounds, delays in regulatory approval meant that the therapy could only be offered to very few patients in Nairobi and surrounding areas. A case report of the Kenyan maggot therapy programme is provided in Chapter 15 and with regard to distribution logistics in Chapter 17 of this book [10, 49].

As discussed under the principle of autonomy, patients are usually dependent on the expertise and advice given by doctors. In the case of maggot therapy this is no different. For the therapy to be widely adopted, it is necessary for doctors, nurses, and the greater healthcare system to endorse maggot therapy and to include it in their treatment 'toolbox'. Prejudicial dislike or disregard for maggot therapy among healthcare professionals is still widespread, especially in jurisdictions where the therapy is new or has not been widely used in the past (personal

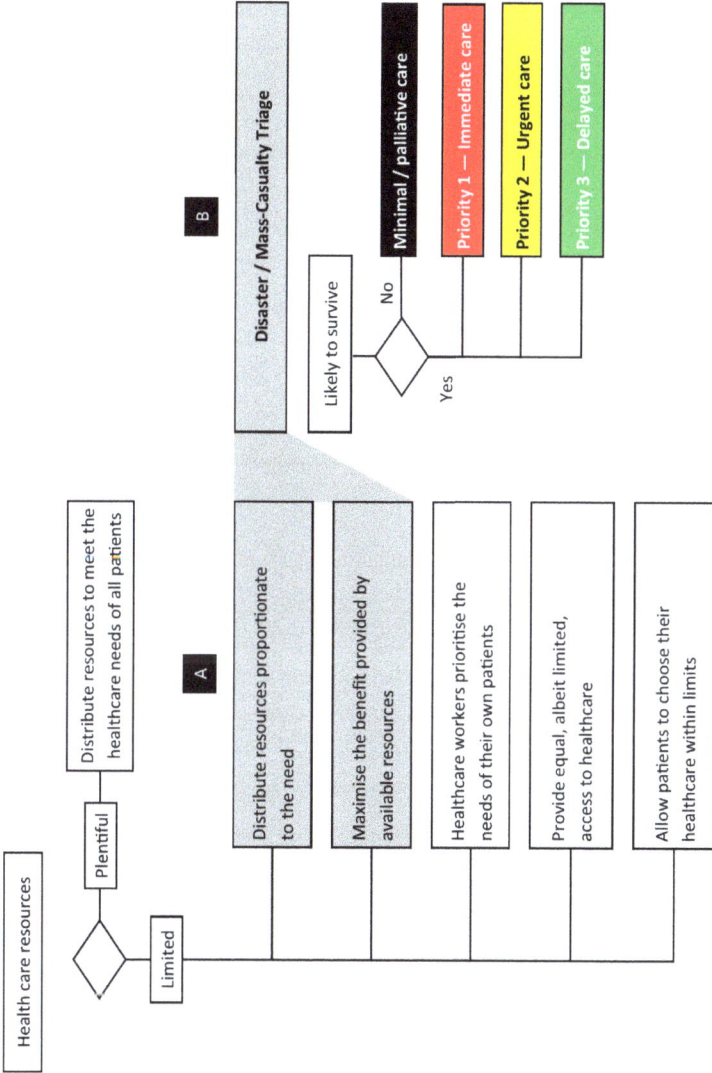

Figure 19.1 Abbreviated and simplified ethical framework for the provision of care in resource-constrained healthcare settings [35, 46]. Strategies for ethical healthcare provision in Column A may apply to any number of situations where resources are limited. However, the utilitarian approach of proportionate distribution that maximises benefit applies specifically to disaster triage (Column B). CC BY-NC.

observation). This, along with aggressive lobbying and marketing by manufacturers of competing wound care products, means that many patients miss out on affordable and highly efficacious maggot therapy. One might think that practitioners in low-resource healthcare settings would embrace maggot therapy but this is not necessarily the case. It is common in low- and middle-income countries that practitioners manipulate patients to make care decisions in which they have a financial interest [50]. In the case of chronic wound care, physicians may recommend surgical debridement instead of maggot therapy because the treatment incurs more surgeon time and therefore greater income [48]. Therefore, a highly affordable and efficacious therapy such as maggot therapy may struggle to gain wide-spread endorsement in favour of more lucrative treatment options. Key to overcoming these barriers are education campaigns for the public, patients, and healthcare professionals that translate and communicate the mounting clinical evidence in favour of maggot therapy. Winning the hearts and minds of future patients, doctors, and nurses may start as early as primary school when children have not yet formed strong negative opinions of maggots [51].

Supply-chain constraints are also responsible for lack of access to maggot therapy, especially in compromised healthcare settings. Medicinal maggots have a short shelf-life, requiring delivery at a temperature of 6–25°C and application to the wound within 24 to 48 hours of dispatch from the laboratory [52]. During times of disaster, in conflict, or in impoverished regions of the world such rapid and reliable distribution of goods is not possible because of broken and disrupted logistics infrastructures. However, these logistics barriers may be overcome with drone transport [53] and innovative supply-chain solutions that locate medicinal maggot production at the point of care. The latter may be achieved, for example, with mobile laboratories for medicinal maggot production, and through capacity building of isolated communities and medics working in austere care settings [54, 55]. This is because medicinal maggot production is a relatively simple process and does not necessarily depend on high-tech equipment or special expertise. Production and supply may be taken up by communities or entrepreneurs that seek an income from breeding and selling medicinal maggots. This economic incentive may further motivate service delivery even in austere settings. However, there is also a chance that treatment becomes unaffordable to the very poor, thus reinforcing healthcare injustices. Such entrepreneurs should be given advice on business models that allow producers and practitioners to cross-subsidise the treatment of the poor through charging wealthy patients higher fees.

Summary

This chapter concludes the present book on maggot therapy but it could have easily been the introductory chapter. Ethical considerations are central to all aspects of healthcare service delivery. Through this lens, maggot therapy can be seen as one of the countless medicines, devices, and therapies that are equally subject to ethical standards. However, the use of living organisms in place of inanimate drugs and devices sets maggot therapy apart from other wound care therapies. Maggots may conjure up feelings ranging from fascination to discomfort or even disgust. Therefore, to appropriately seek true, informed consent, providers of maggot therapy must pay closer attention to patient sensitisation and education. Moreover, the use of living organisms as a therapy adds another layer of complexity. In addition to regular biomedical ethics along the lines of the four principles discussed above, there are animal ethics issues that demand consideration. Unfortunately, little is known about the capacity of invertebrate animals such as flies and their larvae to experience distress and pain, but the question of suffering is central to animal ethics. Consequently, it is incumbent on maggot producers and therapists to be precautious and minimise any potential human and insect suffering.

Even with the best intentions, producers and clinicians may need to compromise on ethics because healthcare professionals are not always completely free to practice according to best-practice ethical standards and principles. Health and safety laws and regulations, and health service providers guided by religious faiths may take a different view on ethical conduct [56]. For example, a Jain patient may object on religious grounds to the killing of a living being such as a maggot [57]. The solution to this could be releasing used maggots after maggot therapy, rather than disposing of them along with the dressing waste. However, for public health and practicality reasons, this is clearly not possible.

Wound care waste is considered infectious waste because soiled dressings, including medicinal maggots, are usually contaminated with pathogens. Therefore, this waste must be collected and disposed of safely, which invariably leads to maggots being killed in the process.

These limitations highlight the need for greater consideration of ethical issues in maggot therapy. It is my hope that both practitioners and scholars are encouraged to engage in this debate and eventually contribute to the development of ethical methods and practices in medicinal maggot production and maggot-assisted wound care.

References

1. Mexican Association for Wound Care and Healing. *Clinical Practice Guidelines for the Treatment of Acute and Chronic Wounds with Maggot Debridement Therapy.* 2010. https://s3.amazonaws.com/aawc-new/memberclicks/GPC_larvatherapy.pdf.

2. Amnesty International, *Codes of Ethics and Declarations Relevant to the Health Professions: An Amnesty International Compilation of Selected Ethics and Human Rights Texts and Other Standards.* 2009, London: Amnesty International.

3. Beauchamp, T.L. and J.F. Childress, *Principles of Biomedical Ethics.* 2001, New York: Oxford University Press.

4. Garber et al., *Guide for the Care and Use of Laboratory Animals, Eighth Edition.* 2010, Washington, D.C.: The National Academy Press.

5. National Health and Medical Research Council, *Australian Code for the Care and Use of Animals for Scientific Purposes, 8th edition.* 2013, National Health and Medical Research Council: Canberra.

6. Kilkenny, C., et al., *Improving Bioscience Research Reporting: The ARRIVE Guidelines for Reporting Animal Research.* Osteoarthritis and Cartilage, 2010. 20(4): pp. 256–260, https://doi.org/10.1016/j.joca.2012.02.010.

7. Freelance, C.B., *To Regulate or Not to Regulate? The Future of Animal Ethics in Experimental Research with Insects.* Science and Engineering Ethics, 2019. 25(5): pp. 1339–1355, https://doi.org/10.1007/s11948-018-0066-9.

8. Stadler, F., *The Maggot Therapy Supply Chain: A Review of the Literature and Practice.* Med Vet Entomol, 2020. 34(1): pp. 1–9, https://doi.org/10.1111/mve.12397.

9. Stadler, F., *Packaging Technology*, in *A Complete Guide to Maggot Therapy: Clinical Practice, Therapeutic Principles, Production, Distribution, and Ethics*, F. Stadler (ed.). 2022, Cambridge: Open Book Publishers, pp. 349–362, https://doi.org/10.11647/OBP.0300.16.

10. Stadler, F., *Distribution Logistics*, in *A Complete Guide to Maggot Therapy: Clinical Practice, Therapeutic Principles, Production, Distribution, and Ethics*, F. Stadler (ed.). 2022, Cambridge: Open Book Publishers, pp. 363–382, https://doi.org/10.11647/OBP.0300.17.

11. Sherman, R., *Medicinal Maggot Application and Maggot Therapy Dressing Technology*, in *A Complete Guide to Maggot Therapy: Clinical Practice, Therapeutic Principles, Production, and Ethics*, F. Stadler (ed.). 2022, Cambridge: Open Book Publishers, pp. 79–96, https://doi.org/10.11647/OBP.0300.05.

12. Sherman, R., *Indications, Contraindications, Interactions, and Side-effects of Maggot Therapy*, in *A Complete Guide to Maggot Therapy: Clinical Practice, Therapeutic Principles, Production, and Ethics*, F. Stadler (ed.). 2022, Cambridge: Open Book Publishers, pp. 63–78, https://doi.org/10.11647/OBP.0300.04.

13. Sherman, R. and F. Stadler, *Wound Aetiologies, Patient Characteristics, and Healthcare Settings Amenable to Maggot Therapy*, in *A Complete Guide to Maggot Therapy: Clinical Practice, Therapeutic Principles, Production, Distribution, and Ethics*, F. Stadler (ed.). 2022, Cambridge: Open Book Publishers, pp. 39–62, https://doi.org/10.11647/OBP.0300.03.

14. Nigam, Y. and M.R. Wilson, *Maggot Debridement*, in *A Complete Guide to Maggot Therapy: Clinical Practice, Therapeutic Principles, Production, Distribution, and Ethics*, F. Stadler (ed.). 2022, Cambridge: Open Book Publishers, pp. 143–152, https://doi.org/10.11647/OBP.0300.08.

15. Nigam, Y. and M.R. Wilson, *The Antimicrobial Activity of Medicinal Maggots*, in *A Complete Guide to Maggot Therapy: Clinical Practice, Therapeutic Principles, Production, Distribution, and Ethics*, F. Stadler (ed.). 2022, Cambridge: Open Book Publishers, pp. 153–174, https://doi.org/10.11647/OBP.0300.09.

16. Nigam, Y. and M.R. Wilson, *Maggot-assisted Wound Healing*, in *A Complete Guide to Maggot Therapy: Clinical Practice, Therapeutic Principles, Production, Distribution, and Ethics*, F. Stadler (ed.). 2022, Cambridge: Open Book Publishers, pp. 175–194, https://doi.org/10.11647/OBP.0300.10.

17. Pianka, E.R., *R-selection and K-selection*. The American Naturalist, 1970. 104(940): p. 592–597, https://doi.org/10.1086/282697.

18. Rueda, L.C., et al., *Lucilia sericata Strain from Colombia: Experimental Colonization, Life Tables and Evaluation of Two Artificial Diets of the Blowfly Lucilia sericata (Meigen) (Diptera: Calliphoridae), Bogota, Colombia Strain*. Biological Research, 2010. 43(2): pp. 197–203, https://dx.doi.org/10.4067/S0716-97602010000200008.

19. Mackerras, M.J., *Observations on the Life-histories, Nutritional Requirements and Fecundity of Blowflies*. Bulletin of Entomological Research, 1933. 24: pp. 353–362, https://dx.doi.org/10.1017/S0007485300031680.

20. SolasCure. *SolasCure*. 2021. https://solascure.com/.

21. Close, B., et al., *Recommendations for Euthanasia of Experimental Animals: Part 1*. Laboratory Animals, 1996. 30(4): pp. 293–316, https://doi.org/10.1258/002367796780739871.

22. Cooper, J.E., *Anesthesia, Analgesia, and Euthanasia of Invertebrates*. ILAR Journal, 2011. 52(2): pp. 196–204, https://doi.org/10.1093/ilar.52.2.196.

23. Lewbart, G.A. and C. Mosley, *Clinical Anesthesia and Analgesia in Invertebrates*. Journal of Exotic Pet Medicine, 2012. 21(1): pp. 59–70, https://doi.org/10.1053/j.jepm.2011.11.007.

24. Wound Healing and Management Node Group, *Recommended Practice: Wound Debridement — Larval Therapy*. Wound Practice and Research, 2014. 22(1): pp. 48–49.

25. Richards, C.S. and M.H. Villet, *Data Quality in Thermal Summation Development Models for Forensically Important Blowflies*. Medical and Veterinary Entomology, 2009. 23(3): pp. 269–276, https://doi.org/10.1111/j.1365-2915.2009.00819.x.

26. Rabêlo, K.C.N., et al., *Bionomics of Two Forensically Important Blowfly Species Chrysomya megacephala and Chrysomya putoria (Diptera: Calliphoridae) Reared on Four Types of Diet*. Forensic Science International, 2011. 210(1–3): pp. 257–262, https://doi.org/10.1016/j.forsciint.2011.03.022.

27. SA Health. *Fact Sheet. Coral Handling Safety Tips for Aquarium Owners*. https://www.sahealth.sa.gov.au/wps/wcm/connect/public+content/sa+health+internet/resources/coral+handling+safety+tips+for+aquarium+owners.

28. UNEP, *Compendium of Technologies for Treatment/Destruction of Healthcare Waste*. 2012, United Nations Environment Programme Division of Technology, Industry and Economics International Environmental Technology Centre: Osaka, Japan. https://www.uncrd.or.jp/content/documents/04_Chandak-UNEP%20IETC.pdf.

29. Stadler, F. and P. Takáč, *Medicinal Maggot Production*, in *A Complete Guide to Maggot Therapy: Clinical Practice, Therapeutic Principles, Production, Distribution, and Ethics*, F. Stadler (ed.). 2022, Cambridge: Open Book Publishers, pp. 289–330, https://doi.org/10.11647/OBP.0300.14.

30. Thomas, K., *Overview and Introduction to Advance Care Planning*, in *Advance Care Planning in End of Life Care*. 2017, Oxford: Oxford University Press, pp. 1–18. http://doi.org/10.1093/oso/9780198802136.003.0001.

31. Benbow, M., *Ethics and Wound Management*. Journal of Community Nursing, 2006. 20(3): pp. 24, 26, 28.

32. Chadwick, P., et al., *Appropriate Use of Larval Debridement Therapy in Diabetic Foot Management: Consensus Recommendations*. Diabetic Foot Journal, 2015. 18(1): pp. 37–42.

33. Petherick, E.S., et al., *Patient Acceptability of Larval Therapy for Leg Ulcer Treatment: A Randomised Survey to Inform the Sample Size Calculation of a Randomised Trial*. BMC Medical Research Methodology, 2006. 6: 43, https://doi.org/10.1186/1471-2288-6-43.

34. NSW Health. *Consent to Medical and Healthcare Treatment Manual*. 2020. https://www.health.nsw.gov.au/policies/manuals/Pages/consent-manual.aspx.

35. Gillon, R., *Medical Ethics: Four Principles Plus Attention to Scope*. BMJ, 1994. 309(6948): pp. 184–188, https://doi.org/10.1136/bmj.309.6948.184.

36. Dau, A.A., S. Tloba, and M.A. Daw, *Characterization of Wound Infections among Patients Injured during the 2011 Libyan Conflict*. Eastern Mediterranean Health Journal = La Revue De Santé De La Méditerranée Orientale = Al-Majallah Al-Ṣiḥḥīyah Li-Sharq Al-Mutawassiṭ, 2013. 19(4): pp. 356–361, http://applications.emro.who.int/emhj/v19/04/EMHJ_2013_19_4_356_361.pdf.

37. Eardley, W.G.P., et al., *Infection in Conflict Wounded*. Philosophical Transactions. Biological Sciences, 2011. 366(1562): pp. 204–218, https://doi.org/10.1098/rstb.2010.0225.

38. Sen, C.S., *Human Wounds and Its Burden: An Updated Compendium of Estimates*. Advances in Wound Care, 2019. 8(2): pp. 39–48, https://doi.org/10.1089/wound.2019.0946.

39. Wuthisuthimethawee, P., et al., *Wound Management in Disaster Settings*. World Journal of Surgery, 2015. 39(4): pp. 842–853, https://doi.org/10.1007/s00268-014-2663-3.

40. Ali, S.M., et al., *The Personal Cost of Diabetic Foot Disease in the Developing World — A Study from Pakistan*. Diabetic Medicine 2008. 25(10): pp. 1231–1233, https://doi.org/10.1111/j.1464-5491.2008.02529.x.

41. Fleischmann, W., M. Grassberger, and R. Sherman, *Maggot Therapy. A Handbook of Maggot-Assisted Wound Healing*. 2004, Stuttgart: Georg Thieme Verlag.

42. Mirabzadeh, A., et al., *Maggot Therapy for Wound Care in Iran: A Case Series of the First 28 Patients*. Journal of Wound Care, 2017. 26(3): pp. 137–143, https://doi.org/10.12968/jowc.2017.26.3.137.

43. PIC/S, *Guide to Good Manufacturing Practice for Medicinal Products — Annexes*. 2017, Pharmaceutical Inspection Convention Pharmaceutical Inspection Co-operation Scheme. https://picscheme.org/en/publications?tri=gmp#zone.

44. Chan, Q.E., M.A. Hussain, and V. Milovic, *Eating out of the Hand, Maggots — Friend or Foe?* Journal of Plastic, Reconstructive and Aesthetic Surgery, 2012. 65(8): pp. 1116–1118, https://doi.org/10.1016/j.bjps.2012.01.014.

45. Stadler, F., R.Z. Shaban, and P. Tatham, *Maggot Debridement Therapy in Disaster Medicine*. Prehospital and Disaster Medicine, 2016. 31(1): pp. 79–84, https://doi.org/10.1017/S1049023X15005427.

46. Bazyar, J., et al., *The Principles of Triage in Emergencies and Disasters: A Systematic Review*. Prehospital and Disaster Medicine, 2020. 35(3): pp. 305–313, https://doi.org/10.1017/S1049023X20000291.

47. Whitaker, I.S., et al., *Larval Therapy from Antiquity to the Present Day: Mechanisms of Action, Clinical Applications and Future Potential*. Postgraduate Medical Journal, 2007. 83(980): pp. 409–413, https://doi.org/10.1136/pgmj.2006.055905.

48. Stadler, F., *Supply Chain Management for Maggot Debridement Therapy in Compromised Healthcare Settings*. 2018. Unpublished doctoral dissertation, Griffith University, Queensland, https://doi.org/10.25904/1912/3170.

49. Takáč, P., et al., and F. Stadler, *Establishment of a Medicinal Maggot Production Facility and Treatment Programme in Kenya*, in *A Complete Guide to Maggot Therapy: Clinical Practice, Therapeutic Principles, Production, Distribution, and Ethics*, F. Stadler (ed.). 2022, Cambridge: Open Book Publishers, pp. 289–330, https://doi.org/10.11647/OBP.0300.14.

50. Ghosh, B.N., *Rich Doctors and Poor Patients: Market Failure and Health Care Systems in Developing Countries*. Journal of Contemporary Asia, 2008. 38(2): pp. 259–276, https://doi.org/10.1080/00472330701546525.

51. Humphreys, I., P. Lehane, and Y. Nigam, *Could Maggot Therapy Be Taught in Primary Schools?* Journal of Biological Education, 2020: pp. 1–11, https://doi.org/10.1080/00219266.2020.1748686.

52. Čičková, H., et al., *Growth and Survival of Bagged Lucilia sericata Maggots in Wounds of Patients Undergoing Maggot Debridement Therapy*. Evidence-based Complementary and Alternative Medicine, 2013. https://doi.org/10.1155/2013/192149.

53. Stadler, F. and P. Tatham, *Drone-assisted Medicinal Maggot Distribution in Compromised Healthcare Settings*, in *A Complete Guide to Maggot Therapy: Clinical Practice, Therapeutic Principles, Production, Distribution, and Ethics*, F. Stadler (ed.). 2022, Cambridge: Open Book Publishers, pp. 383–402, https://doi.org/10.11647/OBP.0300.18.

54. MedMagLabs. *MedMagLabs*. http://medmaglabs.com.

55. Sherman, R.A. and M.R. Hetzler, *Maggot Therapy for Wound Care in Austere Environments*. Journal of Special Operations Medicine, 2017. 17(2): pp. 154–162.

56. Williams, J., R. *World Medical Association Medical Ethics Manual*. 2015. https://www.wma.net/wp-content/uploads/2016/11/Ethics_manual_3rd_Nov2015_en.pdf.

57. Braun, W., *Jainism*, in *World Religions for Healthcare Professionals*, S. Ssorajjakool, et al. (eds). 2017, Florence, United Kingdom: Taylor & Francis Group.

About the Team

Alessandra Tosi was the managing editor for this book.

Melissa Purkiss performed the copy-editing and proofreading.

Katy Saunders designed the cover. The cover was produced in InDesign using the Fontin font.

Luca Baffa typeset the book in InDesign and produced the paperback and hardback editions. The text font is Tex Gyre Pagella; the heading font is Californian FB. Luca produced the EPUB, AZW3, PDF, HTML, and XML editions — the conversion is performed with open source software such as pandoc (https://pandoc.org/) created by John MacFarlane and other tools freely available on our GitHub page (https://github.com/OpenBookPublishers).

This book need not end here...

Share

All our books — including the one you have just read — are free to access online so that students, researchers and members of the public who can't afford a printed edition will have access to the same ideas. This title will be accessed online by hundreds of readers each month across the globe: why not share the link so that someone you know is one of them?

This book and additional content is available at:

https://doi.org/10.11647/OBP.0300

Donate

Open Book Publishers is an award-winning, scholar-led, not-for-profit press making knowledge freely available one book at a time. We don't charge authors to publish with us: instead, our work is supported by our library members and by donations from people who believe that research shouldn't be locked behind paywalls.

Why not join them in freeing knowledge by supporting us: https://www.openbookpublishers.com/section/104/1

Like Open Book Publishers

Follow @OpenBookPublish

Read more at the Open Book Publishers **BLOG**

You may also be interested in:

Non-Communicable Disease Prevention
Best Buys, Wasted Buys and Contestable Buys
Wanrudee Isaranuwatchai, Rachel A. Archer, Yot Teerawattananon and Anthony J. Culyer (eds)

https://doi.org/10.11647/OBP.0195

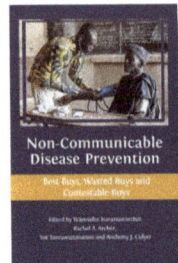

Animals and Medicine
The Contribution of Animal Experiments to the Control of Disease
Jack Botting

https://doi.org/10.11647/OBP.0055

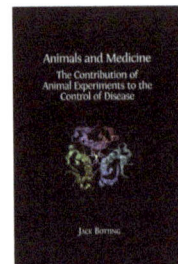

Undocumented Migrants and Healthcare
Eight Stories from Switzerland
Marianne Jossen

https://doi.org/10.11647/OBP.0139

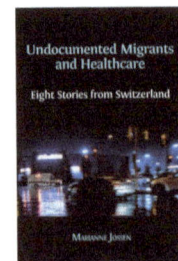

www.ingramcontent.com/pod-product-compliance
Lightning Source LLC
Chambersburg PA
CBHW042312210326
41598CB00042B/7366